Latent Bipolar Disorder

Taiane de Azevedo Cardoso
Ives Cavalcante Passos • Flavio Kapczinski
Editors

Latent Bipolar Disorder

Springer

Editors
Taiane de Azevedo Cardoso
Institute for Mental and Physical Health
and Clinical Translation (IMPACT)
School of Medicine
Deakin University
Geelong, VIC, Australia

Ives Cavalcante Passos
Psychiatry Department
Federal University of Rio Grande do Sul
Porto Alegre, Rio Grande do Sul, Brazil

Flavio Kapczinski
Psychiatry Department
Federal University of Rio Grande do Sul
Porto Alegre, Rio Grande do Sul, Brazil

ISBN 978-3-032-01296-8 ISBN 978-3-032-01297-5 (eBook)
https://doi.org/10.1007/978-3-032-01297-5

This Springer imprint is published by the registered company Springer Nature Switzerland AG
The registered company address is: Gewerbestrasse 11, 6330 Cham, Switzerland

We dedicate this book to those who live with bipolar disorder and to the families who walk beside them—seeking understanding, compassion, and better treatments for their loved ones.

Foreword

Bipolar disorder generally does not begin autochthonously, a lightning bolt out of a clear blue sky. In many people who go on to the develop the disorder, there is a latent or prodromal or at-risk period. However, it is challenging to detect them, because the presence of the latent or prodromal periods can only be definitively known post hoc after the development of frank manic or hypomanic episodes. Additionally, their phenotype is characterised by non-specific features that might signal the onset of several disorders as well as being non-specific transient distress symptoms. Such non-specific symptoms span mood swings and temperamental traits, anxiety, sleep-wake cycle disturbances, behavioural disinhibition and features of depression, particularly in adolescents and young adults. These symptoms form part of many high prevalence disorders including other affective disorders, emerging personality disorder, neurodevelopmental disorders like attention deficit hyperactivity disorder, and addictive disorders. This diagnostic uncertainty is greatest at the earliest stages of these disorders. To complicate things further, comorbidity is normative. And many of these disorders share risk factors like childhood adversity.

There are several imperatives for the accurate and timely detection of at-risk states. Firstly, there is a body of evidence suggesting that earlier treatment is associated with better clinical outcomes. This evidence is greatest for lithium but there is tentative evidence for atypical antipsychotics and psychotherapy as well. Early intervention in bipolar disorder is only really feasible in the earliest stages of the disorder as there is relative preservation of brain structure and cognition during the latent or at-risk stage. Progressive changes typically commence after the first episode. There is an early window for preventive interventions in those with at-risk or latent bipolar states. Lithium remains best evidenced to ameliorate neuroprogression. However, its side effects and the tentative specificity of the latent or prodromal stage limit its application to people after a threshold first manic episode. If there is clinical suspicion that an index presentation is a likely bipolar latent stage or prodrome, clinicians should avoid those medications that are potentially iatrogenic, especially antidepressants or stimulants, which can aggravate rapid cycling and trigger mania.

Importantly, elements of phenomenology assist in the detection of the probable latent stage or prodrome. Depression is one of the most common initial presentations of the prodrome and at-risk states. Bipolar depression is more likely to present with atypical symptoms. These include hypersomnia, anergia or marked fatigue and psychomotor retardation. Other features more common in bipolar than unipolar presentations include multiple discrete episodes, psychosis, abrupt onset and offset, an early age of onset and a seasonal pattern. These features have been termed the probabilistic signature of bipolar depression. In people with a family history of bipolar disorder, these probabilistic features were associated with a seven times greater risk of developing bipolar disorder than depressed individuals without the signature elements. Also, antidepressant-induced elation as well as treatment resistance can indicate an increased risk of transition to bipolar disorder.

Detection of latent or prodromal bipolar disorder should catalyse earlier care. This includes non-specific elements, such as psychotherapy and lifestyle modification. More specific psychological therapies include sleep-wake cycle and social rhythm regulation psychoeducation, and family focused interventions. These are safe in latent or risk states and may minimise relapse risk. Clinicians should aim to identify and manage subthreshold mania, cyclothymia or attenuated bipolar-like syndromes. Bipolar-specific interventions including lamotrigine, atypical antipsychotics or lithium may be indicated if there are significant and impairing symptoms.

The occurrence of emerging manic-like phenomena are the best predictors of early transition to full-threshold mania. However, the challenge is that once mania is recognised, the diagnosis is made. The clinical conundrum is that people do not note or present for care with mild hypomanic symptoms because they are non-impairing and mild, and even desirable. Also, clinicians often do not routinely enquire as to their presence.

In this context, the book by Taiane de Azevedo Cardoso, Ives Cavalcante Passos and Flavio Kapczinski is a valuable and clinically useful addition to the resources for clinicians managing this population. It contains chapters from leading authorities in the field covering topics including definitions of latent bipolar disorder, its epidemiology, what we can learn from cohort studies, and covers differential diagnosis as well as special populations including women's mental health and latent stage disorder. It also covers the vexed issues of suicidality and trauma, why the disorder may disproportionately target most talented and gifted and summarises treatment strategies including pharmacotherapy and psychotherapy. The authors need to be congratulated for addressing this major unmet need in the management of a common and disabling disorder.

Deakin University and Barwon Health
Institute for Mental and Physical Health
and Clinical Translation (IMPACT), School of Medicine
Geelong, VIC, Australia

Michael Berk

Contents

Chapter 1
What Is Latent Bipolar Disorder?

Taiane de Azevedo Cardoso, Ives Cavalcante Passos, and Flavio Kapczinski

1.1 Introduction

Bipolar disorder (BD) is a chronic mental health disorder that affects about 2% of the worldwide population [1]. The peak age at onset is in young adulthood (19.5 years old) [2], and individuals suffering from BD are more likely to present with a poor quality of life [3], cognitive impairment [4], functional impairment [5], and suicide risk [6], as compared to individuals without the condition.

The severe clinical course of BD may be a consequence of a long duration without appropriate treatment due to delayed diagnosis. A recent systematic review and meta-analysis, including 59 studies, showed that there is a median of 3.5 years delay in help seeking (the time between the age at onset of any mood symptoms and the age at seeking formal help), a median of 6.7 years delay in BD diagnosis (the time between the age at onset of a mood episode and age at diagnosis of BD), and a median of 5.9 years delay in treatment (time between the age at diagnosis of BD and age at initiation of a clinical guideline recommended treatment for BD) [7]. The long delay between the initial symptoms and the appropriate diagnosis and treatment emphasizes that it is paramount to better understand the clinical manifestation of latent BD to promote a better prognosis for patients suffering from BD.

T. de Azevedo Cardoso (✉)
Institute for Mental and Physical Health and Clinical Translation (IMPACT), School of Medicine, Deakin University, Geelong, VIC, Australia

I. C. Passos · F. Kapczinski
Psychiatry Department, Federal University of Rio Grande do Sul, Porto Alegre, Rio Grande do Sul, Brazil

T. de Azevedo Cardoso et al. (eds.), *Latent Bipolar Disorder*,
https://doi.org/10.1007/978-3-032-01297-5_1

Thus, the aim of this chapter is to describe the predictors of BD, as well as the definitions of latent BD and the future directions in the field.

1.2 Early Identification in BD: What Is Known So Far

A review discussing the areas of uncertainties and unmet needs in the field of bipolar disorder discussed the importance of improving the identification of at-risk populations [8]. A major goal of modern medicine has been to prevent diseases through early identification and management of risk factors. For example, lifestyle interventions were found to be potentially effective in preventing and managing cardiovascular disease risk factors [9]. However, the identification of at-risk populations in psychiatry, and specifically in BD, has been challenging.

A recent systematic review describing the risk of developing bipolar disorder I-II (BD-I/II) in individuals at clinical high risk for BD showed that the development of BD-I/II ranged from 7.1% to 23.4% after 2 years among individuals at clinical high risk for BD [10]. Predictors of the development of BD included an earlier age of onset of mood symptoms and a family history of mania/hypomania [10]. Family history of BD is a well-known risk factor for the development of BD. Family studies indicated that individuals with a family history of BD have a 10 times greater risk of having BD as compared to individuals without a family history of BD [11]. Considering this strong genetic component, researchers have conducted prospective cohort studies following offspring of parents with BD and comparing their clinical characteristics with offspring of parents without BD, seeking for potential markers that could precede the development of BD.

1.2.1 Contributions from the Offspring Cohort Studies

The Canadian High-Risk Offspring Cohort is an open prospective cohort study that started in 1996 and followed 279 high-risk offspring (offspring of parents with BD or recurrent major depressive disorder) and 87 controls (offspring of parents with no lifetime major psychiatric disorder) [12]. The follow-up duration varied from 1 to 21 years for high-risk offspring, given the open cohort design [12]. In the first 15 years of follow-up, the study included 207 offspring of parents with BD and found that the mean age at onset of the first major mood episode was 17 years. There were no reports of a major mood episode occurring before the age of 12. Importantly, the first episode was a major depressive episode in most cases (90%) [13]. The findings of the largest follow-up (up to 21 years) showed that high-risk offspring presented greater functional impairment as compared to controls [12]. High-risk offspring had an 8.39 times increased risk to develop major depressive disorder, a 35.35 times increased risk to develop sleep disorder, a 9.77 times increased risk to develop subthreshold depressive symptoms, and an 11.15 times increased risk to develop subthreshold hypomanic symptoms as compared to controls [12]. High-risk offspring also presented an earlier age at onset of depressive disorders, substance use disorder, and subthreshold symptoms of depression and hypomania as compared to controls [12]. The onset of BD tended to be in late adolescence or early adulthood (median = 20.73 years; range = 12.37–30.25) [12]. This study described the trajectory of high-risk offspring in four stages: stage 0: individuals are well, but they have a family history; stage 1: individuals present with non-mood disorders, including sleep disorders, anxiety disorders, ADHD, and behavioral disorders; stage 2: individuals present minor mood disorders, including adjustment disorders, depression not otherwise specified, mood disorder not otherwise specified, dysthymia, and cyclothymia; stage 3: individuals present major depressive disorder, single or recurrent; and stage 4: individuals develop bipolar disorder, including bipolar disorder I and II, bipolar disorder not otherwise specified, and schizoaffective bipolar disorder [12]. A recent systematic review and meta-analysis discussed the importance of sleep markers in the early identification of BD [14]. The meta-analysis showed that offspring of parents with BD had greater daytime sleepiness as compared to the offspring of parents without BD. The systematic review also showed that offspring of parents with BD had an increased likelihood of experiencing an adverse sleep pattern (e.g., shorter sleep duration and sleep disorders), as compared to offspring of parents without BD. Finally, some findings indicated that decreased sleep, difficulty falling asleep, and overall sleep problems might be predictors for the development of BD [14].

The Dutch Bipolar Offspring Study was established in 1997 and followed 140 offspring of parents with BD for up to 22 years. The assessments were conducted at five timepoints (baseline and 1-, 5-, 12-, and 22-year follow-up) [15]. The main findings showed that the lifetime prevalence of any mood disorders at baseline was 27%, while the lifetime prevalence of any mood disorders at the follow-up of 12 years was 54%, indicating that the lifetime prevalence of any mood disorders doubled in the follow-up of 12 years and that half of the Dutch bipolar offspring cohort had developed a mood disorder when they were at a mean age of 28 years [16]. Regarding BD specifically, the lifetime prevalence of bipolar spectrum disorders was 4% at baseline and 13% at the follow-up of 12 years [16]. Interestingly, in almost all participants with bipolar spectrum disorders, the illness started with a depressive episode [16]. Finally, the mean age at onset of the first mood episode was 14.6 years, and onset of the first manic or hypomanic episode followed on average 5.3 years later [16]. Findings from the 22-year follow-up showed that no new BD onsets occurred since the 12-year follow-up, indicating that the risk for developing BD in offspring of parents with BD is highest during adolescence and young adulthood [15]. These findings may also suggest that offspring of parents with BD appear to be beyond the window of high risk for BD after 30 years old [15]. It is important to note that the main limitation of the Dutch Bipolar Offspring Study is the lack of a control group. Therefore, although the study brings relevant findings about the clinical trajectories of offspring of parents with BD, it does not show how the trajectories of these individuals differ from the trajectories of offspring of parents without BD.

The Pittsburgh Bipolar Offspring Study is the largest existing study seeking to understand the development and course of psychopathology among offspring of parents with bipolar disorder. This study recruited 391 offspring of parents with BD aged 6–18 and 248 offspring of community controls [17]. The main findings showed that the strongest predictors of the new-onset bipolar spectrum were anxiety/depressive symptoms, affective lability, and subsyndromal manic symptoms [17].

A recent systematic review aimed at describing the incidence and predictors of transitioning to BD among high-risk individuals included 23 publications of 16 cohorts and showed that the conversion to BD was between 8 and 25% (follow-up length varied from 1 to 21 years among the studies included) [18]. The findings indicate that subthreshold (hypo)manic symptoms and elevated depressive symptoms are potential predictors for the conversion to BD among high-risk individuals [18].

Based on these findings, a recent editorial brought an important reflection to the attention of clinicians: (1) adolescence is a critical period for incident cases of BD, particularly in those with a family history; (2) it is essential to assess the history of mania and hypomania in all youth, but especially those with a family history; (3) early adulthood is associated with a peak in psychopathology burden in these at-risk individuals, which decreases somewhat in the following decade; and (4) there is a later spike of major depressive disorder in these at-risk offspring, but time will tell if this is truly heterotypic transmission or will eventually lead to BD onset [19]. Figure 1.1 shows the main clinical predictors for the development of BD among offspring of parents with BD.

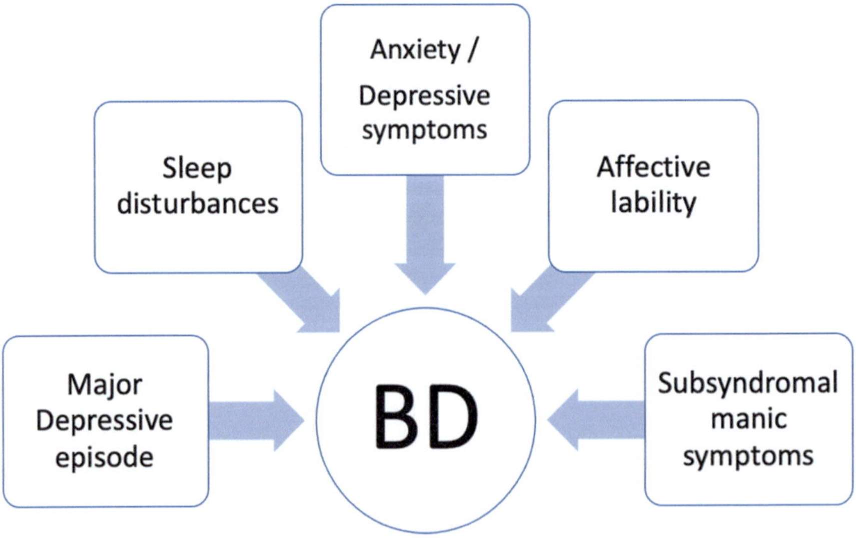

Fig. 1.1 Clinical predictors for the development of bipolar disorder (BD) among offspring of parents with BD

1.2.2 Predictors of Conversion from MDD to BD: Findings from Longitudinal Studies

Considering that most cases will have a major depressive episode as their first episode, it is important to investigate what the predictors are for the conversion from MDD to BD. A systematic review describing the rate and predictors of conversion from unipolar depression to BD included 31 studies and showed that the yearly rate of conversion to BD was 3.9% in the first year after study entry with a diagnosis of unipolar disorder, 3.1% in years 1–2, 1.0% in years 2–5, and 0.8% in years 5–10 [20], indicating that the rate of conversion to BD decreases with time. The risk factors for the conversion from unipolar to bipolar disorder investigated, were the following: gender, age at onset of unipolar disorder, number of depressive episodes, treatment resistance to antidepressants, family history of bipolar disorder, the prevalence of psychotic depression, the prevalence of chronic depression, and severity of depression [20]. The authors did not identify risk factors that were consistently or mainly confirmed to predict conversion across studies. For instance, although gender was evaluated as a risk factor in 6 studies, none found that there was a statistically significant difference in conversion rates between genders [20]. Younger age at onset was found to be associated with conversion in most of the studies (57.1%; 4 out of 7). The higher number of depressive episodes was associated with conversion only in one study (out of 4 studies included) [20]. Family history of BD was a significant predictor of conversion in half of the studies included assessing it (2 out of 4) [20]. Psychotic depression was a significant predictor in the majority of the studies assessing it (66.6%; 4 out of 6) [20]. Two studies assessed whether chronic depression was associated with conversion, and the findings were inconclusive: one study found that chronic depression increased the risk of conversion, while the other found that chronic depression decreased the risk for conversion [20]. Only one study investigated the effect of treatment resistance to antidepressants on conversion to BD and showed that treatment resistance to antidepressants increased the risk of conversion to BD [20]. Among two studies including severity of depression as a risk factor, one found that increased severity increased the risk of conversion, whereas the other found no effect [20].

Another systematic review describing the rates and predictors of transition to BD in prospective follow-up studies of people with MDD included 56 publications and found that the greatest risk of transition was in the first 5 years of follow-up [21]. The main predictors of conversion from MDD to BD were the following: family history of BD (OR = 2.89, 95% CI: 2.01–4.14, N = 7), earlier age of onset of depression (g = −0.33, SE = 0.05, N = 6) and presence of psychotic symptoms (OR = 4.76, 95% CI: 1.79–12.66, N = 5) [21].

A recent study including 130,793 adolescents and young adults aged 10–29 years who were diagnosed with MDD found that the rate of conversion to BD was 13.80% (95% confidence interval: 13.54–14.06%) during the 11-year follow-up [22]. The significant predictors of conversion from MDD to BD were the following: younger age of diagnosis with MDD, moderate and high antidepressant resistance, obesity, psychiatric comorbidities (attention-deficit/hyperactivity disorder, substance use disorder, and cluster B and C personality disorder), a family history of mental disorders (schizophrenia and mood disorders), lower monthly income, and more mental health visits to the clinic each year [22]. Another recent study following 585 adults diagnosed with MDD found that the rate of conversion from MDD to BD in a follow-up of three years was 12.4% [23]. This study showed that risk for conversion from MDD to BD was 3.41-fold higher in subjects who reported lifetime cocaine use at baseline as compared to individuals who did not report lifetime cocaine use at baseline, after adjusting for demographic and clinical confounders, indicating that lifetime cocaine use is a potential predictor of conversion from MDD to BD [23]. Figure 1.2 is showing the clinical predictors for the development of BD among individuals diagnosed with MDD.

1.3 Latent Bipolar Disorder: Definitions and Future Directions

The terminology "latent bipolar disorder" was first introduced to discuss cases where individuals with depression who had been unresponsive to antidepressant therapy were introduced to lithium as an adjunctive treatment to the antidepressants, and when lithium was discontinued, these individuals were at a greater risk of developing bipolar disorder [24]. This concept was later integrated into staging models proposed for BD to describe the subset of individuals who are at risk to develop BD [25, 26]. The staging model proposed by Kapczinski and colleagues [26] includes a latent phase defined by a family history of BD and the presence of mood and anxiety

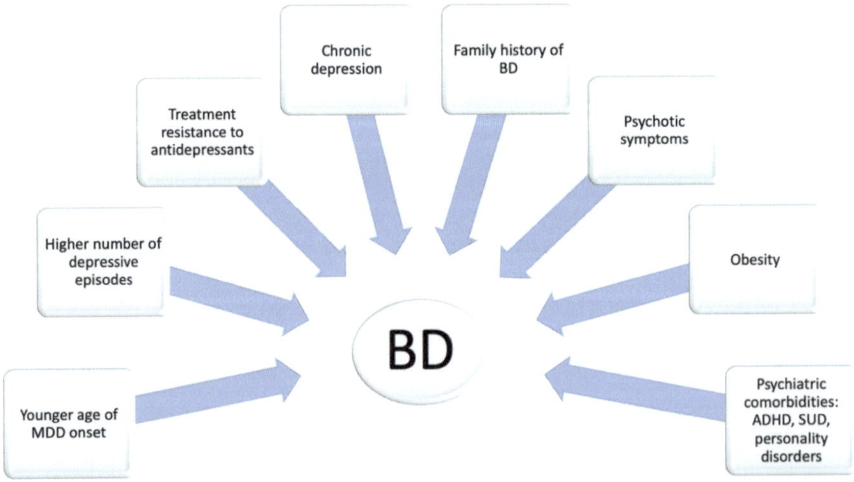

Fig. 1.2 Clinical predictors for the development of bipolar disorder (BD) among individuals diagnosed with major depressive disorder (MDD)

symptoms without meeting criteria for threshold bipolar disorder [26]. McNamara et al. [25] proposed a staging model, describing two stages that precede mania onset [25]. Stage I includes putative risk factors (history of BD in first-degree relatives, physical/sexual abuse, psychosocial stress, substance use/abuse, stimulant medications, and n-3 fatty acid deficiency) [25]. Stage 2 II includes the clinical features (ADHD, unipolar depression, hypomania, anger/irritability, and anxiety) [25]. Latent BD has been discussed as a clinical dilemma, given its complexity [27], and researchers have emphasized that operational criteria for the identification of latent BD are a major unmet need in the field of mental health [28].

Table 1.1 shows the two criteria developed to date aimed at identifying individuals at risk of developing BD. Bechdolf et al. [29] developed an ultra-high-risk criterion for BD, named "bipolar at-risk (BAR)" [29]. This set of criteria was established based on the risk factors to develop BD described in the literature. To be classified as an ultra-high risk for BD, the individual must be aged between 15 and 25 years and meet criteria for at least one of the three following groups in the last 12 months: (1) *Subthreshold mania:* a period of abnormally and persistently elevated, expansive or irritable mood, and at least two additional (hypo)manic symptoms that persists for at least 2 consecutive days but less than 4 days; (2) *Depression + Cyclothymic features:* Depression is characterized by depressed mood, or loss of interest or pleasure, and at least two additional depressive symptoms that persist for at least 1 week. Cyclothymic features are characterized by numerous episodes with subthreshold manic symptoms not meeting group 1 criteria and numerous episodes with depressive symptoms (e.g., subthreshold mania as defined in group I only for 4 h within a 24-hour period and at least 4 cumulative lifetime days meeting the criteria); and (3) *Depression + Genetic Risk:* Depression is characterized by depressed mood, or loss of interest or pleasure, and at least two additional depressive symptoms that persist for at least 1 week. Genetic risk is defined as having a first-degree relative with BD. When validating the BAR criteria, the authors showed that the rates of conversion to BD were greater in the BAR group (22.7%, $n = 5$) than in the non-BAR group (0.7%, $n = 1$, $p < 0.001$) in a sample of youth seeking mental health treatment, who were followed up for an average of 265.5 days. Although the sample size is small, these findings indicate that the BAR criteria are useful to identify latent BD [29].

Table 1.1 Developed criteria to identify individuals at risk of developing BD

Bipolar-At-Risk (BAR) [29]	Bipolar-At-Risk State (BARS) [30]
Age: 15–25 years	Age: 15–35 years
Group 1: Subthreshold mania	Group 1: Subthreshold mania
Group 2: Depression + Cyclothymic features	Group 2: Depression + Cyclothymic features
Group 3: Depression + Genetic risk	Group 3: Depression + Genetic risk
	Group 4: Cyclothymic features + Genetic risk
	Group 5: Subthreshold mixed episode
	Group 6: Mood swings

The BAR criteria were further refined in 2018. Fusar-Poli et al. [30] proposed an expansion on the age range (15–35 years) and the addition of three groups to the already existing groups listed in the BAR criteria [30]. The three new groups included in these refined criteria are the following: (1) *Cyclothymic features + genetic risk*, (2) *Subthreshold mixed episode*: subthreshold mania and depressed mood nearly every day but less than five consecutive days, and (3) *Mood swings*: recent onset mood instability. The refinement of the criteria was informed by evidence indicating that subthreshold mixed episodes and mood swings may represent prodromal features of bipolar disorder. These new criteria were named Bipolar-At-Risk State (BARS). The authors have also developed a semi-structured interview, the Semi-structured Interview for Bipolar-At-Risk States (SIBARS). The SIBARS interview was developed for youths aged 15–35 and comprehended 5 domains: (1) Subthreshold Mania, (2) Depression, (3) Cyclothymic Features, (4) Genetic Risk, and (5) Mood Swings. In a sample of 205 participants (32 meeting the BAR criteria and 173 not meeting the BAR criteria), the authors showed that individuals meeting the BAR criteria had an increased risk of developing BD compared to individuals not meeting the BAR criteria (Hazard Ratio [HR]: 5.30, 95% Confidence Interval [CI]: 1.679–16.757], $p = 0.004$) in a follow-up of a median of 1692 days. However, the accuracy was poor (Harrell's $C = 0.659$). The BARS criteria were tested in the same sample of 205 participants (41 meeting the BARS criteria and 164 not meeting the BARS criteria), and the authors found that individuals meeting the BARS criteria had an increased risk of developing BD compared to individuals not meeting the BARS criteria (HR: 12.364, 95% CI: 3.694–41.379], $p < 0.001$). The accuracy was adequate (Harrell's $C = 0.777$). Finally, the accuracy and clinical utility of the SIBARS interview were considered adequate in a prospective study including 71 participants [30].

The criteria proposed to date are interesting and a starting point on establishing a formal classification to identify latent BD. However, some key features discussed earlier in this chapter are missing in the currently available criteria, such as sleep patterns, psychotic symptoms, substance use, and other psychiatric comorbidities (e.g., ADHD and personality disorders). In addition, the limited combination of features (e.g., depression + genetic risk and cyclothymic features + genetic risk) does not encompass the complex manifestation of symptoms seen in BD. Therefore, developing operational criteria Developed criteria for the identification of latent bipolar disorder still need further refinement. A more individualized approach, potentially enhanced by AI-driven techniques (e.g., the development of risk calculators), is necessary to refine these criteria.

References

1. Merikangas KR, Jin R, He JP, et al. Prevalence and correlates of bipolar spectrum disorder in the world mental health survey initiative. Arch Gen Psychiatry. 2011; https://doi.org/10.1001/archgenpsychiatry.2011.12.

2. Solmi M, Radua J, Olivola M, et al. Age at onset of mental disorders worldwide: large-scale meta-analysis of 192 epidemiological studies. Mol Psychiatry. 2022; https://doi.org/10.1038/s41380-021-01161-7.
3. Pascual-Sánchez A, Jenaro C, Montes-Rodríguez JM. Quality of life in euthymic bipolar patients: a systematic review and meta-analysis. J Affect Disord. 2019; https://doi.org/10.1016/j.jad.2019.05.032.
4. Dickinson T, Becerra R, Coombes J. Executive functioning deficits among adults with Bipolar Disorder (types I and II): a systematic review and meta-analysis. J Affect Disord. 2017; https://doi.org/10.1016/j.jad.2017.04.010.
5. Léda-Rêgo G, Bezerra-Filho S, Miranda-Scippa Â. Functioning in euthymic patients with bipolar disorder: a systematic review and meta-analysis using the functioning assessment short test. Bipolar Disord, 101111/bdi12904. 2020;
6. Pompili M, Gonda X, Serafini G, Innamorati M, Sher L, Amore M, Rihmer Z, Girardi P. Epidemiology of suicide in bipolar disorders: a systematic review of the literature. Bipolar Disord. 2013; https://doi.org/10.1111/bdi.12087.
7. Scott J, Graham A, Yung A, Morgan C, Bellivier F, Etain B. A systematic review and meta-analysis of delayed help-seeking, delayed diagnosis and duration of untreated illness in bipolar disorders. Acta Psychiatr Scand. 2022; https://doi.org/10.1111/acps.13490.
8. Bauer M, Andreassen OA, Geddes JR, Vedel KL, Lewitzka U, Schulze TG, Vieta E. Areas of uncertainties and unmet needs in bipolar disorders: clinical and research perspectives. Lancet Psychiatry. 2018; https://doi.org/10.1016/S2215-0366(18)30253-0.
9. Lim GP, Appalasamy JR, Ahmad B, Quek KF, Ramadas A. Peer-led lifestyle interventions for the primary prevention of cardiovascular disease in community: a systematic review of randomised controlled trials. BMC Public Health. 2024; https://doi.org/10.1186/s12889-024-18328-w.
10. de Pablo GS, et al. Predicting bipolar disorder I/II in individuals at clinical high-risk: results from a systematic review. J Affect Disord. 2023;325:778–86.
11. Merikangas KR, Chakravarti A, Moldin SO, et al. Future of genetics of mood disorders research. Biol Psychiatry. 2002; https://doi.org/10.1016/s0006-3223(02)01471-3.
12. Duffy A, Goodday S, Keown-Stoneman C, Grof P. The emergent course of bipolar disorder: observations over two decades from the Canadian high-risk offspring cohort. Am J Psychiatry. 2019; https://doi.org/10.1176/appi.ajp.2018.18040461.
13. Duffy A, Alda M, Hajek T, Grof P. Early course of bipolar disorder in high-risk offspring: prospective study. Br J Psychiatry. 2009;195:457–8.
14. Aguiar KR, Cabelleira MBB, Jansen K, de Azevedo Cardoso T. Sleep alterations as a predictor of bipolar disorder among offspring of parents with bipolar disorder: a systematic review and meta-analysis. Trends Psychiatry Psychother. 2021; https://doi.org/10.47626/2237-6089-2021-0256.
15. FGL H, Mesman E, MHJ H. Beyond the window of risk? The Dutch bipolar offspring study: 22-year follow-up. J Am Acad Child Adolesc Psychiatry. 2024; https://doi.org/10.1016/j.jaac.2024.05.024.
16. Mesman E, Nolen WA, Reichart CG, Wals M, Hillegers MH. The Dutch bipolar offspring study: 12-year follow-up. Am J Psychiatry. 2013; https://doi.org/10.1176/appi.ajp.2012.12030401.
17. Hafeman DM, Merranko J, Axelson D, et al. Toward the definition of a bipolar Prodrome: dimensional predictors of bipolar spectrum disorders in at-risk youths. Am J Psychiatry. 2016; https://doi.org/10.1176/appi.ajp.2015.15040414.
18. Keramatian K, Chakrabarty T, Saraf G, Yatham LN. Transitioning to bipolar disorder: a systematic review of prospective high-risk studies. Curr Opin Psychiatry. 2022; https://doi.org/10.1097/YCO.0000000000000762.
19. Hafeman DM. Editorial: following offspring of parents with bipolar disorder into middle adulthood: risk windows relevant to child psychiatrists. J Am Acad Child Adolesc Psychiatry. 2024; https://doi.org/10.1016/j.jaac.2024.08.009.

20. Kessing LV, Willer I, Andersen PK, Bukh JD. Rate and predictors of conversion from unipolar to bipolar disorder: a systematic review and meta-analysis. Bipolar Disord. 2017; https://doi.org/10.1111/bdi.12513.
21. Ratheesh A, Davey C, Hetrick S, Alvarez-Jimenez M, Voutier C, Bechdolf A, PD MG, Scott J, Berk M, Cotton SM. A systematic review and meta-analysis of prospective transition from major depression to bipolar disorder. Acta Psychiatr Scand. 2017; https://doi.org/10.1111/acps.12686.
22. Kung FH, Tsai CK, Cheng CM, Tsai SJ, Su TP, Chen TJ, Bai YM, Liang CS, Chen MH. Diagnostic conversion to bipolar disorder among adolescents and young adults with major depressive disorder: a nationwide longitudinal study. Eur Child Adolesc Psychiatry. 2024; https://doi.org/10.1007/s00787-024-02401-1.
23. de Azevedo Cardoso T, Jansen K, Mondin TC, Pedrotti MF, de Lima Bach S, da Silva RA, de Mattos Souza LD, Balanzá-Martínez V, Frey BN, Kapczinski F. Lifetime cocaine use is a potential predictor for conversion from major depressive disorder to bipolar disorder: a prospective study. Psychiatry Clin Neurosci. 2020; https://doi.org/10.1111/pcn.13012.
24. Faedda GL, Tondo L, Baldessarini RJ. Lithium discontinuation: uncovering latent bipolar disorder? Am J Psychiatry. 2001;158:1337–9.
25. McNamara RK, Nandagopal JJ, Strakowski SM, DelBello MP. Preventative strategies for early-onset bipolar disorder: towards a clinical staging model. CNS Drugs. 2010;24:983–96.
26. Kapczinski F, Dias VV, Kauer-Sant'Anna M, Frey BN, Grassi-Oliveira R, Colom F, Berk M. Clinical implications of a staging model for bipolar disorders. Expert Rev Neurother. 2009;9:957–66.
27. Gitlin MJ. Diagnosing latent bipolar disorder: a clinical dilemma. Bipolar Disord. 2018;20:300–2.
28. Kapczinski F, Montezano BB, de Azevedo Cardoso T. Latent bipolar disorder. Lancet. 2023;401:2109.
29. Bechdolf A, Nelson B, Cotton SM, et al. A preliminary evaluation of the validity of at-risk criteria for bipolar disorders in help-seeking adolescents and young adults. J Affect Disord. 2010; https://doi.org/10.1016/j.jad.2010.06.016.
30. Fusar-Poli P, De Micheli A, Rocchetti M, Cappucciati M, Ramella-Cravaro V, Rutigliano G, Bonoldi I, McGuire P, Falkenberg I. Semistructured interview for bipolar at risk states (SIBARS). Psychiatry Res. 2018; https://doi.org/10.1016/j.psychres.2018.03.074.

Chapter 2
Epidemiology of Bipolar Disorder

Lars Vedel Kessing

2.1 Introduction

Mood disorders have received considerable attention in psychiatric epidemiology over the last 25 years, including the five-site United States National Institutes of Mental Health Epidemiologic Catchment Area Study (*ECA*), the US National Comorbidity Survey (*NCS*), the National Psychiatric Morbidity Survey of Great Britain, and most recently, the World Mental Health Survey (*WMH*) across many countries. Thus, there is substantial data from around the world on the epidemiology of mood disorders. In addition, many of the population-based case registers and twin registries have also paid particular interest to mood disorders, and some of these registers have the additional advantage of being able to consider genetic as well as environmental risk factors.

Depressive disorder and bipolar disorder hold large similarities in pathogenesis, course of illness, and outcomes, and it is estimated that approximately one percent of patients convert from depressive disorder to bipolar disorder per year as patients develop hypomanic or manic episodes [1, 2], approximating 20–40% during the lifetime course.

The following is an updated version of an overview of "epidemiology of mood disorders" in the *New Oxford Textbook of Psychiatry* by the author Kessing [3], focusing on bipolar disorder only.

L. V. Kessing (✉)
Psychiatric Center Copenhagen and Department of Clinical Medicine, University of Copenhagen, Copenhagen, Denmark
e-mail: lars.vedel.kessing@regionh.dk

T. de Azevedo Cardoso et al. (eds.), *Latent Bipolar Disorder*,
https://doi.org/10.1007/978-3-032-01297-5_2

2.2 Impact of Bipolar Disorder on Societies

Bipolar disorder is a common mental disease that imposes a high societal burden in terms of morbidity, mortality, lost productivity, and costs [4]. The Global Burden of Disease study, which is a comprehensive assessment of disability and mortality from diseases and injuries from 1990 onwards, highlights the importance of mood disorders, including bipolar disorder, for the world. According to the Global Burden of Disease study, the incidence, prevalence, and years lived with disability (YLDs) for bipolar disorder all increased from 1990 to 2019 [5]. The incidence of bipolar disorder increased by 48%, from 3.06 million in 1990 to 4.53 million globally in 2017, and it is estimated that in 2019, 40 million people experienced bipolar disorder [6].

In the United States, the estimated total annual national economic burden of bipolar disorder was more than $195 billion in 2018, with approximately 25% attributed to direct medical costs, while indirect costs due to unemployment, lost work productivity for patients/caregivers, etc. accounted for 72–80% of the national economic burden. Using the measure of disability-adjusted life years (DALY), the World Health Organization (WHO) revealed that bipolar disorder was the sixth leading cause of disease burden in the world in 1990. In 2010, mental and substance abuse disorders accounted for 7% of all DALYs worldwide, and within mental and substance abuse disorders, depressive disorder accounted for 40% and bipolar disorder for 7% of the DALYs [7]. Together mood disorders burden society with the highest healthcare costs of all psychiatric and neurological disorders [8]. One DALY represents the loss of a healthy year of life and aggregates the years of life lived with disability (YLD) with the years of life lost due to premature mortality (YLL). For bipolar disorder, the DALYs increased by 54.4%, from 6.02 million in 1990 to 9.29 million in 2017 [9]. These estimations have contributed to shifting international focus toward mood disorders as a leading cause of burden in their own right and also in comparison to more recognized physical disorders.

2.3 Diagnostic Issues

While classical bipolar disorder, with episodes of euphoric mania interspersed with episodes of depression, is one of the clearest clinical syndromes in psychiatry, the boundaries of bipolar disorder remain contested. As case definition is central to epidemiology, all the contested boundaries of bipolar disorder could influence prevalence rates and our understanding of risk factors. Some of the major boundary issues for bipolar disorder include the overlap of bipolar disorder with psychotic features with schizoaffective disorder and schizophrenia and the overlap of bipolar disorder with unipolar depressive disorder when patients who present primarily with depression have brief or mild episodes of hypomania. There is also an overlap of bipolar disorder with apparent personality disorder, especially Cluster B personality disorders such as borderline and narcissism, and the issue of when hyperthymic personality merges into bipolar disorder. When bipolar disorder is comorbid with alcohol or substance abuse, there are also important diagnostic issues.

Another important issue in determining caseness of bipolar disorder for epidemiological surveys is symptom pattern and duration. A number of the diagnostic instruments for assessing bipolarity in population surveys limit the questions on mania to a type of symptom profile characterized by euphoria, grandiosity, increased energy, and decreased sleep. Whether the commonly used epidemiology interviews adequately detect those individuals who have manic episodes characterized by irritability, anger, and activation is very debatable. The other key diagnostic issue is what criteria are used to categorize the minimum duration for hypomania: is four days too long, or is even 2 days too long? Furthermore, as insight is sometimes impaired in hypomania and mania, and as these are low-prevalence disorders, the accuracy of case detection of bipolar disorders in populations remains an issue for further research.

2.4 Prevalence and Incidence

Prior population studies, such as the ECA and its related cross-national studies and the NCS, reported that the lifetime prevalence of bipolar I disorder varied from 0.3% to 1.5% [10, 11]. Subsequent studies such as the NCS replication study [12] report data on both bipolar I and bipolar II disorder and find lifetime (and 12-month) prevalence estimates of 1.0% (0.6%) for bipolar I, 1.1% (0.8%) for bipolar II, and 2.4% (1.4%) for subthreshold bipolar disorder. Broader definitions of mania/hypomania have resulted in lifetime prevalence rates increasing to about 4% or even higher [13]. In bipolar disorder I, the prevalence in males and females is similar. This is in contrast to the reasonably consistent female excess found in bipolar II disorder and depressive disorder.

The combined incidence of bipolar disorder I and II is estimated to be 10–30 per 100,000 year (0.01–0.03% per year).

2.5 Comorbidity

In the NCS, all identified bipolar I individuals suffered from at least one, and often up to three or more, comorbid disorders [12]. The most common comorbid disorders included the full range of anxiety disorders, alcohol and drug dependence, and antisocial behaviors.

Clinical studies find that bipolar patients with comorbid substance dependence are less adherent to prescribed mood stabilizers and have more frequent hospital readmissions. Stimulant abuse/dependence rates are especially increased in bipolar disorder.

Individuals with bipolar disorder have the full range of anxiety disorders, including phobias, panic disorder, and obsessive-compulsive disorder.

A controversial area of comorbidity with bipolar disorder is that of childhood attention deficit disorder. Early studies have suggested high comorbidity between attention deficit disorder and child and adolescent mania/bipolar disorder [14, 15], whereas longitudinal data [16–19] as well as studies with more careful diagnostic sorting of symptoms [17, 20] have revealed lower comorbidity and supported the differentiation of child and adolescent mania/bipolar disorder from hyperkinetic disorder/attention deficit disorder. As argued by Arnold and colleagues, "Indeed, if one automatically count such symptoms as hyperactivity and impaired attention toward both disorders without noting association with mood episodes, and especially if one does not require episodicity for bipolar disorder it may artificially inflate the comorbidity rate" [20]. In this way, longitudinal results seem to confirm the observation that even though the symptoms may not be so different between mania and ADHD, the clinical presentation and the illness course, with an episodic course in bipolar disorder and a more chronic course in ADHD, differ between the disorders [18, 21].

2.6 Risk Factors for Bipolar Disorders

In considering the risk factors for bipolar disorder, it is useful to separate risk factors into those that are risk factors for lifetime vulnerability (e.g., genetic factors) and those that are risk factors for the onset of an episode of depression or mania (e.g., life events). Thus, in determining risk factors for lifetime vulnerability, genetic factors constitute the largest single risk factor. Bipolar disorder is one of the psychiatric disorders with the highest heritability, at about 70–80% [22].

However, if one is considering who is vulnerable to an episode of mania over the next six months, genetic factors will play a relatively smaller part, and predictions may be best based on other factors such as past history, childbirth, the presence of subsyndromal affective symptoms and cognitive deviances, being treated for depression with antidepressant medication, and the approach of spring or summer.

Although organic factors, such as some type of central nervous system damage, are unusual risk factors in young adults, in late-onset bipolar disorder (age of onset more than 50 years), organic disease of the central nervous system is an increasing factor for the development of mania.

2.7 Age of Onset and Course of Illness

Early-onset bipolar I disorder is more familial and is associated with a higher genetic risk in bipolar disorder. Different population studies show that the mean age of onset of bipolar disorder varies from 17 to 30 years, but there seem to be differences between Europe and the United States. European data suggest a mean age in the late twenties, whereas the United States data suggest a mean age in the early twenties. Reasons for these substantial differences are not known but may include greater genetic loading due to a higher risk of affective illness in those who migrated from Europe to the United States, a higher rate of assortative mating in the United States as well as various genetic mechanisms, including anticipation and gene–environment interactions that may also differ in importance between the United States and Europe. Further, the increasing overweight among children and adolescents has been suggested as a contributing factor, being more prevalent in the United States.

Nevertheless, as age of onset is not normally distributed, the mean is a slightly misleading variable; while the mean age of onset may be in the twenties, for a substantial proportion of patients, age of onset is the teenage years.

The majority of first episodes in bipolar I disorder are depressive: approximately 85% of patients have a depressive first episode, 10% a manic episode, and 3–5% a mixed episode. Typically, the duration of depressive episodes is between 2 and 5 months although longer durations are often seen. The duration of manic episodes averages around two months.

Long-term studies suggest that the vast majority of patients with bipolar disorder I, approximating 90–100%, will develop more episodes after the first manic episode. The course of illness is heterogeneous—some will develop few episodes and some many—but on average the risk of recurrence increases with the number of prior affective episodes, suggesting a clinical progression of the illness [23–25]. Long-term studies also show that despite treatment, patients with bipolar disorder type I or II suffer from affective symptoms of some severity approximately half of their lifetime. Over the course of illness, 80% of affective episodes are of the depressive type and 20% of the manic or mixed type for bipolar disorder type I. The presence of even milder affective symptoms is associated with decreased quality of life and functional and cognitive problems.

2.8 Social, Functional, and Cognitive Outcomes

Approximately 40–60% of patients with bipolar disorder present with persistent cognitive deficits in the remitted state and across several cognitive domains, including attention, verbal learning, and executive function [26, 27]. Such cognitive deficits may be prevalent even among healthy relatives of patients with bipolar disorder or early in the course of illness [27]. There is robust evidence from several studies that patients' persistent cognitive dysfunction is a key contributor to their socio-occupational disability independent of mood symptoms [28–30]. Functional impairment is prevalent in bipolar disorder, with unemployment rates 4- and ten-fold higher than in the general population [31]. Approximately two-thirds of the patients are unable to regain premorbid levels of social and vocational functioning following a single episode [32], and verbal memory and executive function seem moderately related to employment outcome [33].

Patients with bipolar disorder have a two to three times increased risk of developing dementia in the long run [34–36], and there are some suggestions that the risk of developing dementia may increase with the number of episodes in patients with depressive disorder and in patients with bipolar disorder [37]. Long-term treatment with lithium may decrease the risk of developing dementia [38–40], further supporting a link between bipolar disorder and dementia.

2.9 Undiagnosed Bipolar Disorder and Use of Health Services

There is often an interval between the onset of mood episodes and seeking help (median 3.5 years), and it may take 5–7 years for a bipolar patient to receive both the correct diagnosis and be prescribed mood-stabilizing medication, resulting in an extended period of untreated illness [41].

Receiving a correct bipolar diagnosis at initial assessment is complicated by few depressed patients seeking help for hypomanic/manic episodes and more seeking assistance only for their depressive episodes, while viewing any hypomanic/manic episodes as neither harmful nor problematic nor particularly pathological. In combination with assessment nuances, this leads to an estimated 20–40% of bipolar patients being misdiagnosed as having a unipolar depressive disorder and administered antidepressant medication that can worsen the longitudinal course of bipolar disorder principally by causing more switching or more mixed states [42]. Further, the proportion of undiagnosed bipolar disorder in epidemiological samples diagnosed with depressive disorder is high, quantified as up to half of identified depressive cases depending on the sensitivity of the criteria from which bipolar disorder can be accurately recognized as well as practice and referral nuances [42].

In the ECA study, 39% of those with bipolar I or bipolar II disorders received outpatient psychiatric treatment within 1 year, and about 10% would receive inpatient treatment within a 6-month period. In the NCS study, 45% of those with bipolar disorder had received psychiatric treatment in the previous 12 months, although 93% reported lifetime treatment for their bipolar disorder. However, both of these studies suggest that more than half the individuals with bipolar disorder are not currently in psychiatric treatment.

Misdiagnosis or delayed help-seeking has been considered a major contributor to poor outcome in bipolar disorder, with 80% of undiagnosed patients experiencing psychosocial problems impacting their relationships, employment, finances, and health. Further consequences of inappropriately treated bipolar disorder include an increased risk of suicide, longer hospitalizations, poorer social functioning, and general deterioration of the condition.

2.10 Use of Pharmacotherapy

Major changes have taken place since the year 2000 in prescription patterns for bipolar disorder in mental care in Western countries in general [43, 44]. Nationwide and other population-based longitudinal pharmacoepidemiological studies on prescription patterns have shown that lithium is prescribed less and antiepileptics and atypical antipsychotics are prescribed substantially more in recent years. Especially the prescription of the anticonvulsant lamotrigine and the atypical antipsychotic quetiapine has increased substantially (from 0% to 3% in the year 2000 to approximately 40% of all patients in the year 2011 [43]). In many areas of the world, lithium has gone from being the first drug prescribed as maintenance therapy for bipolar disorder to being replaced by atypical antipsychotics or antiepileptics [44]. The use of antidepressants has been constantly high in Western countries, approximating 70–80% of all patients since the year 2000 [43, 45]. Combination therapy of mood stabilizers (lithium, antiepileptics, and antipsychotics) and also antidepressants has increased substantially during the last decade.

Overall, the development in prescription patterns during the last decades is not in accordance with the evidence and recommendations in international guidelines in relation to the use of lithium [44, 46–50] and antidepressants [48, 51–54] in bipolar disorder. Changes in study populations do not seem to explain the changes in prescription pattern and use [43]. The high rates of combination therapy reflect that in real life, patients responses and remission rates are low with monotherapy for acute episodes, and relapse rates are high during maintenance monotherapy therapy [55].

2.11 Adherence to Treatment

Pharmacoepidemiological studies have consistently shown that adherence to medication is a major clinical challenge in the treatment of bipolar disorder. As much as half of the patients do not take medication or take it in other durations and doses than prescribed, although randomized trials show that group-based psychoeducation can substantially add to improved adherence.

2.12 Risk Factors for Affective Episodes in Patients with Bipolar Disorder

A range of other biological factors are particularly relevant risk factors to the onset of episodes of illness, but they may contribute a relatively small part to lifetime vulnerability. Many women have their first episode of depression or mania in the postpartum period. There is substantial evidence that seasonal patterns influence the onset of manic and depressive episodes. There are consistent findings of an excess of manic episodes in late spring and early summer. To date, however, the nature of the environmental factors that influence this late spring, early summer peak of manic episodes is less clear.

There is also substantial evidence that disruptions of normal biological rhythms may precipitate the onset of manic or depressive episodes. This has been documented in relation to international travel involving east–west or west–east travel with disruption of circadian rhythms. Disruption of circadian rhythms through shift work or other factors, which disrupt the normal sleep cycles, may also be important triggers to the onset of episodes of mania.

Adverse life events have been well documented to be precipitants of manic episodes, as well as depression. It appears that life events are more likely prior to the first or second episode of mania and are less likely later in the course of illness.

2.13 Life Expectancy, Mortality, and Causes of Death

Standardized mortality rates (SMR) among patients with bipolar disorder have consistently been found to be increased 2–3 times compared to the general population [56–58], and life expectancy has been reported to be decreased 8 to 12 years for patients with bipolar disorder compared to the general population [59]. The increased mortality is related to increased mortality due to suicide [56, 60], unintentional injuries [56, 58], and comorbid general medical illnesses, including cardiovascular disease [56–58, 61], diabetes [56, 62, 63], and chronic obstructive pulmonary disease [56, 64].

The standardized mortality ratio (SMR) for completed suicide is estimated to be between 10 and 15 [65]. The lifetime risk of suicide may have been overestimated in some prior studies due to incomplete follow-up in selected samples or rather short-term follow-up of patients with first-time treated mental disorders [66]. The absolute risk of committing suicide within 36 years after the first psychiatric contact has been estimated to be 8% for men and 5% for women [66]. Suicide is a prevalent reason for lost life years, specifically during adolescence and early and mid-adulthood, and the risk clearly decreases with age [67]. Among 15-year-old patients with bipolar disorder, suicide accounted for 23–24% of all lost life years, decreasing to 0–5% for patients aged 75 years of age [67]. However, rather surprisingly, natural causes of death are already the most prevalent reason for lost life years from adolescence and increase substantially during early and mid-adulthood, i.e., from age 15 years and during the twenties, thirties, and forties [67]. For 15–year-old boys with bipolar disorder, natural causes of death have been found to account for 58% of 12 lost life years, and for 15–year-old girls, natural causes account for 67% of 9 lost life years, increasing to 74% and 80% for 45-year-old men and women, respectively [67].

Reasons for the increased mortality due to comorbid general medical illness in bipolar disorder may include unhealthy lifestyle, decreased healthcare, adverse pharmacological effects, and biological factors [68]. In relation to biological factors, accelerated aging has recently been proposed as a mechanism explaining the increased prevalence of comorbid medical illness due to disparate pathophysiological changes observed in bipolar disorder, such as brain structural alterations, cognitive deficits, oxidative stress imbalance, amyloid metabolism, immunological deregulation, immunosenescence, neurotrophic deficiencies, and telomere shortening [69]. It is well established that in addition to being differentially affected by chronic medical disorders, the age of onset of chronic medical disorders is much earlier when compared to individuals in the general population [70].

2.14 Impact of Bipolar Disorder on Societies and the Need for Early Intervention Studies

The Global Burden of Disease study highlights the importance of mood disorders, including bipolar disorder, for the world. According to the Global Burden of Disease study, the incidence, prevalence, and years lived with disability (YLDs) for bipolar disorder all increased from 1990 to 2019 [5]. It is estimated that in 2019, 40 million people experienced bipolar disorder (https://www.who.int/news-room/fact-sheets/detail/mental-disorders). For bipolar disorder, the disability-adjusted life years (DALY) increased by 54.4%, from 6.02 million in 1990 to 9.29 million in 2017 [9]. These estimations have contributed to shifting international focus toward mood disorders as a leading cause of burden in their own right and also in comparison to more recognized physical disorders.

As bipolar disorders are associated with long-term deficits in social, functional, and cognitive outcomes and a substantially decreased life expectancy, there is a need for future studies on early and lifestyle interventions [71]. A randomized trial has shown that early intervention, combining optimized pharmacological treatment and psychoeducation, following the onset of bipolar disorder substantially improves the outcome of the bipolar illness [72], and specifically so among young adults below 25 years of age [73].

References

1. Angst J, Sellaro R, Stassen HH, Gamma A. Diagnostic conversion from depression to bipolar disorders: results of a long-term prospective study of hospital admissions. J Affect Disord. 2005;84:149–57.
2. Bukh JD, Andersen PK, Kessing LV. Rates and predictors of remission, recurrence and conversion to bipolar disorder after the first lifetime episode of depression-a prospective 5-year follow-up study. Psychol Med. 2016;46:1151–61.
3. Kessing LV. Epidemiology of mood disorders. In: Goodwin GM, Geddes JR, editors. The new Oxford textbook of psychiatry. 3rd ed. Oxford: Oxford University Press; 2017.

4. Bessonova L, Ogden K, Doane MJ, O'sullivan AK, Tohen M. The economic burden of bipolar disorder in the United States: a systematic literature review. Clinicoecon Outcomes Res. 2020;12:481–97.
5. Lai J, Li S, Wei C, Chen J, Fang Y, Song P, Hu S. Mapping the global, regional and national burden of bipolar disorder from 1990 to 2019: trend analysis on the global burden of disease study 2019. Br J Psychiatry. 2024;224:36–46.
6. World Health Organization. Mental disorders. 2022. https://www.who.int/news-room/fact-sheets/detail/mental-disorders. Assessed 5 Apr 2024.
7. Whiteford HA, Degenhardt L, Rehm J, Baxter AJ, Ferrari AJ, Erskine HE, Charlson FJ, Norman RE, Flaxman AD, Johns N, Burstein R, Murray CJ, Vos T. Global burden of disease attributable to mental and substance use disorders: findings from the global burden of disease study 2010. Lancet. 2013;382:1575–86.
8. Olesen J, Gustavsson A, Svensson M, Wittchen HU, Jonsson B. The economic cost of brain disorders in Europe. Eur J Neurol. 2012;19:155–62.
9. He H, Hu C, Ren Z, Bai L, Gao F, Lyu J. Trends in the incidence and DALYs of bipolar disorder at global, regional, and national levels: results from the global burden of disease study 2017. J Psychiatr Res. 2020;125:96–105.
10. Kessler RC, Rubinow DR, Holmes C, Abelson JM, Zhao S. The epidemiology of DSM-III-R bipolar I disorder in a general population survey. Psychol Med. 1997;27:1079–89.
11. Weissman MM, Bland RC, Canino GJ, Faravelli C, Greenwald S, Hwu HG, Joyce PR, Karam EG, Lee CK, Lellouch J, Lepine JP, Newman SC, Rubio-Stipec M, Wells JE, Wickramaratne PJ, Wittchen H, Yeh EK. Cross-national epidemiology of major depression and bipolar disorder. JAMA. 1996;276:293–9.
12. Merikangas KR, Akiskal HS, Angst J, Greenberg PE, Hirschfeld RM, Petukhova M, Kessler RC. Lifetime and 12-month prevalence of bipolar spectrum disorder in the National Comorbidity Survey replication. Arch Gen Psychiatry. 2007;64:543–52.
13. Hoertel N, Le SY, Angst J, Dubertret C. Subthreshold bipolar disorder in a U.S. national representative sample: prevalence, correlates and perspectives for psychiatric nosography. J Affect Disord. 2013;146:338–47.
14. Geller B, Luby J. Child and adolescent bipolar disorder: a review of the past 10 years. J Am Acad Child Adolesc Psychiatry. 1997;36:1168–76.
15. Geller B, Sun K, Zimerman B, Luby J, Frazier J, Williams M. Complex and rapid-cycling in bipolar children and adolescents: a preliminary study. J Affect Disord. 1995;34:259–68.
16. Craney JL, Geller B. A prepubertal and early adolescent bipolar disorder-I phenotype: review of phenomenology and longitudinal course. Bipolar Disord. 2003;5:243–56.
17. Fahrendorff AM, Pagsberg AK, Kessing LV, Maigaard K. Psychiatric comorbidity in patients with pediatric bipolar disorder: a systematic review. Acta Psychiatr Scand. 2023;148:110–32.
18. Kessing LV, Vradi E, Kragh AP. Diagnostic stability in pediatric bipolar disorder. J Affect Disord. 2015b;172:417–21.
19. Youngstrom EA, Birmaher B, Findling RL. Pediatric bipolar disorder: validity, phenomenology, and recommendations for diagnosis. Bipolar Disord. 2008;10:194–214.
20. Arnold LE, Demeter C, Mount K, Frazier TW, Youngstrom EA, Fristad M, Birmaher B, Findling RL, Horwitz SM, Kowatch R, Axelson DA. Pediatric bipolar spectrum disorder and ADHD: comparison and comorbidity in the LAMS clinical sample. Bipolar Disord. 2011;13:509–21.
21. Carlson GA, Klein DN. How to understand divergent views on bipolar disorder in youth. Annu Rev Clin Psychol. 2014;10:529.
22. Lohoff FW, Berrettini WH. Genetics of bipolar disorder. In: Yatham L, Maj M, editors. Bipolar disorder: clinical and neurobiological foundations. Wiley-Blackwell; 2010.
23. Kessing LV. Course and cognitive outcome in major affective disorder. Dissertation for doctor of medical science (DMSc), 2001. Dan Med J. 2015;62(B5160):1–44.
24. Kessing LV. Longitudinal course and clinical progression in bipolar disorder: an updated systematic review. In: Passos IC, Kapczinski F, Berk M, editors. Bipolar disorder: an evidence-based clinical guide. Cham: Springer; 2024.

25. Kessing LV, Andersen PK. Predictive effects of previous episodes on the risk of recurrence in depressive and bipolar disorders. Curr Psychiatry Rep. 2005;7:413–20.
26. Burdick KE, Russo M, Frangou S, Mahon K, Braga RJ, Shanahan M, Malhotra AK. Empirical evidence for discrete neurocognitive subgroups in bipolar disorder: clinical implications. Psychol Med. 2014;44:3083–96.
27. Kjærstad HL, Poulsen E, Vinberg M, Kessing LV, Miskowiak KW. Differential trajectory of cognitive functions in neurocognitive subgroups of newly diagnosed patients with bipolar disorder and their unaffected first-degree relatives: a longitudinal study. J Affect Disord. 2022;311:115–25.
28. Depp CA, Mausbach BT, Harmell AL, Savla GN, Bowie CR, Harvey PD, Patterson TL. Meta-analysis of the association between cognitive abilities and everyday functioning in bipolar disorder. Bipolar Disord. 2012;14:217–26.
29. Martinez-aran A, Vieta E, Torrent C, Sanchez-moreno J, Goikolea JM, Salamero M, Malhi GS, Gonzalez-pinto A, Daban C, Alvarez-grandi S, Fountoulakis K, Kaprinis G, Tabares-seisdedos R, Ayuso-mateos JL. Functional outcome in bipolar disorder: the role of clinical and cognitive factors. Bipolar Disord. 2007;9:103–13.
30. Mur M, Portella MJ, Martinez-aran A, Pifarre J, Vieta E. Influence of clinical and neuropsychological variables on the psychosocial and occupational outcome of remitted bipolar patients. Psychopathology. 2009;42:148–56.
31. Sletved KSO, Ziersen SC, Andersen PK, Vinberg M, Kessing LV. Socio-economic functioning in patients with bipolar disorder and their unaffected siblings: results from a nation-wide population-based longitudinal study. Psychol Med. 2023;53:706–13.
32. Huxley N, Baldessarini RJ. Disability and its treatment in bipolar disorder patients. Bipolar Disord. 2007;9:183–96.
33. Tse S, Chan S, NG KL, Yatham LN. Meta-analysis of predictors of favorable employment outcomes among individuals with bipolar disorder. Bipolar Disord. 2014;16:217–29.
34. Kessing LV, Nilsson FM. Increased risk of developing dementia in patients with major affective disorders compared to patients with other medical illnesses. J Affect Disord. 2003;73:261–9.
35. Kessing LV, Olsen EW, Mortensen PB, Andersen PK. Dementia in affective disorder: a case-register study. Acta Psychiatr Scand. 1999;100:176–85.
36. Velosa J, Delgado A, Finger E, Berk M, Kapczinski F, de Azevedo Cardoso T. Risk of dementia in bipolar disorder and the interplay of lithium: a systematic review and meta-analyses. Acta Psychiatr Scand. 2020;141:510–21.
37. Kessing LV, Andersen PK. Does the risk of developing dementia increase with the number of episodes in patients with depressive disorder and in patients with bipolar disorder? J Neurol Neurosurg Psychiatry. 2004;75:1662–6.
38. Gerhard T, Devanand DP, Huang C, Crystal S, Olfson M. Lithium treatment and risk for dementia in adults with bipolar disorder: population-based cohort study. Br J Psychiatry. 2015;207:46–51.
39. Kessing LV, Forman JL, Andersen PK. Does lithium protect against dementia? Bipolar Disord. 2010;12:87–94.
40. Kessing LV, Sondergard L, Forman JL, Andersen PK. Lithium treatment and risk of dementia. Arch Gen Psychiatry. 2008;65:1331–5.
41. Scott J, Graham A, Yung A, Morgan C, Bellivier F, Etain B. A systematic review and meta-analysis of delayed help-seeking, delayed diagnosis and duration of untreated illness in bipolar disorders. Acta Psychiatr Scand. 2022;146:389–405.
42. Mccraw S, Parker G, Graham R, Synnott H, Mitchell PB. The duration of undiagnosed bipolar disorder: effect on outcomes and treatment response. J Affect Disord. 2014;168:422–9.
43. Kessing LV, Vradi E, Andersen PK. Nationwide and population-based prescription patterns in bipolar disorder. Bipolar Disord. 2016;18:174–82.
44. Shuy YK, Santharan S, Chew QH, Sim K. International trends in lithium use for pharmacotherapy and clinical correlates in bipolar disorder: a scoping review. Brain Sci. 2024;14:102.

45. Haeberle A, Greil W, Russmann S, Grohmann R. Mono- and combination drug therapies in hospitalized patients with bipolar depression. Data from the European drug surveillance program AMSP. BMC Psychiatry. 2012;12:153.
46. Goodwin GM. Evidence-based guidelines for treating bipolar disorder: revised second edition-recommendations from the British Association for Psychopharmacology. J Psychopharmacol. 2009;23:346–88.
47. Grunze H, Vieta E, Goodwin GM, Bowden C, Licht RW, Moller HJ, Kasper S. The world federation of societies of biological psychiatry (WFSBP) guidelines for the biological treatment of bipolar disorders: update 2012 on the long-term treatment of bipolar disorder. World J Biol Psychiatry. 2013;14:154–219.
48. NICE. Bipolar disorder: the assessment and management of bipolar disorder in adults, children and young people in primary and secondary care. NICE clinical guideline 185. 2015.
49. Severus E, Taylor MJ, Sauer C, Pfennig A, Ritter P, Bauer M, Geddes JR. Lithium for prevention of mood episodes in bipolar disorders: systematic review and meta-analysis. Int J Bipolar Disord. 2014;2:15.
50. Yatham LN, Kennedy SH, Parikh SV, Schaffer A, Bond DJ, Frey BN, Sharma V, Goldstein BI, Rej S, Beaulieu S, Alda M, Macqueen G, Milev RV, Ravindran A, O'donovan C, Mcintosh D, Lam RW, Vazquez G, Kapczinski F, Mcintyre RS, Kozicky J, Kanba S, Lafer B, Suppes T, Calabrese JR, Vieta E, Malhi G, Post RM, Berk M. Canadian network for mood and anxiety treatments (CANMAT) and International society for bipolar disorders (ISBD) 2018 guidelines for the management of patients with bipolar disorder. Bipolar Disord. 2018;20:97–170.
51. Grunze H, Vieta E, Goodwin GM, Bowden C, Licht RW, Moller HJ, Kasper S. The world federation of societies of biological psychiatry (WFSBP) guidelines for the biological treatment of bipolar disorders: update 2010 on the treatment of acute bipolar depression. World J Biol Psychiatry. 2010;11:81–109.
52. Pacchiarotti I, Bond DJ, Baldessarini RJ, Nolen WA, Grunze H, Licht RW, Post RM, Berk M, Goodwin GM, Sachs GS, Tondo L, Findling RL, Youngstrom EA, Tohen M, Undurraga J, Gonzalez-pinto A, Goldberg JF, Yildiz A, Altshuler LL, Calabrese JR, Mitchell PB, Thase ME, Koukopoulos A, Colom F, Frye MA, Malhi GS, Fountoulakis KN, Vazquez G, Perlis RH, Ketter TA, Cassidy F, Akiskal H, Azorin JM, Valenti M, Mazzei DH, Lafer B, Kato T, Mazzarini L, Martinez-aran A, Parker G, Souery D, Ozerdem A, Mcelroy SL, Girardi P, Bauer M, Yatham LN, Zarate CA, Nierenberg AA, Birmaher B, Kanba S, El-Mallakh RS, Serretti A, Rihmer Z, Young AH, Kotzalidis GD, Macqueen GM, Bowden CL, Ghaemi SN, Lopez-jaramillo C, Rybakowski J, Ha K, Perugi G, Kasper S, Amsterdam JD, Hirschfeld RM, Kapczinski F, Vieta E. The international society for bipolar disorders (ISBD) task force report on antidepressant use in bipolar disorders. Am J Psychiatry. 2013;170:1249–62.
53. Sidor MM, Macqueen GM. Antidepressants for the acute treatment of bipolar depression: a systematic review and meta-analysis. J Clin Psychiatry. 2011;72:156–67.
54. Yatham LN, Kennedy SH, Parikh SV, Schaffer A, Beaulieu S, Alda M, O'donovan C, Macqueen G, Mcintyre RS, Sharma V, Ravindran A, Young LT, Milev R, Bond DJ, Frey BN, Goldstein BI, Lafer B, Birmaher B, Ha K, Nolen WA, Berk M. Canadian network for mood and anxiety treatments (CANMAT) and International society for bipolar disorders (ISBD) collaborative update of CANMAT guidelines for the management of patients with bipolar disorder: update 2013. Bipolar Disord. 2013;15:1–44.
55. Kessing LV, Hellmund G, Andersen PK. Predictors of excellent response to lithium: results from a nationwide register-based study. Int Clin Psychopharmacol. 2011;26:323–8.
56. Crump C, Sundquist K, Winkleby MA, Sundquist J. Comorbidities and mortality in bipolar disorder: a Swedish national cohort study. JAMA Psychiatry. 2013;70:931–9.
57. Laursen TM, Munk-olsen T, Nordentoft M, Mortensen PB. Increased mortality among patients admitted with major psychiatric disorders: a register-based study comparing mortality in unipolar depressive disorder, bipolar affective disorder, schizoaffective disorder, and schizophrenia. J Clin Psychiatry. 2007;68:899–907.

58. Osby U, Brandt L, Correia N, Ekbom A, Sparen P. Excess mortality in bipolar and unipolar disorder in Sweden. Arch Gen Psychiatry. 2001;58:844–50.
59. Kessing LV, Vradi E, Andersen PK. Life expectancy in bipolar disorder. Bipolar Disord. 2015a;17:543–8.
60. Harris EC, Barraclough B. Suicide as an outcome for mental disorders. A meta-analysis. Br J Psychiatry. 1997;170:205–28.
61. Weiner M, Warren L, Fiedorowicz JG. Cardiovascular morbidity and mortality in bipolar disorder. Ann Clin Psychiatry. 2011;23:40–7.
62. Calkin CV, Gardner DM, Ransom T, Alda M. The relationship between bipolar disorder and type 2 diabetes: more than just co-morbid disorders. Ann Med. 2013;45:171–81.
63. Mcintyre RS, Konarski JZ, Misener VL, Kennedy SH. Bipolar disorder and diabetes mellitus: epidemiology, etiology, and treatment implications. Ann Clin Psychiatry. 2005;17:83–93.
64. Laursen TM, Munk-olsen T, Gasse C. Chronic somatic comorbidity and excess mortality due to natural causes in persons with schizophrenia or bipolar affective disorder. PLoS One. 2011;6:e24597.
65. Rihmer Z, Fawcett J. Suicide and bipolar disorder. In: Yatham LN, Maj M, editors. Clinical and neurobiological foundations. John Wiley & Sons, Ltd; 2010.
66. Nordentoft M, Mortensen PB, Pedersen CB. Absolute risk of suicide after first hospital contact in mental disorder. Arch Gen Psychiatry. 2011;68:1058–64.
67. Kessing LV, Vradi E, Mcintyre RS, Andersen PK. Causes of decreased life expectancy over the life span in bipolar disorder. J Affect Disord. 2015c;180:142–7.
68. Roshanaei-Moghaddam B, Katon W. Premature mortality from general medical illnesses among persons with bipolar disorder: a review. Psychiatr Serv. 2009;60:147–56.
69. Rizzo LB, Costa LG, Mansur RB, Swardfager W, Belangero SI, Grassi-Oliveira R, Mcintyre RS, Bauer ME, Brietzke E. The theory of bipolar disorder as an illness of accelerated aging: Implications for clinical care and research. Neurosci Biobehav Rev. 2014;42C:157–69.
70. Mcintyre RS, Jerrell JM. Metabolic and cardiovascular adverse events associated with antipsychotic treatment in children and adolescents. Arch Pediatr Adolesc Med. 2008;162:929–35.
71. Ratheesh A, Hett D, Ramain J, Wong E, Berk L, Conus P, Fristad MA, Goldstein T, Hillegers M, Jauhar S, Kessing L, Miklowitz DJ, Murray G, Scott J, Tohen M, Yatham LN, Young AH, Berk M, Marwaha S. A systematic review of interventions in the early course of bipolar disorder I or II: a report of the International Society for Bipolar Disorders Taskforce on early intervention. Int J Bipolar Disord. 2023;11
72. Kessing LV, Hansen HV, Hvenegaard A, Christensen EM, Dam H, Gluud C, Wetterslev J. Treatment in a specialised out-patient mood disorder clinic v. standard out-patient treatment in the early course of bipolar disorder: randomised clinical trial. Br J Psychiatry. 2013;202:212–9.
73. Kessing LV, Hansen HV, Christensen EM, Dam H, Gluud C, Wetterslev J. Do young adults with bipolar disorder benefit from early intervention? J Affect Disord. 2014:152–4. 403-408

Chapter 3
Bipolar Disorder Offspring Cohorts: Clinical Implications

Maj Vinberg

3.1 Background

A familial history of bipolar disorder matters. Genetic and environmental risk factors interact, and bipolar disorder is influenced by exposure to multiple factors (physical, psychological, and social) [1]. Already, Kraepelin [2] noted that the most potent risk factor was a family history of bipolar disorder, and decades of family studies have revealed a solid familial contribution to bipolar disorders. The first high-risk family studies were conducted in Germany after the First World War as a follow-up to Kraepelin and colleagues' valuable initial research [3, 4]. A comprehensive review of family and twin studies was published in Goodwin and Jamison's second edition of the textbook Manic-depressive Illness, Bipolar Disorders and Recurrent Depression [5]. In summary, 14 family studies conducted between 1921 and 1952 were identified, but data from three German studies were not available, leaving 11 studies analyzing data on a total of 5515 first-degree relatives of manic-depressive patients, and the overall risk of manic-depressive illness in the offspring was estimated to be 12.3%. Further, 32 studies were conducted between 1960 and 2006, covering 12,245 first-degree relatives of bipolar, bipolar I, bipolar II, major depressive disorder, and control probands. These studies found an 11.9% risk of bipolar illness in first-degree relatives of bipolar probands versus 1.0% in relatives of control probands.

The original version of the chapter has been revised. A correction to this chapter can be found at https://doi.org/10.1007/978-3-032-01297-5_18

M. Vinberg (✉)
Department of Clinical Medicine, Psychiatry University of Copenhagen, Copenhagen, Denmark

Psychiatric Centre North Zealand, Copenhagen University Hospital - Mental Health Services CPH, 1The Early Multimodular Prevention and Intervention Research Institution (EMPIRI), Copenhagen, Denmark
e-mail: maj.vinberg@regionh.dk

T. de Azevedo Cardoso et al. (eds.), *Latent Bipolar Disorder*,
https://doi.org/10.1007/978-3-032-01297-5_3

3.2 The Genetics of Latent Bipolar Disorder

Twin studies with concordance rates for bipolar disorder of 0.36–0.80 in MZ twins and 0.04–0.19 in DZ twins [6] repeatedly have understated that bipolar disorder has a high genetic penetrance. Register studies [7] and meta-analyses have further replicated that the offspring of affected parents have a strongly elevated relative risk of bipolar disorder and lifetime risk of developing any mental disorder [8, 9]. Further nationwide register studies have confirmed the risk in offspring aged 0–18. A Danish population-based sample of all individuals hospitalized or in outpatient clinic contact for the first time with bipolar affective disorder showed that individuals with a first-degree relative with bipolar affective disorder had a 13.63 times greater risk (95% confidence interval, 11.81–15.71) of developing bipolar affective disorder [10]. A nationwide Swedish study found that children of parents with bipolar disorder had two to three times higher risks of all psychiatric diagnoses, except for bipolar disorder, for which the risk was 11-fold [11].

Together, these studies report high rates of psychopathology in offspring, although the onset of bipolar I disorder is still relatively rare among offspring with a parent with bipolar disorder. Evidence from twin, family, and adoption studies indicates a strong genetic predisposition to bipolar disorder and, further, a close transdiagnostic relationship between bipolar disorder, unipolar disorder, and schizophrenia. Overall, these studies have identified that individuals with a family history of bipolar disorder are at a higher risk of developing the disorder themselves. The genetics of bipolar disorder are still complex and involve a combination of genetic and environmental factors. Hence, the genetics of latent bipolar disorders are presumably even more complicated, and the intergenerational heritability makes it even more difficult to disentangle bipolar disorders. The genetic scores derived from genome-wide association studies thus explain only a fraction of the heritability estimates obtained from whole-genome studies on single populations, known as the "hidden heritability" puzzle. Multiple lines of evidence suggest that the roles of genetic and environmental factors depend on each other. Gene x environment interactions may also underlie the paradox of strong environmental factors in a highly heritable disorder such as bipolar disorder, the low estimates of shared environmental influences in twin studies, and the heritability gap between twin and molecular heritability estimates. The offspring of parents with bipolar disorder seem overall to be more vulnerable to the effects of prenatal and postnatal environmental exposures, suggesting that the expression of genetic liability depends on the environment [12, 13].

Consequently, genetics alone do not determine the development of bipolar disorder. Environmental factors, such as stress, substance abuse, life events, and social support, also play a crucial role in the manifestation of the disorder. The interaction between genetic susceptibility and environmental triggers is thought to influence the onset and course of bipolar disorder. Being at familial risk for bipolar disorders further seems to lower the threshold for subclinical psychopathology due to the pooling of multiple illness-related genes and innate hyper-reactivity to stress. Genes predisposing to bipolar disorders may hence be transmitted to offspring without expression of the phenotype, and bipolar disorders probably result from many interacting genes being influenced by environmental factors [12]. Multiple genes are believed to contribute to the risk of developing bipolar disorder, each with a small effect. These genes may impact various biological pathways related to mood regulation, neurotransmitter function, DNA methylation, and circadian rhythms. Several candidate genes may play a role in bipolar disorder, such as the CACNA1C gene, which is involved in calcium channel signaling [13]. A genome-wide association study of 41,917 bipolar disorder cases and 371,549 European-ancestry controls identified 64 associated genomic loci. Bipolar disorder risk alleles were enriched in synaptic signaling pathways and brain-expressed genes, particularly those with a high specificity of expression in neurons of the prefrontal cortex and hippocampus [14]. However, genetic studies still need to be translated into clinical practice. They may benefit from a more detailed phenotypic description and clustering of these, including familial risk, as in a recent systematic review of characteristics indexing genetic differences in bipolar disorder. Moderate to strong evidence for a positive association of age at onset, subtype (bipolar I versus bipolar II), psychotic symptoms, and manic symptoms with familial/genetic risk of bipolar disorder was revealed [13]. Overall, while progress has been made in understanding the genetic basis of bipolar disorder, further research is needed to uncover the specific genetic mechanisms underlying the condition and how these interact with environmental factors to influence disease risk and presentation.

There is considerable interest in the familial transmission of psychiatric illness. However, many studies still examine single disorders, e.g., schizophrenia, bipolar disorder, and anxiety disorder, and are based on a cross-sectional snapshot of clinical states and other risk markers [12]. It also seems that the earliest expressions of psychopathology include a nonspecific mixture of affective dysregulation, aberrant resistance, motivational changes, and anxiety states. It is not possible to disentangle the gene-specific trajectories from the environmental trajectories. Still, although there is considerable insight into the genetic puzzles that underlie the development and onset of bipolar disorder, no treatments are available targeting the genetic pathways. However, the environmental impact can be influenced and modified. Unveiling the environmental risk and resilience factors is, therefore, a pragmatic focus, e.g., reducing the environmental stressors, e.g., descaling familial stress or early exposure to smoking, alcohol, and cannabis.

Bipolar disorder, hence, runs in families and has a potentially significant negative impact on the health and longevity of both those with the disorder and their family [15]. Still, the specific factors that are transmitted intergenerational are unknown. Family studies or high-risk studies provide an essential research field: the studies of high-risk samples, which focus on subgroups at increased risk for a disorder due to a family history [16, 17]. In these studies, comparisons are made between those with and without familial risk [18] and between high-risk persons who develop a condition of interest and high-risk persons who remain free of the condition [19].

Further, up to 70% of patients with bipolar disorder have their onset before the age of 25, and the mean time from first hypomanic or manic episodes to diagnosis is approximately 6–8 years [20]. The developmental transition from childhood to adulthood is a crucial period for the early prevention of the onset of psychiatric disorders, as both psychological and neurobiological maturation processes increase the risk of developing psychopathology [21]. Yet, there is a gap in the hospital system where child and adolescent psychiatry cease and adult psychiatry begins, creating an additional hole in clinical knowledge and experience in assessing and treating modifiable and important multimodal risk factors and early psychopathological presentations in high-risk adolescents. Individuals with latent bipolar disorders thus risk falling in between, hence missing a vital window of possibilities for early preventive intervention. Additionally, there is a clinical knowledge and experience gap in evaluating and treating modifiable risk factors and early psychopathological presentations in high-risk adolescents.

3.3 Longitudinal Studies of Offspring of Patients with Bipolar Disorder

Longitudinal studies of offspring from childhood until early adulthood thus provide a unique possibility to get a deeper insight into early psychopathology and to establish early interventions that may hold or reverse this process. High-risk studies further offer a way of analyzing relatively rare outcomes. They can provide insight into inherited vulnerability, potential risk factors, the early clinical manifestations and intermediate causal pathways, and facilitate the identification of prodromal stages without the confounding effects of the changes associated with the burden of the illness [22]. These studies can provide essential information to guide prevention and notably initiate early treatment that seems to hinder a more severe progression of the disorder [23–25]. Such studies are crucial to discover robust risk and resilience factors.

Several prospective clinical studies of high-risk subjects, including bipolar probands and their offspring, have been following children into adulthood, providing fine-grained data. Please see the overview of follow-up assessments regarding risk factors for the onset of bipolar disorders based on offspring studies (Table 3.1). Together, these studies report high rates of psychopathology in offspring, although the onset of bipolar I disorder is still relatively rare among offspring with a parent with bipolar disorder.

Another approach is to follow discordant twins [18, 42] or siblings and offspring together, as done in, e.g., the Bipolar Onset study [43], mainly including whole siblings as high-risk participants. Finally, several register-based studies, mainly from Scandinavia, have explored the impact of being a first-degree relative to a proband with bipolar disorder [11]. A Danish register study revealed that children of parents with bipolar disorder were indistinguishable from the reference group

Table 3.1 Longitudinal studies of offspring of parents with bipolar disorders

Study and year	Offspring Number, mean age at follow-up	Controls Number, mean age at follow-up	Follow-up time	Main findings, risk factors
Birmaher et al. 2021 [26]	116 13.0	45 13.8	9.6	Most offspring of BD parents did not develop BD, but they were at specific high risk for developing BD, particularly those with preschool ADHD and early-onset parental BD. Lower socioeconomic status, younger parental mood disorder onset, and younger parental age at offspring's birth were significant predictors of BD onset.
Hafeman et al. 2023 [27]	113 13.3			Risk factors Preschool irritability and sleep problems.
De la Serna et al. 2021 [28]	90 13.9 (3.2)	107 13.9 (3.2)	2.0	The prevalence of psychopathology and comorbidity was higher in BD offspring; there were no differences in functioning.
Duffy et al. 2019 [29] Goodday et al. 2019 [30]	279 16.5 (6.3)	87 14.71 (2.2)	7.7 6.1	Cumulative incidence rate of BD in offspring = 24.5%, median onset age is 20.7. Risk factors Childhood anxiety and sleep disorders Avoidant coping strategies increased the risk, while higher self-esteem significantly decreased the risk.
Egeland et al. 2012 [31]	115 Approx. 23.4	106 Approx. 24.1	16.0	Sensitivity, crying, hyper-alertness, anxiety/worry, and somatic complaints. During school years, parents reported mood (sad) and energy changes (low, not high), decreased sleep, and fearfulness as key symptoms.
Eraso-Osorio et al. 2021 [32]	131 20.5 (6.0)	150 20.4 (6.9)	4.0	Bipolar offspring had greater risk for presenting subthreshold symptoms and definitive psychiatric disorders, affective disorders, psychotic disorders, and externalizing disorders. In addition, the Bipolar Offspring group had a younger age of onset for psychoactive substance consumption and lower overall functioning.

(continued)

Table 3.1 (continued)

Study and year	Offspring Number, mean age at follow-up	Controls Number, mean age at follow-up	Follow-up time	Main findings, risk factors
Giacomi et al. 2023 [33]	31 with onset inclusion age 10.2	33 Not onset inclusion age 8.3	16.2	Higher scores on three temperament dimensions: "rhythmicity of habits" (regularity in performing daily habits), "task-orientation" (high persistence and low distractibility), and "approach to novelty" (tendency to approach new objects and persons).
Helmink et al. 2024 [34]	100 Offspring 38.3	0	22.0	The risk for homotypic transmission of BD in offspring of parents with BD is highest during adolescence. The heterotypic risk for mood disorder onset and recurrences continues over the life course.
Koenders et al. 2020 [35]	28.1		12.0	Severe mood disorders are often preceded by milder psychopathology. Emotional maltreatment was significantly associated with the onset of mood disorder.
Kemner et al. 2015 [36]			12.0	The first mood episode was associated with more stressful life events and a passive coping style.
Hemager et al. 2023 [37]	105 11.9	181 11.9	4.0	Familial high risk of bipolar disorder displayed social functioning comparable to controls except for impaired coping skills.
Krantz et al. 2023 [38]				Lower levels of stimulation and support in their homes than controls.
Burton et al. 2023 [39]				Children with a familial high risk of bipolar disorder showed no motor developmental differences.
Soehner et al. 2019 [40]	269 15.9	217 15.9	3.8	Offspring of probands with BD have greater exposure to independent and neutral life events than offspring of healthy controls. Greater frequency and severity of stressful life events were associated with Axis I disorder in offspring of both BD and non-BD affected probands.
Levensohn et al. 2017 [41]	227		3.6	Poor sleepers had twice the odds of developing BP than good and variable sleepers.

BD bipolar disorder

regarding school grades. However, the offspring of mothers with BD had a slightly increased risk of any physical contact, and they had more than double the risk of death than individuals without severe parental mental illness [44, 45]. The mentioned register study from Sweden found that the offspring of bipolar probands had significantly increased risks of several somatic conditions, low school grades, criminal behavior, victimization, accidents, and suicidal behavior [11].

The studies confirm that a family history of bipolar disorders increases the risk of psychopathology, and up to 40–60% of offspring of parents with mood disorders will eventually develop psychiatric symptoms, most commonly anxiety and depression. Most studies confirm the previously described enhanced risk of onset of bipolar disorders. High-risk studies of first-degree relatives of patients with bipolar disorder have provided insights into the pathological processes that occurred before the onset of full-blown mood disorder and revealed that subclinical anxiety, hypomanic and depression symptoms, stress reactions, severe life events, childhood trauma, sleep disturbances, circadian rhythm dysfunction, metabolic syndrome, and decreased functioning all belong to early-stage syndromes and seem to act as predictors for the onset of psychiatric illness [46–52].

Overall, all the above-mentioned studies reveal similar patterns of risk factors withstanding on five pillows, as illustrated below and in Fig. 3.1.

1. Genetic and familial risk.
2. Psychopathology, affective instability, sleep disturbances, cognitive problems, anxiety, and minor mood symptoms.
3. Environmental risk, overall functioning, sociodemographics, childhood trauma, and severe life events.
4. Psychological risk factors, emotional regulation, coping style, and personality traits.
5. Physical risk factors, physical complaints and disease, dietary habits, smoking, sedentary lifestyle, and alcohol and substance use.

An essential risk marker is global functioning. Decreased overall functioning is a core feature in adolescents at high familial risk, meaning that many at-risk adolescents need educational and economic support. It's important to note that 50% will continue to have lifelong impaired functioning [46, 47]. Assessing functioning, including personal hygiene, exercise, good eating, reading ability, and performing more complex home tasks, e.g., cleaning, cooking, and shopping, are essential. All tasks are required for independent living and represent the basis for other activities, including work and leisure [48]. Therefore, functional outcomes are recommended as outcomes and primary research targets in high-risk studies.

3.4 The Clinical Relevance of the Described Findings and Practical Recommendations for Healthcare Providers and Families

Bipolar disorder can be seen as the end state of a long process. In 1993, Fava and Kellner introduced the concept of staging to psychiatric classification and developed staging models for several psychiatric disorders, including bipolar and

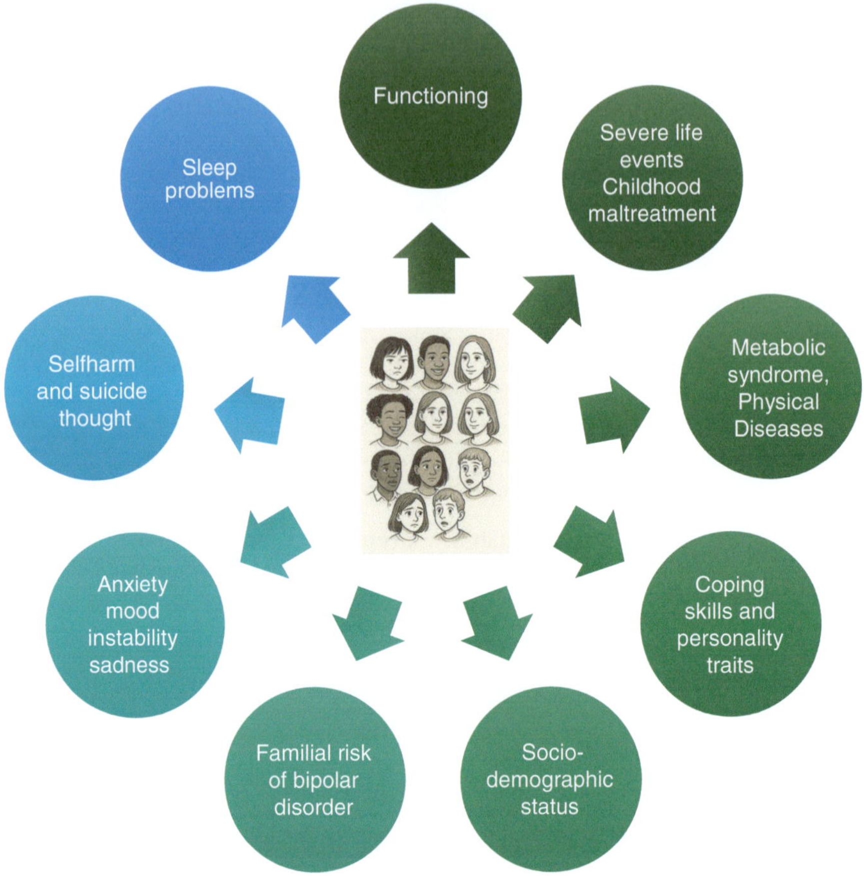

Fig. 3.1 Overview of risk factors for onset of bipolar disorders

unipolar disorders [53]. The staging model is based on longitudinal rather than cross-sectional observations and characterizes disorders according to severity, development, and features and potentially allows the clinician to select different treatments for earlier stages [54]. However, familial risk may not necessarily apply to a single disorder; it may instead represent a vulnerability to a spectrum of psychiatric disorders [55]. As psychiatric disorders have overlapping etiologies and co-aggregate in families, the present research may move from using traditional, descriptive diagnoses to clinical entities or categories that seem more closely related to the underlying workings of the brain. However, this broader approach is debatable, as it may be more likely to characterize distinct pathways only if conducted in narrowly defined subgroups of individuals at high risk for specific illnesses [56]. An important objective in psychiatry would be to shift from the traditional focus on treating end-stage illness to intervening in the earlier stages, as already happens in other medical areas.

Overall, the described literature points towards the possibility of determining the risk of latent bipolar disorders. These findings add weight to the clinical arguments for earlier and more thorough psychiatric assessment using all available information, including multiple informants and neuropsychological testing in individuals with a family history of bipolar disorder. The aim is to achieve earlier diagnosis and more accessible admission to preventive, tailored interventions and, when needed, early psychiatric treatment [49, 57]. For example, cognitive impairment substantially impacts functional outcomes, e.g., affecting the offspring's school performance. Another highly clinically significant finding is that up to 50% of patients with bipolar disorders report severe life events, including childhood trauma. The impact of being at familial risk also seems to include that the offspring are at risk for developing prolonged and pathological reactions that may blur the clinical picture when exposed to severe adverse events [58]. Further, it is essential to note that the impact of familial risk seems to persist over time, and the impact should not be limited to adolescence and early adulthood but should be lifetime, likely with differentiated age-specific strategies [7].

Several researchers have suggested different risk calculators for assessing offspring based on the longitudinal data from the high-risk cohorts [59–61]. Hence, actively using risk assessment, also supported by the Task Force Report from the International Society for Bipolar Disorder (ISBD) [62], could ensure that high-risk individuals have easy access to psychiatric assessment. A relevant clinical approach includes an assessment of the offspring as part of the treatment offered to the parents with bipolar disorder. It will depend on the parents with bipolar disorder's willingness to include their children in their treatment; however, based on qualitative interviews, parents with bipolar disorder express a massive wish for professional support and involvement [63].

Children of parents with bipolar disorder, hence, have clinical relevance in terms of increased risk for developing mental illness. Understanding this risk is crucial for healthcare providers and families in providing appropriate support and interventions. Clinically, parents with bipolar disorder often have several questions concerning their children's mental health, so the following are practical recommendations for healthcare providers and families.

The first approach is to pave the way for early identification, e.g., through regular assessments. The healthcare system could offer a regular screening of children of parents with bipolar disorder for early signs of mood disturbances or behavioral changes to promote early identification and intervention that may mitigate the progression of potential mood disorders. This approach allows for tracking changes in mood, behavior, or cognitive functioning, and, importantly, it detects symptoms early and facilitates timely interventions. Whether these assessments should include genetic counselling may still be too early. However, families with a history of bipolar disorder often have speculations and concerns due to the genetic risk. They may benefit from genetic counselling to understand the hereditary implications of the condition and information about the risk factors, inheritance patterns, and available testing options.

The second approach is to initiate early psychological treatment, including psychoeducation, for the families, helping the children by helping their parents with bipolar disorders and optimizing the treatments offered to target mothers and, importantly, also fathers, including perinatal services. This approach includes educating them about early signs of mental illness, early symptoms, triggers, and treatment options, which can empower them to recognize warning signs and provide practical support to their children. Psychoeducation can also reduce stigma and enhance family communication. A systematic review included seven articles (participants in total 138) of young people aged under 30 years with a family history of bipolar disorder. Overall, it was concluded that there is a lack of randomized trials exploring whether a psychological intervention may delay or prevent the onset of bipolar disorder [64]. An important target is encouraging a healthy lifestyle that includes regular physical activity, balanced nutrition, sufficient sleep, and stress management techniques to support overall mental and physical well-being in at-risk offspring.

The third approach is the possibility to initiate early medical treatment. Studies exploring the effects of pharmacological treatment in latent bipolar disorder are sparse, and the number of studies (below ten), the sample sizes (participants, in total 299), and the number of RCTs are small to modest [65]. There has only been one recent study from 2017 [66], whereas most studies were over ten years old. The latter study was the only one to report a positive effect in reducing manic symptoms in a double-blinded, controlled 12-week study. A search on ClinicalTrials.gov identifies several planned or ongoing studies. However, most of them have passed marked completion or report recruitment difficulties. Finally, the above-described approaches depend on easy access to mental health services, ensuring that at-risk offspring have access to mental health services, including therapy, counselling, or psychiatric care if needed. Prompt intervention can improve outcomes and quality of life for children at risk.

Overall, practical recommendations call for an early intervention approach to improve coping strategies and reduce exposure to childhood trauma and severe life events, as well as to prompt comprehensive psychiatric help and, if necessary, medical treatment. Such an approach helps prevent psychopathology from going untreated for lengthy periods and might halt the onset and progression of disorders, as well as potentially being more effective [67]. However, these hypotheses must be tested in a randomized clinical research design to determine whether the suggested monitoring, diagnosis, and treatment approach would benefit social, clinical, and economic outcomes.

3.5 Future Perspectives

By implementing these practical recommendations, healthcare providers and families can work together to support the mental health and well-being of offspring with a familial risk of bipolar disorder and their families. Cross-disciplinary and cross-sectional collaborations, early intervention, family support, and easy, non-stigmatizing access to a supportive healthcare system are vital in managing the clinical implications of being the offspring of patients with bipolar disorders [68, 69]. Prevention strategies assessing and targeting latent bipolar disorder are a promising avenue that needs to be explored in well-designed randomized study designs. These studies should include longer-term follow-up and may implement a range of outcomes relating to the offspring, the parents with bipolar disorder, and the whole family's function and well-being. An important research question is whether you can balance the latent risk forwards and backwards, thus not just passing the threshold for illness onset but also going backwards to identify latent risks or gain resilience.

3.6 Clinical Relevance

Primary selective prevention strategies targeting young adults are highly warranted. Providing new evidence about tailored treatment strategies in youth at familial risk will move the field and change the outcome for at-risk youth throughout their lifetime. As proven successful in other disciplines, such as cardiovascular health and other physical diseases, psychiatry practice would benefit from applying a more systematic, progressive prevention strategy.

3.7 Clinical Considerations

- When treating the parents, include treating the children using the clinical access to the parents with bipolar disorder and their co-parents.
- Emphasize the treatment as a whole family treatment offer, as this approach is comprehensive and beneficial for all family members.
- Include knowledge of risk factors, e.g., use risk calculators.
- Act when the at-risk offspring clinically passes the risk threshold.
- Keep an integrated approach and use a lower- and higher-intensity intervention continuum.
- Emphasize respecting and understanding the offspring and the family by avoiding pathologizing.
- Monitor the offspring's overall functioning.
- Help the parents by helping their children and vice versa.

References

1. Craddock N, Sklar P. Genetics of bipolar disorder. Lancet. 2013;381(9878):1654–62.
2. Kraepelin E. Manic-depressive insanity and paranoia. Edinburgh: Thoemmes Press; 1921.

3. Zerbin-Rudin E, Kendler KS. Ernst Rudin (1874–1952) and his genealogic-demographic department in Munich (1917–1986): an introduction to their family studies of schizophrenia. Am J Med Genet. 1996;67(4):332–7.
4. Kendler KS, Zerbin-Rudin E. Abstract and review of "Studien Uber Vererbung und Entstehung Geistiger Storungen. I. Zur Vererbung und Neuentstehung der Dementia praecox." (Studies on the inheritance and origin of mental illness: I. To the problem of the inheritance and primary origin of dementia praecox). 1916. Am J Med Genet. 1996;67(4):338–42.
5. Goodwin J. Manic-depressive illness. New York/Oxford: Oxford University Press; 1990.
6. Polderman TJ, Benyamin B, de Leeuw CA, Sullivan PF, van Bochoven A, Visscher PM, et al. Meta-analysis of the heritability of human traits based on fifty years of twin studies. Nat Genet. 2015;47(7):702–9.
7. Vedel Kessing L, Ziersen SC, Andersen PK, Vinberg M. A nationwide population-based longitudinal study mapping psychiatric disorders during lifetime in siblings to patients with bipolar disorder. Acta Psychiatr Scand. 2021;282:18–25.
8. Uher R, Pavlova B, Radua J, Provenzani U, Najafi S, Fortea L, et al. Transdiagnostic risk of mental disorders in offspring of affected parents: a meta-analysis of family high-risk and registry studies. World Psychiatry. 2023;22(3):433–48.
9. Lau P, Hawes DJ, Hunt C, Frankland A, Roberts G, Mitchell PB. Prevalence of psychopathology in bipolar high-risk offspring and siblings: a meta-analysis. Eur Child Adolesc Psychiatry. 2018;27(7):823–37.
10. AAE T, Laursen TM, Munk-Olsen T, Ranning A, Mortensen PB, Plessen KJ, et al. Incidence of child and adolescent mental disorders in children aged 0–17 with familial high risk for severe mental illness: a Danish register study. Schizophr Res. 2018;197:298–304.
11. Takami Lageborn C, Zhou M, Boman M, Sjolander A, Larsson H, BM D'O, et al. Childhood and adolescence outcomes in offspring to parents with bipolar disorder: the impact of lifetime parental comorbidity, parental sex, and bipolar subtype. J Child Psychol Psychiatry. 2024;
12. Scaini G, Valvassori SS, Diaz AP, Lima CN, Benevenuto D, Fries GR, et al. Neurobiology of bipolar disorders: a review of genetic components, signaling pathways, biochemical changes, and neuroimaging findings. Braz J Psychiatry. 2020;42(5):536–51.
13. van Loo HM, de Vries YA, Taylor J, Todorovic L, Dollinger C, Kendler KS. Clinical characteristics indexing genetic differences in bipolar disorde: a systematic review. Mol Psychiatry. 2023;28(9):3661–70.
14. Mullins N, Forstner AJ, O'Connell KS, Coombes B, JRI C, Qiao Z, et al. Genome-wide association study of more than 40,000 bipolar disorder cases provides new insights into the underlying biology. Nat Genet. 2021;53(6):817–29.
15. Madsen LH, Sletved KSO, Kessing LV, Vinberg M. Physical health status in first-degree relatives of patients with bipolar disorder, a systematic review. Nord J Psychiatry. 2022;76(6):433–41.
16. Salazar de Pablo G, Cabras A, Pereira J, Castro Santos H, de Diego H, Catalan A, et al. Predicting bipolar disorder I/II in individuals at clinical high-risk: results from a systematic review. J Affect Disord. 2023;325:778–86.
17. Sandstrom A, MacKenzie L, Pizzo A, Fine A, Rempel S, Howard C, et al. Observed psychopathology in offspring of parents with major depressive disorder, bipolar disorder and schizophrenia. Psychol Med. 2020;50(6):1050–6.
18. Vinberg M. A comparison of psychopathology, socio-economic status, cognitive function, personality traits and salivary cortisol in twins with and without a co-twin history of affective disorder. Dan Med Bull. 2007;54:69–78.
19. Stapp EK, Mendelson T, Merikangas KR, Wilcox HC. Parental bipolar disorder, family environment, and offspring psychiatric disorders: a systematic review. J Affect Disord. 2020;268:69–81.
20. Dagani J, Signorini G, Nielssen O, Bani M, Pastore A, Girolamo G, et al. Meta-analysis of the interval between the onset and management of bipolar disorder. Can J Psychiatr. 2017;62(4):247–58.

21. Yang R, Curtis J, Jensen C, Levy P, Chown K, Lappin JM. Detection and intervention in emerging youth mental health issues: outcomes from the first year of the CASPAR service. Early Interv Psychiatry. 2020;
22. Duffy A, Carlson GA. How does a developmental perspective inform us about the early natural history of bipolar disorder? J Can Acad Child Adolesc Psychiatry. 2013;22(1):6–12.
23. Bender RE, Alloy LB. Life stress and kindling in bipolar disorder: review of the evidence and integration with emerging biopsychosocial theories. Clin Psychol Rev. 2011;31(3):383–98.
24. Shapero BG, Weiss RB, Burke TA, Boland EM, Abramson LY, Alloy LB. Kindling of life stress in bipolar disorder: effects of early adversity. Behav Ther. 2017;48(3):322–34.
25. Kessing LV, Hansen HV, Christensen EM, Dam H, Gluud C, Wetterslev J, et al. Do young adults with bipolar disorder benefit from early intervention? J Affect Disord. 2014;152–154:403–8.
26. Birmaher B, Merranko J, Hafeman D, Goldstein BI, Diler R, Levenson JC, et al. A longitudinal study of psychiatric disorders in offspring of parents with bipolar disorder from preschool to adolescence. J Am Acad Child Adolesc Psychiatry. 2021;60(11):1419–29.
27. Hafeman DM, Merranko J, Joseph HM, Goldstein TR, Goldstein BI, Levenson J, et al. Early indicators of bipolar risk in preschool offspring of parents with bipolar disorder. J Child Psychol Psychiatry. 2023;64(10):1492–500.
28. De la Serna E, Ilzarbe D, Sugranyes G, Baeza I, Moreno D, Rodríguez-Toscano E, et al. Lifetime psychopathology in child and adolescent offspring of parents diagnosed with schizophrenia or bipolar disorder: a 2-year follow-up study. Eur Child Adolesc Psychiatry. 2021;30(1):117–29.
29. Duffy A, Goodday S, Keown-Stoneman C, Grof P. The emergent course of bipolar disorder: Observations over two decades from the Canadian high-risk offspring cohort. Am J Psychiatry. 2019;176(9):720–9.
30. Goodday SM, Bentall R, Jones S, Weir A, Duffy A. Coping strategies and self-esteem in the high-risk offspring of bipolar parents. Aust N Z J Psychiatry. 2019;53(2):129–35.
31. Egeland JA, Endicott J, Hostetter AM, Allen CR, Pauls DL, Shaw JA. A 16-year prospective study of prodromal features prior to BPI onset in well Amish children. J Affect Disord. 2012;142(1–3):186–92.
32. Eraso-Osorio JJ, Palacio-Ortiz JD, Quintero-Cadavid CP, Estrada-Jaramillo S, Andrade-Carrillo R, Gómez-Cano S, et al. High risk for psychiatric disorders in bipolar offspring. A four years prospective study. Rev Colomb Psiquiatr (Engl Ed). 2021;50(4):273–84.
33. Giacomo FD, Strippoli MF, Castelao E, Amoussou JR, Gholam M, Ranjbar S, et al. Risk factors for mood disorders among offspring of parents with bipolar disorder: findings from a discordant-sibling study. Psychiatry Res. 2023;330:115615.
34. Helmink FGL, Mesman E, MHJ H. Beyond the window of risk? The Dutch bipolar offspring study: 22-Year Follow-up. J Am Acad Child Adolesc Psychiatry. 2024;
35. Koenders MA, Mesman E, Giltay EJ, Elzinga BM, Hillegers MHJ. Traumatic experiences, family functioning, and mood disorder development in bipolar offspring. Br J Clin Psychol. 2020;59(3):277–89.
36. Kemner SM, Mesman E, Nolen WA, Eijckemans MJ, Hillegers MH. The role of life events and psychological factors in the onset of first and recurrent mood episodes in bipolar offspring: results from the Dutch bipolar offspring study. Psychol Med. 2015;45(12):2571–81.
37. Hemager N, Gregersen M, Christiani CJ, Hjorthøj C, Knudsen CB, Veddum L, et al. Development of social functioning in preadolescent children at familial high-risk of schizophrenia or bipolar disorder: a 4-year follow-up study from age 7 to 11. Psychiatry Res. 2023;327:115397.
38. Krantz MF, Hjorthøj C, Brandt JM, Prøsch ÅK, Rohd SB, Wilms M, et al. Home environment of 11-year-old children born to parents with schizophrenia or bipolar disorder: a controlled, 4-year follow-up study: the Danish high risk and resilience study: VIA 11. Psychol Med. 2023;53(6):2563–73.
39. Burton BK, Krantz MF, Skovgaard LT, Brandt JM, Gregersen M, Søndergaard A, et al. Impaired motor development in children with familial high risk of schizophrenia or bipolar

disorder and the association with psychotic experiences: a 4-year Danish observational follow-up study. Lancet Psychiatry. 2023;10(2):108–18.
40. Soehner AM, Bertocci MA, Levenson JC, Goldstein TR, Rooks B, Merranko J, et al. Longitudinal associations between sleep patterns and psychiatric symptom severity in high-risk and community comparison youth. J Am Acad Child Adolesc Psychiatry. 2019;58(6):608–17.
41. Levenson JC, Soehner A, Rooks B, Goldstein TR, Diler R, Merranko J, et al. Longitudinal sleep phenotypes among offspring of bipolar parents and community controls. J Affect Disord. 2017;215:30–6.
42. Ottesen NM, Meluken I, Scheike T, Kessing LV, Miskowiak KW, Vinberg M. Clinical characteristics, life adversities and personality traits in monozygotic twins with, at risk of and without affective disorders. Front Psych. 2018;9:401. https://doi.org/10.3389/fpsyt.2018.00401.
43. Kessing LV, Munkholm K, Faurholt-Jepsen M, Miskowiak KW, Nielsen LB, Frikke-Schmidt R, et al. The bipolar illness onset study: research protocol for the BIO cohort study. BMJ Open. 2017;7(6):e015462.
44. Ranning A, Benros ME, AAE T, Davidsen KA, Hjorthoj C, Nordentoft M, et al. Morbidity and mortality in the children and young adult offspring of parents with schizophrenia or affective disorders—a nationwide register-based cohort study in 2 million individuals. Schizophr Bull. 2020;46(1):130–9.
45. Ranning A, Laursen T, Agerbo E, Thorup A, Hjorthoj C, JRM J, et al. School performance from primary education in the adolescent offspring of parents with schizophrenia and bipolar disorder- a national, register-based study. Psychol Med. 2018;48(12):1993–2000.
46. Kulkarni NP, Dimick MK, Kennedy KG, Axelson DA, Sakolsky DJ, Diler RS, et al. Controlled study of metabolic syndrome among offspring of parents with bipolar disorder. J Clin Psychiatry. 2024;85(3)
47. Kamali M, Stapp EK, Fullerton JM, Ghaziuddin N, Hulvershorn L, MG MI, et al. Examining the association of familial and social stress, trauma, and support on mood, anxiety, and behavioral symptoms and diagnoses in youth at risk for bipolar disorder and controls. J Affect Disord. 2024;363:79–89.
48. FGL H, Vandeleur CL, Preisig M, STG G, MHJ H, Mesman E. Functional outcomes across development in offspring of parents with bipolar disorder. J Affect Disord. 2023;340:490–505.
49. Vinberg M, Miskowiak K, Kessing LV. Risk markers for affective disorder, a seven-years follow up study of a twin cohort at low and high risk for affective disorder. J Psychiatr Res. 2013;47(5):565–71.
50. Menculini G, Balducci PM, Attademo L, Bernardini F, Moretti P, Tortorella A. Environmental risk factors for bipolar disorders and high-risk states in adolescence: a systematic review. Medicina (Kaunas). 2020;56(12)
51. la Cour Karottki NF, Coello K, Stanislaus S, Melbye S, Kjaerstad HL, Sletved KSO, et al. Sleep and physical activity in patients with newly diagnosed bipolar disorder in remission, their first-degree unaffected relatives and healthy controls. Int J Bipolar Disord. 2020;8(1):16.
52. Lei B, Feng H, Yang L, Wang J, Chen J, Song W, et al. Circadian rhythm dysfunction and psychopathology in the offspring of parents with bipolar disorder: a high-risk study in the Chinese population. Gen Psychiatr. 2024;37(3):e101239.
53. Fava GA, Kellner R. Staging: a neglected dimension in psychiatric classification. Acta Psychiatr Scand. 1993;87(4):225–30.
54. Hartmann JA, Nelson B, Ratheesh A, Treen D, PD MG. At-risk studies and clinical antecedents of psychosis, bipolar disorder and depression: a scoping review in the context of clinical staging. Psychol Med. 2019;49(2):177–89.
55. Rasic D, Hajek T, Alda M, Uher R. Risk of mental illness in offspring of parents with schizophrenia, bipolar disorder, and major depressive disorder: a meta-analysis of family high-risk studies. Schizophr Bull. 2013;
56. Duffy A, Malhi GS, Grof P. Do the trajectories of bipolar disorder and schizophrenia follow a universal staging model? Can J Psychiatr. 2017;62(2):115–22.

57. Duffy A, Grof P. Longitudinal studies of bipolar patients and their families: translating findings to advance individualized risk prediction, treatment and research. Int J Bipolar Disord. 2024;12(1):12.
58. Av Kák Kollsker S, Coello K, Stanislaus S, Melbye S, Lie Kjaerstad H, Stefanie Ormstrup Sletved K, et al. Association between lifetime and recent stressful life events and the early course and psychopathology in patients with newly diagnosed bipolar disorder, first-degree unaffected relatives and healthy controls: cross-sectional results from a prospective study. Bipolar Disord. 2022;24(1):59–68.
59. Birmaher B, Merranko JA, Gill MK, Hafeman D, Goldstein T, Goldstein B, et al. Predicting personalized risk of mood recurrences in youths and young adults with bipolar spectrum disorder. J Am Acad Child Adolesc Psychiatry. 2020;59(10):1156–64.
60. CDG K-S, Goodday SM, Preisig M, Vandeleur C, Castelao E, Grof P, et al. Development and validation of a risk calculator for major mood disorders among the offspring of bipolar parents using information collected in routine clinical practice. EClinicalMedicine. 2021;39:101083.
61. Ratheesh A, Hammond D, Watson M, Betts J, Siegel E, McGorry P, et al. Bipolar at-risk criteria and risk of bipolar disorder over 10 or more years. JAMA Netw Open. 2023;6(9):e2334078.
62. Faedda GL, Baldessarini RJ, Marangoni C, Bechdolf A, Berk M, Birmaher B, et al. An international society of bipolar disorders task force report: precursors and prodromes of bipolar disorder. Bipolar Disord. 2019;21(8):720–40.
63. Johansen M, Wagner CB, Pedersen S, Stokholm J, Vinberg M. How do PARents with Affective disorders perceive their intergenerational risk of mental illness? Results from a qualitative study – PARAMENTAL. Submitted. 2024.
64. Perich T, Mitchell PB. Psychological interventions for young people at risk for bipolar disorder: a systematic review. J Affect Disord. 2019;252:84–91.
65. Møller C, Miskowiak K, Kessing LV, Vinberg M. Pharmacological treatment of individuals at familial risk for bipolar or major depressive disorders: a scoping review. Curr Treat Options Psychiatry. 2022;9:55–72.
66. Findling RL, Youngstrom EA, Rowles BM, Deyling E, Lingler J, Stansbrey RJ, et al. A double-blind and placebo-controlled trial of aripiprazole in symptomatic youths at genetic high risk for bipolar disorder. J Child Adolesc Psychopharmacol. 2017;27(10):864–74.
67. Scott J, Iorfino F, Capon W, Crouse J, Nelson B, Chanen AM, et al. Staging 2.0: refining transdiagnostic clinical staging frameworks to enhance reliability and utility for youth mental health. Lancet Psychiatry. 2024;11(6):461–71.
68. Perich T, Mitchell PB, Vilus B. Stigma in bipolar disorder: a current review of the literature. Aust N Z J Psychiatry. 2022;56(9):1060–4.
69. Furlong M, McGuinness C, Mulligan CM, SL MG, McGilloway S. Family Talk versus usual services in improving child and family psychosocial functioning in families with parental mental illness: a randomised controlled trial and cost analysis. Front Psych. 2024;15:1287378.

Chapter 4
Diagnostic Conversion from Major Depressive Disorder to Bipolar Disorder

Bruno Braga Montezano, Amanda Cunha Ritter, and Karen Jansen

4.1 Introduction

Mood disorders are among the top three causes of disability worldwide [1]. The Lancet Commission on Global Mental Health and Sustainable Development emphasizes that mental health is a fundamental human right and a priority for nations' progress [2]. According to the Global Burden of Disease (GBD) study, mental disorders affected approximately 970.1 million people globally in 2019, with 279.6 million cases of major depressive disorder (MDD) and 39.5 million cases of bipolar disorder (BD) [3]. Both conditions are chronic and debilitating, with overlapping symptoms that often make diagnosis challenging [4].

While understanding the burden of mood disorders is critical, distinguishing unipolar from bipolar depression remains one of the most significant diagnostic challenges in clinical practice. Although current classifications such as the DSM-5-TR clearly distinguish MDD from BD, the clinical reality is more complex [5]. Many

B. B. Montezano
Graduate Program in Psychiatry and Behavioral Sciences, Universidade Federal do Rio Grande do Sul, Porto Alegre, RS, Brazil

Laboratório de Psiquiatria Molecular, Hospital de Clínicas de Porto Alegre (HCPA), Instituto Nacional de Ciência e Tecnologia Translacional em Medicina (INCT-TM), Porto Alegre, RS, Brazil
e-mail: bmontezano@hcpa.edu.br

A. C. Ritter
School of Medicine, Pontifícia Universidade Católica do Rio Grande do Sul, Porto Alegre, RS, Brazil

K. Jansen (✉)
Graduate Program in Health and Behavior, Universidade Católica de Pelotas, Pelotas, RS, Brazil
e-mail: Karen.jansen@ucpel.edu.br

T. de Azevedo Cardoso et al. (eds.), *Latent Bipolar Disorder*,
https://doi.org/10.1007/978-3-032-01297-5_4

patients initially diagnosed with MDD eventually transition to a diagnosis of BD, a phenomenon known as diagnostic conversion. Studies indicate that conversion rates range from 3.9% in the first year after an initial MDD diagnosis to 0.8% between the fifth and tenth years [6]. This transition has significant clinical implications, as a delayed diagnosis of BD is associated with higher rates of treatment resistance, worsening of symptoms, and an increased risk of severe complications such as suicide [7, 8].

Identifying predictors of conversion from MDD to BD is, therefore, a priority in psychiatry. The literature suggests that factors such as early age of onset, family history of BD, treatment resistance to antidepressants, and psychotic features may increase the risk of conversion [9, 10]. However, methodological variability across studies has made it difficult to consistently confirm predictors. Additionally, advances in biomarkers and technologies, such as neuroimaging and machine learning, offer new opportunities to identify at-risk patients and improve early diagnosis.

Understanding the predictors of conversion is not just an academic endeavor but a clinical necessity. These insights can guide monitoring strategies and early interventions, optimizing treatment and reducing the long-term impact for vulnerable patients. This chapter explores the rates, risk factors, and emerging tools to predict the conversion from MDD to BD, contributing to the development of a more precise and personalized diagnostic approach.

4.2 Differential Diagnosis Between MDD and BD

Differentiating MDD from BD remains a significant clinical challenge due to overlapping symptoms, particularly during depressive episodes. However, clinical, neurobiological, and genetic characteristics can help distinguish between these conditions.

Patients with BD often have an earlier onset of depression, typically before age 15, a higher number of lifetime affective episodes, and a greater likelihood of psychiatric hospitalizations. In a study by Judd et al. [11], which followed 146 patients with BD type I over 13 years, depressive symptoms predominated for nearly half the follow-up period, while manic and hypomanic episodes occurred less than 10% of the time. Additionally, symptoms such as hypersomnia, weight gain, psychomotor slowing, and psychosis are more common in BD, whereas unipolar depression typically manifests with insomnia, persistent sadness, and somatic symptoms [12, 13]. Seasonality is also more pronounced in BD, with depressive episodes more frequently occurring in winter [13]. These findings emphasize the need for longitudinal monitoring to identify distinguishing markers.

A family history of bipolar disorder is one of the most robust predictors for distinguishing BD from MDD. A study by Dervic et al. [14] showed that patients with BD type I and II had a significantly higher likelihood of a family history of bipolar disorder compared to patients with MDD, highlighting genetic vulnerability as a key factor.

Recent studies have identified promising biomarkers to differentiate MDD from BD. A systematic review by Siegel-Ramsay et al. [15], analyzing 88 MRI studies, found significant structural and functional differences between the two disorders. Patients with BD showed greater neural connectivity and reduced gray matter volume in the prefrontal cortex and hippocampus. Differences in the default mode network were linked to depressive symptoms in MDD and heightened emotional distractibility in BD.

Additionally, techniques such as electroencephalography (EEG) have demonstrated utility in differential diagnosis. In a study by Galkin and Bokhan [16], differences in bioelectrical activity asymmetry, spectral power, and coherence were observed in patients with BD and MDD. The analysis of evoked potentials revealed greater latency of the P300 component and a reduction in its amplitude in patients with bipolar disorder compared to unipolar depression, making the evoked potentials analysis method more promising for addressing the issue of differential diagnosis [16].

A recent study by Tomasik et al. [17] used metabolomic profiling of dried blood spot samples to differentiate MDD from BD. Individuals with BD exhibited distinct metabolite profiles associated with lifetime manic symptoms. Including biomarkers like these significantly improved diagnostic accuracy in clinical scenarios with limited data.

Other studies have explored computational approaches to improve diagnostic accuracy between unipolar depressive episodes and bipolar depressive episodes. Suen et al. (2021) built classification models using clinical and sociodemographic data, achieving areas under the ROC curve (AUC) ranging from 59% to 84%. Depressive symptoms and anxiety symptoms were the most relevant for tree-based models, while gender, age, negative affect, and anxiety symptoms were significant for regularized regression models [18]. Wollenhaupt-Aguiar et al. (2020) employed machine learning techniques to combine peripheral biomarker measurements and construct signatures to differentiate unipolar depressive episodes and bipolar depressive episodes. They demonstrated a classification performance of 69% (AUC), with sensitivity and specificity of 62% and 66%, respectively, using variables such as interleukin-4, thiobarbituric acid reactive substances, and interleukin-10 [19].

Despite these advances, symptom overlap still requires detailed longitudinal assessments for more accurate diagnoses. Emerging technologies, such as machine learning and molecular biomarkers, hold the potential to complement current clinical criteria and enhance diagnostic accuracy [15, 17]. As research progresses, integrating these tools into clinical practice will be essential to improve diagnostic precision, optimize treatment strategies, and ultimately enhance patient outcomes.

4.3 Rates and Predictors of Conversion from MDD to BD

The conversion from MDD to BD is a clinically significant phenomenon, often occurring within the first few years following the initial diagnosis of MDD. A meta-analysis by Kessing et al. (2017) reported annual conversion rates of 3.9% in the first year, 3.1% between years 1 and 2, 1.0% in years 2–5, and 0.8% in years 5–10 [6]. Similarly, Tse et al. (2021) observed a cumulative conversion rate of 19.5% over 20 years, with an average time to transition of 10.8 years [20]. Kim et al. (2020) reported a 6.46% conversion rate over an average follow-up period of 3.26 years among young adults [21]. Another meta-analysis by Ratheesh et al. (2017) estimated that 22.5% of individuals diagnosed with MDD would transition to BD over 12–18 years, with the highest risk of conversion occurring within the first five years [9]. These findings underscore the importance of close monitoring during this critical window to improve outcomes and guide appropriate interventions.

Several key predictors of conversion have been consistently identified. Among the factors, early onset of depression (age < 30 years) is strongly associated with a higher likelihood of conversion, as demonstrated by Musliner et al. (2018) and Kim et al. (2020) [21, 22]. Ratheesh et al. (2017) reported an adjusted odds ratio of 2.9 for individuals with a family history of BD, one of the most robust predictors [9]. Gender differences have also been observed, with slightly higher cumulative incidences of conversion among females (8.7%) compared to males (7.7%) [22], though no studies have identified a statistically significant gender effect [9].

Clinical characteristics play a pivotal role in predicting conversion. Psychotic symptoms during depressive episodes have been highlighted as significant risk factors [6, 9, 20]. Substance use, particularly cocaine, has emerged as a notable factor associated with conversion. A longitudinal study of adults with MDD reported a 3.4-fold increase in conversion risk among individuals with a history of lifetime cocaine use, even after adjusting for demographic and clinical confounders [23]. There are also studies that demonstrate specific clinical features in individuals with MDD who have a high recurrence rate of depressive episodes, some of which are associated with bipolar disorder. In a study of 2347 patients from the BRIDGE-II-mix database, individuals with high recurrence (>3 depressive episodes) exhibited a greater family history of BD, higher rates of psychotic features, antidepressant-induced manic switches, and comorbidity with borderline personality disorder [24].

Comorbid psychiatric disorders further increase conversion risk and complicate the clinical picture. A study of 130,793 adolescents and young adults identified moderate to high antidepressant resistance, obesity, attention-deficit/hyperactivity disorder (ADHD), substance use disorder, and personality disorders (clusters B and C) as significant predictors [25]. Additionally, Avila et al. (2022) reported that individuals who transitioned to BD displayed greater severity of cluster B personality traits and elevated antisocial and borderline personality symptoms, while showing lower obsessive-compulsive personality traits [26]. These findings align with studies suggesting that personality disorder symptom severity significantly predicts shorter time to hypomanic and major depressive episodes, as well as conversion to BD [27].

Recent advancements in biomarker and neuroimaging research offer promising tools for predicting conversion. Sun et al. (2024) identified abnormalities in dynamic low-frequency fluctuations (dALFF) in brain networks, achieving an area under the curve (AUC) of 72.7% for predicting conversion [28]. Wirowski et al. (2024) highlighted that elevated levels of nerve growth factor (NGF) as a biomarker, particularly when interacting with cocaine use, predict the conversion from MDD to BD, emphasizing the value of integrating neurobiological and clinical data for enhanced predictive accuracy [29].

A study at Johns Hopkins Medicine, which included 21,341 patients, found a higher risk of conversion among individuals initially diagnosed with MDD. Significant conversion rates were also observed among those initially diagnosed with anxiety disorders and ADHD [30]. Psychotic depression and inpatient treatment during depressive episodes further emerged as strong predictors of conversion, underscoring the role of illness severity in the progression of BD.

Treatment resistance to antidepressants, often accompanied by antidepressant-induced manic switches, is another critical predictor. A study examining 3212 patients initially diagnosed with MDD found that 6.69% transitioned to BD, with nearly three-quarters converting to bipolar type II. Among those who converted during antidepressant treatment, significant differences emerged when compared to those with spontaneous BD. The conversion group exhibited higher rates of familial BD (33.7% vs. 21.0%), a greater frequency of prior depressive episodes per year, and elevated levels of suicidality, including a higher incidence of suicide attempts. Furthermore, they demonstrated a greater likelihood of exhibiting a cyclothymic temperament, a history of mood-stabilizer use, and a younger age of onset [31].

In summary, the transition from MDD to BD is influenced by a combination of demographic, genetic, clinical, and neurobiological factors. Early identification and intervention for high-risk individuals, alongside advancements in computational tools and biomarker research, have the potential to refine predictive models and improve clinical outcomes. These findings highlight the importance of integrating multifaceted approaches to address the complexities of mood disorder trajectories.

4.4 Preventing Diagnostic Conversion from MDD to BD

Patients with MDD face an elevated risk of conversion to BD [9], making early intervention a cornerstone of improving clinical outcomes. A systematic review by Saraf et al. (2020) analyzed the effectiveness of psychological and pharmacological treatments in individuals at high risk for BD, defined as young patients with active mood symptoms and a family history of mood disorders [32]. Their findings, based on 16 trials spanning six weeks to five years, highlighted the potential of aripiprazole in reducing mood symptoms and improving functioning in high-risk populations. Psychological interventions also showed promise in improving outcomes related to mood, anxiety, sleep, and functioning. However, the review underscored significant gaps in the literature, with few studies explicitly using conversion to BD as an outcome measure, indicating a need for more targeted research.

Psychotherapeutic interventions provide additional support in managing high-risk individuals. Cognitive Behavioral Therapy (CBT) helps patients manage mood instability, while Interpersonal and Social Rhythm Therapy (IPSRT) stabilizes daily rhythms and sleep patterns, which are often disrupted in individuals predisposed to BD. Family-Focused Therapy (FFT) engages family members to create a supportive environment and reduce stressors, which can exacerbate mood disorders. Pfenning et al. (2014) reviewed psychotherapeutic approaches and found evidence supporting their potential to reduce mood symptoms and delay or prevent conversion to BD [33]. Psychoeducation also plays a critical role, empowering patients to recognize early warning signs and adhere to treatment plans, which has been shown to reduce relapse rates [34].

Lifestyle interventions are equally critical in reducing the risk of conversion and stabilizing mood. It is established that alterations in sleep patterns may serve as an indicator of the onset of BD in at-risk populations [35]. Consequently, there is a need to gain a deeper understanding of sleep health. Regular sleep patterns are essential, as disrupted sleep is a well-documented trigger for mood instability. Maintaining a consistent sleep schedule, creating a restful sleep environment, and limiting exposure to bright light or screens before bedtime are effective strategies [36]. Stress management techniques such as mindfulness meditation, yoga, and relaxation training can help reduce the physiological and emotional impact of stress, which is a significant risk factor for mood episodes [37]. Regular physical activity, such as aerobic exercise or strength training, has been associated with reduced depressive symptoms and improved mood stability [38]. Thus, it is of continued importance to address depressive symptomatology, as the recurrence of depressive episodes is a significant factor in the conversion of bipolar disorder.

Similarly, eating habits can affect mental health, influencing the recurrence or remission of depressive symptoms associated with the overall number of mood episodes and, consequently, the risk of conversion to BD. A balanced diet contributes to mental health. Following a Mediterranean diet, which includes fruits, vegetables, whole grains, lean proteins, and healthy fats, has been linked to improved mood regulation and reduced inflammation. Omega-3 fatty acids, found in fish and nuts, have shown potential benefits in stabilizing mood and reducing depressive episodes [39]. Avoiding alcohol and recreational drugs, particularly cocaine, is crucial, as substance use significantly increases the risk of mood instability and conversion to BD [29].

Structured daily routines further support mood stability, which may serve to protect patients from the recurrence of depressive episodes, by regulating circadian rhythms. Incorporating regular schedules for meals, sleep, exercise, and social activities can prevent the mood disruptions associated with irregular routines. Interventions like IPSRT emphasize the importance of stabilizing these rhythms to reduce relapse rates [36], which have been identified as being linked to a poorer course of MDD and an elevated risk of conversion. Social engagement also plays a pivotal role in preventing mood instability. Participation in community events and group activities and maintaining strong personal relationships can reduce feelings of isolation and improve overall mental health.

Emerging tools such as digital health applications and wearable devices enhance the ability to monitor high-risk patients effectively. These technologies track mood, sleep, and activity patterns, providing early warnings of potential mood destabilization. Machine learning models that integrate clinical, behavioral, and biological data offer further opportunities to refine prediction and prevention strategies [40].

The integration of psychological, pharmacological, and lifestyle interventions creates a comprehensive approach to managing individuals at risk for conversion from MDD to BD. While current evidence highlights the promise of these strategies, significant gaps remain, underscoring the need for more rigorous, long-term studies. By combining evidence-based interventions with advanced monitoring tools, clinicians can better support patients and reduce the long-term impact of BD.

4.5 Neuroprogression and Conversion from MDD to BD

Neuroprogression in bipolar disorder (BD) refers to the gradual deterioration in brain structure, function, and clinical outcomes associated with the recurrence and severity of mood episodes [41]. This concept has been extensively studied in BD but holds significant implications for individuals transitioning from MDD to BD. Evidence suggests that neuroprogression may underlie this diagnostic conversion, highlighting the need for early detection and intervention.

Brain imaging studies have revealed progressive anatomical changes in BD, such as ventricular enlargement and reductions in gray matter volume, particularly in the hippocampus and prefrontal cortex. These changes correlate with the cumulative number of mood episodes and illness duration, reinforcing the hypothesis that repeated episodes contribute to neurodegeneration [42, 43]. Neuroinflammation also plays a critical role, with elevated levels of cytokines like TNF-α and IL-6 identified in late-stage BD. These markers suggest an ongoing systemic inflammatory process that exacerbates neurodegenerative pathways and could accelerate the transition from MDD to BD in vulnerable individuals [44].

The neuroprogressive trajectory of BD has also been linked to cognitive and functional impairments. Cognitive deficits, including impaired memory, executive function, and emotional regulation [45], are more pronounced in individuals with a history of multiple mood episodes [46–48]. These deficits often emerge early in the illness course and worsen with progression, serving as potential markers for conversion.

Clinical staging models provide a framework for understanding this progression. These models suggest that early depressive episodes, particularly in individuals with genetic predispositions to BD, may represent prodromal stages of the disorder. Symptoms such as subthreshold hypomania, mixed features, and psychotic depression are indicative of later staging and may signal an increased risk of conversion

[49]. For example, offspring of patients with BD exhibit a trajectory of non-mood disorders in childhood to mood disorders in adolescence, culminating in BD diagnoses during early adulthood [50].

Furthermore, biological markers such as decreased brain-derived neurotrophic factor (BDNF) levels, increased oxidative stress, and shortened telomeres have been associated with illness progression. These markers reflect underlying neurobiological changes that parallel clinical deterioration. Recent research has also highlighted the role of epigenetic modifications and altered immune responses in driving neuroprogression, underscoring the complexity of mechanisms involved [51].

Longitudinal studies are critical to delineating the relationship between neuroprogression and diagnostic conversion. Monitoring high-risk populations, such as individuals with early-onset depression, familial BD, and recurrent depressive episodes, can provide valuable insights into the stages of neuroprogression. Emerging technologies, including multimodal neuroimaging and machine learning, hold promise for identifying patients at risk and tailoring early interventions to mitigate progression and improve outcomes [43].

In conclusion, neuroprogression offers a compelling framework for understanding the transition from MDD to BD. It emphasizes the importance of addressing the cumulative impact of mood episodes on brain health and leveraging biomarkers and clinical staging to guide prevention strategies. By integrating these insights into clinical practice, we can enhance the early identification and management of individuals at risk for BD, ultimately improving their long-term prognosis.

4.6 Clinical Considerations

- A significant proportion of patients initially diagnosed with MDD may later convert to BD, and it highlights the challenge of early and accurate diagnosis;
- Patients with early-onset depression, a family history of BD, or psychotic symptoms should be closely monitored during the first five years post-MDD diagnosis, a critical period for conversion risk;
- Predictors of conversion from MDD to BD also include substance use, especially a history of cocaine use, and psychiatric comorbidities may also increase the risk of transitioning to BD;
- Early psychotherapeutic interventions help stabilize mood, address early signs of bipolarity, and improve treatment adherence;
- Lifestyle modifications, such as maintaining regular sleep schedules, managing stress, engaging in physical activity, adhering to a Mediterranean diet, and avoiding cocaine and other substances, can significantly reduce the risk of conversion;
- There is a need for refined tools such as risk calculators and multimodal predictive models that can aid early identification of individuals with MDD who are at high risk of conversion to BD.

4.7 Future Perspectives

Advancing the understanding of diagnostic conversion from MDD to BD remains a critical focus in psychiatric research. Key challenges include (a) distinguishing unipolar depression from latent bipolar trajectories during initial presentations, (b) clarifying the role of antidepressants in individuals with early-onset depression and high conversion risk, (c) refining clinical and biological markers that predict conversion to BD, and (d) developing reliable screening tools to identify underlying BD in individuals misdiagnosed with unipolar depression.

Efforts should concentrate on identifying early developmental and clinical risk markers, such as family history of BD, early-onset depressive symptoms, and psychotic features, to construct predictive models of diagnostic conversion. Neurobiological advancements, including biomarkers like BDNF levels and neuroimaging techniques, hold promise in delineating latent bipolar signatures. Incorporating computational tools and machine learning algorithms may enhance diagnostic accuracy and identify patients at highest risk of conversion [52].

Regarding diagnostic conversion prediction, innovation has been helping move the field of identifying who will convert to BD from unipolar cases. A study from Gan et al. [53] aimed to develop a clinical characteristic-based model to predict the diagnosis of bipolar disorder among patients with current major depressive episodes in a 1-year time frame. The model achieved almost 80% accuracy and identified age at first onset, maximum duration of depressive episodes, somatalgia, hypersomnia, diurnal variation of mood, and irritability as predictors. It shows that there is potential for predictive modeling in identification and early intervention for these cases.

Further, longitudinal studies specifically designed to track individuals diagnosed with MDD over time are essential. These studies should aim to map the trajectory from MDD to BD while integrating neuroprogressive changes and evaluating the long-term impact of pharmacological and psychotherapeutic interventions. Emphasizing the critical window of risk within the first five years post-MDD diagnosis is vital for developing early intervention strategies.

The future holds promise for the creation of comprehensive models that incorporate genetic, neurobiological, and clinical data to understand the complex interplay between MDD and BD. By fostering interdisciplinary collaboration and leveraging emerging technologies, the field can move closer to the goal of preventing diagnostic conversion and improving outcomes for at-risk individuals.

References

1. James SL, Abate D, Abate KH, Abay SM, Abbafati C, Abbasi N, et al. Global, regional, and national incidence, prevalence, and years lived with disability for 354 diseases and injuries for 195 countries and territories, 1990–2017: a systematic analysis for the global burden of disease study 2017. Lancet. 2018;392(10159):1789–858.

2. Patel V, Saxena S, Lund C, Thornicroft G, Baingana F, Bolton P, et al. The lancet Commission on global mental health and sustainable development. Lancet. 2018;392(10157):1553–98.
3. GBD 2019 Mental Disorders Collaborators. Global, regional, and national burden of 12 mental disorders in 204 countries and territories, 1990–2019: a systematic analysis for the global burden of disease study 2019. Lancet Psychiatry. 2022;9(2):137–50.
4. Nestsiarovich A, Reps JM, Matheny ME, SL DV, Lynch KE, Beaton M, et al. Predictors of diagnostic transition from major depressive disorder to bipolar disorder: a retrospective observational network study. Transl Psychiatry. 2021;11(1):642.
5. Miola A, Tondo L, Pinna M, Contu M, Baldessarini RJ. Comparison of bipolar disorder type II and major depressive disorder. J Affect Disord. 2023;323:204–12.
6. Kessing LV, Willer I, Andersen PK, Bukh JD. Rate and predictors of conversion from unipolar to bipolar disorder: a systematic review and meta-analysis. Bipolar Disord. 2017;19(5):324–35.
7. Scott J, Leboyer M. Consequences of delayed diagnosis of bipolar disorders. L'Encephale. 2011;37(Suppl):3.
8. Grande I, Berk M, Birmaher B, Vieta E. Bipolar disorder. Lancet. 2016;387(10027):1561–72.
9. Ratheesh A, Davey C, Hetrick S, Alvarez-Jimenez M, Voutier C, Bechdolf A, et al. A systematic review and meta-analysis of prospective transition from major depression to bipolar disorder. Acta Psychiatr Scand. 2017;135(4):273–84.
10. Dobson KG, Vigod SN, Mustard C, Smith PM. Major depressive episodes and employment earnings trajectories over the following decade among working-aged Canadian men and women. J Affect Disord. 2021;285:37–46.
11. Judd LL, Akiskal HS, Schettler PJ, Endicott J, Maser J, Solomon DA, et al. The long-term natural history of the weekly symptomatic status of bipolar I disorder. Arch Gen Psychiatry. 2002;59(6):530.
12. Hirschfeld RM. Differential diagnosis of bipolar disorder and major depressive disorder. J Affect Disord. 2014;169:S12–6.
13. Smith DJ, Craddock N. Unipolar and bipolar depression: different or the same? Br J Psychiatry. 2011;199(4):272–4.
14. Dervic K, Garcia-Amador M, Sudol K, Freed P, Brent DA, Mann JJ, et al. Bipolar I and II versus unipolar depression: clinical differences and impulsivity/aggression traits. Eur Psychiatry. 2015;30(1):106–13.
15. Siegel-Ramsay JE, Bertocci MA, Wu B, Phillips ML, Strakowski SM, Almeida JRC. Distinguishing between depression in bipolar disorder and unipolar depression using magnetic resonance imaging: a systematic review. Bipolar Disord. 2022;24(5):474–98.
16. Galkin SA, Bokhan NA. The differential diagnosis of unipolar and bipolar depression based on EEG signals. Zhurnal Nevrol Psikhiatrii Im SS Korsakova. 2022;122(11):51.
17. Tomasik J, Harrison SJ, Rustogi N, Olmert T, Barton-Owen G, SYS H, et al. Metabolomic biomarker signatures for bipolar and unipolar depression. JAMA Psychiatry. 2024;81(1):101.
18. Suen PJC, Goerigk S, Razza LB, Padberg F, Passos IC, Brunoni AR. Classification of unipolar and bipolar depression using machine learning techniques. Psychiatry Res. 2021;295:113624.
19. Wollenhaupt-Aguiar B, Librenza-Garcia D, Bristot G, Przybylski L, Stertz L, Kubiachi Burque R, et al. Differential biomarker signatures in unipolar and bipolar depression: a machine learning approach. Aust N Z J Psychiatry. 2020;54(4):393–401.
20. Tse AC, Fok ML, Yim LC, Leung MM, Leung CM. Diagnostic conversion to bipolar disorder in unipolar depressed patients in Hong Kong: A 20-year follow-up study. J Affect Disord. 2021;286:94–8.
21. Kim H, Kim Y, Baek JH, Fava M, Mischoulon D, Nierenberg AA, et al. Predictive factors of diagnostic conversion from major depressive disorder to bipolar disorder in young adults ages 19–34: a nationwide population study in South Korea. J Affect Disord. 2020;265:52–8.
22. Musliner KL, Østergaard SD. Patterns and predictors of conversion to bipolar disorder in 91 587 individuals diagnosed with unipolar depression. Acta Psychiatr Scand. 2018;137(5):422–32.

23. Cardoso TA, Jansen K, Mondin TC, Moreira FP, Bach SL, Silva RA, et al. Lifetime cocaine use is a potential predictor for conversion from major depressive disorder to bipolar disorder: a prospective study. Psychiatry Clin Neurosci. 2020;74(8):418–23.
24. Mazzarini L, Kotzalidis GD, Piacentino D, Rizzato S, Angst J, Azorin JM, et al. Is recurrence in major depressive disorder related to bipolarity and mixed features? Results from the BRIDGE-II-Mix study. J Affect Disord. 2018;229:164–70.
25. Kung FH, Tsai CK, Cheng CM, Tsai SJ, Su TP, Chen TJ, et al. Diagnostic conversion to bipolar disorder among adolescents and young adults with major depressive disorder: a nationwide longitudinal study. Eur Child Adolesc Psychiatry. 2024;33(10):3625–35.
26. Bartz De Ávila G, Montezano BB, Dias De Mattos Souza L, De Azevedo Cardoso T, Azevedo Da Silva R, Mondin TC, et al. Personality disorders as predictors for the conversion from major depressive disorder to bipolar disorder: a prospective cohort study. Psychiatry Res Commun. 2022;2(3):100068.
27. Ng TH, Burke TA, Stange JP, Walshaw PD, Weiss RB, Urosevic S, et al. Personality disorder symptom severity predicts onset of mood episodes and conversion to bipolar I disorder in individuals with bipolar spectrum disorder. J Abnorm Psychol. 2017;126(3):271–84.
28. Sun H, Yan R, Hua L, Xia Y, Chen Z, Huang Y, et al. Abnormal stability of spontaneous neuronal activity as a predictor of diagnosis conversion from major depressive disorder to bipolar disorder. J Psychiatr Res. 2024;171:60–8.
29. Wirowski N, Lobato AS, Bender LV, TDA C, Mondin TC, Souza LDDM, et al. Serum biomarkers, lifetime substance use and conversion to bipolar disorder. L'Encéphale. 2024; S0013700624001969
30. Li K, Rodriguez KM, Zandi P, Goes FS. Who transitions to bipolar disorder? A comparison of major depressive disorder, anxiety, and ADHD. J Affect Disord. 2025;371:6–12.
31. Tondo L, Miola A, Pinna M, Contu M, Baldessarini RJ. Antidepressant-associated diagnostic change from major depressive to bipolar disorder. Acta Psychiatr Scand. 2024;150(3):126–37.
32. Saraf G, Moazen-Zadeh E, Pinto JV, Ziafat K, Torres IJ, Kesavan M, et al. Early intervention for people at high risk of developing bipolar disorder: a systematic review of clinical trials. Lancet Psychiatry. 2021;8(1):64–75.
33. Pfennig A, Correll CU, Marx C, Rottmann-Wolf M, Meyer TD, Bauer M, et al. Psychotherapeutic interventions in individuals at risk of developing bipolar disorder: a systematic review. Early Interv Psychiatry. 2014;8(1):3–11.
34. Colom F, Vieta E, Reinares M, Martínez-Arán A, Torrent C, Goikolea JM, et al. Psychoeducation efficacy in bipolar disorders: beyond compliance enhancement. J Clin Psychiatry. 2003;64(9):1101–5.
35. de Aguiar KR, Cabelleira MD, Montezano BB, Jansen K, de Azevedo Cardoso T. Sleep alterations as a predictor of bipolar disorder among offspring of parents with bipolar disorder: a systematic review and meta-analysis. Trends Psychiatry Psychother Impr. 2021;43(4):256–69.
36. Frank E, Kupfer DJ, Thase ME, Mallinger AG, Swartz HA, Fagiolini AM, et al. Two-year outcomes for interpersonal and social rhythm therapy in individuals with bipolar I disorder. Arch Gen Psychiatry. 2005;62(9):996.
37. Segal ZV, JMG W, Teasdale JD, Kabat-Zinn J. Mindfulness-based cognitive therapy for depression. New York, NY: The Guilford Press; 2012.
38. Mammen G, Faulkner G. Physical activity and the prevention of depression. Am J Prev Med. 2013;45(5):649–57.
39. Jacka FN, O'Neil A, Opie R, Itsiopoulos C, Cotton S, Mohebbi M, et al. A randomised controlled trial of dietary improvement for adults with major depression (the 'SMILES' trial). BMC Med. 2017;15(1):23.
40. Meehan AJ, Lewis SJ, Fazel S, Fusar-Poli P, Steyerberg EW, Stahl D, et al. Clinical prediction models in psychiatry: a systematic review of two decades of progress and challenges. Mol Psychiatry. 2022;27(6):2700–8.

41. Kapczinski NS, Mwangi B, Cassidy RM, Librenza-Garcia D, Bermudez MB, Kauer-Sant'anna M, et al. Neuroprogression and illness trajectories in bipolar disorder. Expert Rev Neurother. 2017;17(3):277–85.
42. Kapczinski F, Frey BN, Kauer-Sant'Anna M, Grassi-Oliveira R. Brain-derived neurotrophic factor and neuroplasticity in bipolar disorder. Expert Rev Neurother. 2008;8(7):1101–13.
43. Grewal S, McKinlay S, Kapczinski F, Pfaffenseller B, Wollenhaupt-Aguiar B. Biomarkers of neuroprogression and late staging in bipolar disorder: a systematic review. Aust N Z J Psychiatry. 2023;57(3):328–43.
44. Fries GR, Walss-Bass C, Bauer ME, Teixeira AL. Revisiting inflammation in bipolar disorder. Pharmacol Biochem Behav. 2019;177:12–9.
45. Miola A, Cattarinussi G, Antiga G, Caiolo S, Solmi M, Sambataro F. Difficulties in emotion regulation in bipolar disorder: a systematic review and meta-analysis. J Affect Disord. 2022;302:352–60.
46. Semkovska M, Quinlivan L, O'Grady T, Johnson R, Collins A, O'Connor J, et al. Cognitive function following a major depressive episode: a systematic review and meta-analysis. Lancet Psychiatry. 2019;6(10):851–61.
47. Kriesche D, CFJ W, Tschentscher N, Engel RR, Karch S. Neurocognitive deficits in depression: a systematic review of cognitive impairment in the acute and remitted state. Eur Arch Psychiatry Clin Neurosci. 2023;273(5):1105–28.
48. Cardoso T, Bauer IE, Meyer TD, Kapczinski F, Soares JC. Neuroprogression and cognitive functioning in bipolar disorder: a systematic review. Curr Psychiatry Rep. 2015;17(9):75.
49. Kapczinski F, Magalhães PVS, Balanzá-Martinez V, Dias VV, Frangou S, Gama CS, et al. Staging systems in bipolar disorder: an international society for bipolar disorders task force report. Acta Psychiatr Scand. 2014;130(5):354–63.
50. Raouna A, Osam CS, MacBeth A. Clinical staging model in offspring of parents with bipolar disorder: a systematic review. Bipolar Disord. 2018;20(4):313–33.
51. Barbé-Tuana FM, Parisi MM, Panizzutti BS, Fries GR, Grun LK, Guma FT, et al. Shortened telomere length in bipolar disorder: a comparison of the early and late stages of disease. Rev Bras Psiquiatr. 2016;38(4):281–6.
52. Silva Ribeiro J, Pereira D, Salagre E, Coroa M, Santos Oliveira P, Santos V, et al. Risk calculators in bipolar disorder: a systematic review. Brain Sci. 2020;10(8):525.
53. Gan Z, Diao F, Wei Q, Wu X, Cheng M, Guan N, et al. A predictive model for diagnosing bipolar disorder based on the clinical characteristics of major depressive episodes in Chinese population. J Affect Disord. 2011;134(1–3):119–25.

Chapter 5
Differential Diagnosis Between Unipolar Depression and Bipolar Depression

Giovanna Maiolli Signori, Carolina de Moura Marolli, Rodrigo Martins Teixeira, Gabriel Gonçalves Veloso, Pedro Kazlauckas Lucas, and Ives Cavalcante Passos

5.1 Introduction

Mood disorders primarily encompass bipolar disorder and major depressive disorder, both of which overlap depressive symptoms, posing a diagnostic challenge [1]. Bipolar disorder is a prevalent and disabling psychiatric illness, affecting 2% of the global population [2, 3]. Approximately half and three quarters of patients with bipolar disorder type I and type II, respectively, initially experience depressive episodes [2]. Furthermore, the accurate diagnosis and treatment of bipolar disorder are delayed by about 9 years [3].

G. M. Signori
Laboratory of Molecular Psychiatry, Centro de Pesquisa Experimental (CPE) and Centro de Pesquisa Clínica (CPC), Hospital de Clínicas de Porto Alegre (HCPA), Porto Alegre, RS, Brazil

Universidade Luterana do Brasil (ULBRA), Canoas, RS, Brazil

C. de Moura Marolli
Universidade de Ciências da Saúde de Porto Alegre (UFCSPA), Porto Alegre, RS, Brazil

R. M. Teixeira · G. G. Veloso
Universidade Federal do Rio Grande do Sul (UFRGS), Porto Alegre, RS, Brazil

P. K. Lucas
Laboratory of Molecular Psychiatry, Centro de Pesquisa Experimental (CPE) and Centro de Pesquisa Clínica (CPC), Hospital de Clínicas de Porto Alegre (HCPA), Porto Alegre, RS, Brazil

Universidade Federal do Rio Grande do Sul (UFRGS), Porto Alegre, RS, Brazil

I. C. Passos (✉)
Psychiatry Department, Federal University of Rio Grande do Sul, Porto Alegre, Rio Grande do Sul, Brazil

T. de Azevedo Cardoso et al. (eds.), *Latent Bipolar Disorder*,
https://doi.org/10.1007/978-3-032-01297-5_5

The distinction between bipolar and unipolar depression is important since the misdiagnosis can lead to poor prognosis and manic switch in patients with bipolar disorder [3]. Additionally, early diagnosis is essential for effective treatment and to prevent long-term complications, improve prognosis, and reduce the risk of suicide [1, 4]. The aim of the present chapter is to review the literature on the differential diagnosis between unipolar and bipolar depression, exploring diagnostic criteria, symptoms, genetic factors, and other risk factors. By the end of the chapter, the reader will be more informed and prepared to deal with this clinical challenge and improve the quality of life of patients with mood disorders.

5.2 Diagnostic Criteria for Major Depressive Disorder and Bipolar Disorder

According to DSM-5-TR, bipolar disorder is characterized by alternating episodes of depression and mania in type I or depression and hypomania in type II. It is worth mentioning that a single manic episode without a history of depressive episodes can also characterize bipolar disorder type I. Episodes of mania and hypomania are characterized by discrete periods of elevated or irritable mood, increased energy, and heightened activity that represent a noticeable change from usual behavior. In bipolar I disorder, the symptoms are severe enough to require the patient to be hospitalized or cause impairment in social or professional functioning [5, 6]. Major depressive disorder is defined by a major depressive episode and the absence of a history of manic or hypomanic episodes. However, the presence of manic/hypomanic symptoms may still be compatible with the diagnosis of major depressive disorder, characterizing the specifier “with mixed features.” Therefore, it is crucial to evaluate if the symptoms fulfill the criteria for a hypomanic episode to accurately distinguish between major depressive disorder and bipolar II disorder. A major depressive episode consists of a period of at least two weeks with depressed mood or loss of interest or pleasure in daily activities for most of the day, almost every day. In addition, the individual must experience at least four (or three, if the individual presents with both depressed mood and loss of interest) additional symptoms during the period, such as changes in appetite, sleep, and psychomotor activity. The episode must be accompanied by clinically significant distress or impairment in social, professional, or other important functioning [3].

Bipolar disorder may be misdiagnosed as major depressive disorder due to the prominence of depression in the presentation of the illness. It is worth noting that the first episode of bipolar disorder is often depressive, and depressive symptoms are the most frequent in the long-term course of bipolar disorder. Additionally, depression is the main reason for individuals to seek help. In episodes of major depression, investigating the history of previous episodes of mania or hypomania is necessary [3].

It is unlikely that individuals will initially complain of hypomania because they do not recognize the symptoms or consider hypomania desirable, as, by definition, it does not cause significant harm. However, other people may feel disturbed by the behavior in hypomanic episodes. In this sense, clinical information obtained through an objective anamnesis provided by other people, such as close friends or relatives, are often useful in establishing the diagnosis of bipolar II disorder. Another difficulty in establishing a hypomanic episode may be confusion with the several days of euthymia and restoration of energy and activity that may come after remission of a major depressive episode. Furthermore, individuals with hypomania with mixed features may not characterize their symptoms as hypomania, experiencing them as depression with increased energy or irritability [3].

According to the DSM-5-TR, bipolar disorder typically begins with a depressive episode and is not recognized until a hypomanic episode appears, which happens in around 12% of people initially diagnosed with major depressive disorder. Many individuals experience several episodes of major depression before the first recognized hypomanic episode, with typically an interval of more than 10 years between the onset of the illness and the diagnosis of bipolar disorder [5, 6].

In children, the literature suggests that 30% of young people who present to clinical practice with prodromal symptoms of major depressive disorder have already experienced symptoms of mania or hypomania [4, 7]. One of the major concerns of treatment with antidepressants is the induction of manic symptoms, psychomotor agitation, and an increase in suicidal behavior. Therefore, there is a need for efforts to identify past episodes of mania or hypomania and differentiate bipolar from unipolar disorder in clinical and research settings [4, 8–10]. Below, the table presents the diagnostic criteria for manic and hypomanic episodes, as outlined in DSM-5-TR [5] (Table 5.1).

5.3 Genetics and Family History

Genetic processes significantly affect the predisposition to bipolar disorder, with heritability estimated at 60–80% [11, 12]. According to the DSM-5-TR, while the risk of the disorder is 1% in the general population, in patients with first-degree relatives with bipolar disorder, the risk can reach up to 10%. Studies demonstrate that the presence of a family history of bipolar disorder was 44.7% in individuals with bipolar II disorder and 15.3% in major depressive disorder [6, 9]. Still, the heredity mechanism is not Mendelian and involves multiple genes that interact with each other, the environment, and random factors. There are also studies that suggest that bipolar disorder shares a genetic origin with schizophrenia, and manic and depressive tendencies are inherited separately [9].

One of the most distinctive features between bipolar disorder and major depressive disorder is a family history of psychiatric illnesses. Nevertheless, this isolated factor cannot be solely relied upon for diagnostic purposes due to the higher prevalence of major depressive disorder compared to bipolar disorder, which makes it a clinical feature with low specificity for identification purposes [9]. Studies suggest that the depressive disorder has a heritability of 30–50% [13], while the heritability of bipolar disorder is up to 80% [11]. Furthermore, major depressive disorder demonstrated familial aggregation, with first-degree relatives having a 1.84-fold higher risk of developing depressive disorders compared to the general population [13]. In

Table 5.1 Diagnostic criteria for manic and hypomanic episodes—DSM-5-TR

Manic episode	Hypomanic episode
(A) A distinct period of abnormally and persistently elevated, expansive, or irritable mood and abnormally and persistently increased goal-directed activity or energy, lasting at least 1 week and present most of the day, nearly every day (or any duration if hospitalization is necessary).	(A) A distinct period of abnormally and persistently elevated, expansive, or irritable mood and abnormally and persistently increased activity or energy, lasting at least 4 consecutive days and present most of the day, nearly every day.
(B) During the period of mood disturbance and increased energy or activity, three (or more) of the following symptoms (four if the mood is only irritable) are present to a significant degree and represent a noticeable change from usual behavior: Inflated self-esteem or grandiosity. Decreased need for sleep. More talkative than usual or pressure to keep talking. Flight of ideas or subjective experience that thoughts are racing. Distractibility, as reported or observed. Increase in goal-directed activity or psychomotor agitation. Excessive involvement in activities that have a high potential for painful consequences.	(B) During the period of mood disturbance and increased energy and activity, three (or more) of the following symptoms (four if the mood is only irritable) have persisted, represent a noticeable change from usual behavior, and have been present to a significant degree: Inflated self-esteem or grandiosity. Decreased need for sleep. More talkative than usual or pressure to keep talking. Flight of ideas or subjective experience that thoughts are racing. Distractibility, as reported or observed. Increase in goal-directed activity or psychomotor agitation. Excessive involvement in activities that have a high potential for painful consequences.
(C) The mood disturbance is sufficiently severe to cause marked impairment in social or occupational functioning or to necessitate hospitalization to prevent harm to self or others, or there are psychotic features.	(C) The episode is associated with an unequivocal change in functioning that is uncharacteristic of the individual when not symptomatic.
(D) The episode is not attributable to the physiological effects of a substance or to another medical condition.	(D) The disturbance in mood and the change in functioning are observable by others. The episode is not attributable to the physiological effects of a substance (e.g., a drug of abuse, a medication, or other treatment).
	(E) The episode is not severe enough to cause marked impairment in social or occupational functioning or to necessitate hospitalization. If there are psychotic features, the episode is, by definition, manic.

(continued)

Table 5.1 (continued)

Manic episode	Hypomanic episode
Note: A full manic episode that emerges during antidepressant treatment (e.g., medication, electroconvulsive therapy) but persists at a fully syndromal level beyond the physiological effect of that treatment is sufficient evidence for a manic episode and, therefore, a bipolar I diagnosis.	*Note*: A hypomanic episode that emerges during antidepressant treatment (e.g., medication, electroconvulsive therapy) but persists at a fully syndromal level beyond the physiological effect of that treatment is sufficient evidence for a hypomanic episode diagnosis. However, caution is indicated so that one or two symptoms (particularly increased irritability, edginess, or agitation following antidepressant use) are not taken as sufficient for diagnosis of a hypomanic episode nor necessarily indicative of a bipolar diathesis.

addition, a meta-analysis of adolescents with bipolar I disorder showed that their first-degree relatives had a 5.96-fold higher risk of bipolar I disorder than the average population [1].

5.4 Trauma in Bipolar and Unipolar Disorder

The etiology of bipolar disorder has focused on genetic influences, providing evidence of a strong genetic component. On the other hand, there is emerging evidence that bipolar disorder is also influenced by certain environmental factors, especially early traumatic experiences [14]. Traumatic events significantly influence bipolar disorder, being 2.6 times more prevalent in adults with the disorder than in those without. These events not only aggravate the illness but also lead to earlier onset, increased episodes of psychosis and depression, higher recurrence rates, and elevated risks of suicidal tendencies [15].

Negative experiences significantly affect the central nervous system and can lead to various structural and functional changes in the brain. These changes particularly impact areas like the hippocampus and amygdala, which play a crucial role in the onset of bipolar and depressive disorders [16]. Chronic stress associated with traumas is correlated with the dysregulation of the hypothalamic-pituitary-adrenal axis and inflammatory markers [17, 18], alterations in the volume and in the structure of central brain structures, and other lasting neural adaptations. Delineation of transdiagnostic mechanisms may connect trauma to various forms of psychopathology later in life [19].

Adolescence and childhood are periods of mental vulnerability for the development of future psychiatric disorders. It is important to adopt trauma intervention measures [20]. Adverse childhood experiences are known environmental risk factors for bipolar disorders, for example, sexual abuse, physical neglect, parental loss, bullying, and collective violence [20–22]. There is a threefold increase in the likelihood of developing a mental disorder when a person is exposed to multiple traumas [20]. Multiple traumatic experiences in a patient, especially in childhood, result in more severe disorders, earlier symptom onset, more depressive episodes, and more suicide attempts compared to patients without these experiences [23].

Bipolar disorder has been associated with a history of post-traumatic stress disorder. These patients were more likely to develop symptoms of hypomanic or manic episodes and bipolar II disorder [24]. These traumatic experiences throughout life are associated with a more severe, symptomatic bipolar disorder, increased morbidity, accelerated illness progression, and suicidal tendency [17, 24]. Moreover, childhood sexual abuse is more prevalent in patients with bipolar disorder (11.5%) than in those with unipolar disorder (1.1%) [25]. Sexual abuse increases the risk of bipolar disorder by triggering a cascade of neurobiological events that result in persistent sensitization of the central nervous system and alterations in brain structure or function [14]. This trauma is associated with a more severe course of the disease, faster cycling frequencies, and increased suicide attempts [25, 26]. It is important to highlight that the presence of trauma is strongly associated with worse cerebral functioning in these patients. Therefore, clinical management and treatment should be addressed with trauma-focused psychotherapy [21].

5.5 Prodromal Symptoms and Longitudinal Trajectory of Bipolar Disorder and Major Depressive Disorder

Besides risk factors such as family history and traumatic experiences, longitudinal studies are trying to determine if specific symptom presentations before the disease meets full diagnostic criteria are more closely related to one disorder than the other [27]. One significant difference between these disorders is the age of onset of the first mood episode. While the first episodes in bipolar disorder typically occur before the age of 25, the median onset for major depressive disorder is around the early thirties [28].

There is strong evidence that subthreshold presentations of hypomania or mania are crucial predictors of bipolar disorder. A cohort of high-risk offspring of individuals with bipolar disorder found that subthreshold manic or hypomanic episodes were associated with the prospectively observed onset of mania/hypomania (hazard ratio = 7.57). This highlights the importance of screening for attenuated forms of mania when treating young patients with mood lability, anxiety, or behavioral disorders [27]. Sleep disturbances may also be a prognostic factor for the development of bipolar disorder, but more evidence is needed [29].

Despite the high rate of comorbidities in unipolar depression [30], studies have found that bipolar disorder is associated with more psychiatric comorbidities than major depressive disorder [1]. Bipolar disorder has a higher prevalence of comorbid mental illnesses, with 65% of individuals having one or more concomitant psychiatric disorders, particularly anxiety disorders (approximately 71%), personality disorders (approximately 36%), and attention-deficit hyperactivity disorder (approximately 10%–20%) [3, 28]. Substance use disorders are highly prevalent in both conditions, but there is a higher prevalence in bipolar disorder. While some studies report a prevalence of around 25% for substance use disorder in major depressive disorder [31], the lifetime prevalence of substance use disorder in bipolar disorder is estimated to be around 56%, with cannabis and cocaine being more substantially involved (20% and 17% comorbidity, respectively) [32]. There is also evidence that the use of cocaine and cannabis is a risk factor for developing bipolar disorder, with frequent cannabis use (at least three times per week) potentially increasing even more the risk [33].

Bipolar disorder, more than unipolar depression, is proposed to begin with a prodromal or latent stage and progress dynamically and longitudinally from an at-risk stage to a late and resistant stage. In childhood, this may manifest as sleep disorders, attention deficit, anxiety disorder, and mood swings, progressing in adolescence to an increased risk of adjustment disorders, mood symptoms, impulsivity, and substance use disorders, with suicidality emerging as a stronger prodromal sign and being cited as the main feature predicting this condition [34]. This sequence of symptoms is less clear for unipolar depression.

Premorbid intelligence quotient (IQ) and school failures are also prodromal factors that may help differentiate both diseases. A 2023 study analyzing data from a cohort of 3580 individuals revealed that a lower IQ (below 70) at age 18 is associated with an increased risk of bipolar disorder, while a higher IQ (above 120) is linked to major depressive disorder. Additionally, an increased number of school failures is associated with major depressive disorder [35].

Moreover, many symptoms in depressive episodes increase the likelihood that the depression is from bipolar disorder, such as atypical symptoms, psychosis, mixed features, abrupt onset, psychomotor retardation, and postpartum depression [36]. These differences will be further explained in the following topic.

5.6 Clinical Differences in Depressive Symptoms in Major Depressive Disorder and Bipolar Depression

Establishing a differential diagnosis between unipolar and bipolar disorder can be difficult when the patient first presents with a depressive episode. As described by the DSM-5-TR, both unipolar and bipolar depression share the same diagnostic criteria [5]. However, it is known that certain refined characteristics of the clinical presentation and course of the disorder may provide useful insights for differential diagnosis [37, 38].

First, it is important to investigate the features of the patient's symptomatology with a comprehensive history of the disease. According to two reviews from the literature [37, 38], the presence of manic spectrum symptoms and psychotic features in a depressive episode increases the likelihood of this being a bipolar depression. Furthermore, as described in the same reviews, mood lability—rather than just sad humor—also raises that probability. Features of an atypical depressive episode

Table 5.2 Differential diagnoses and characteristics associated with bipolar disorder in the context of a depressive episode

	Suggestive of bipolar depression	Suggestive of unipolar depression
Symptomatology	Atypical symptoms (increased appetite, hypersomnia). Mixed features. Psychotic symptoms or catatonia. Abrupt onset and offset of symptoms. Psychomotor retardation. Postpartum depression.	Initial insomnia/reduced sleep. Appetite and/or weight loss. Normal or increased activity levels. Somatic complaints.
Course of illness	Early onset of first depression (<25 years). Multiple prior episodes (≥5 episodes). Treatment-resistant depression. Childhood sexual abuse.	Late onset of first depression (>25 years). Long duration of current episode (>6 months).
Family History	Family history of bipolar disorder	Negative family history of bipolar disorder

(hypersomnia, increased appetite, and weight gain) increase it as well. Another important factor is suicidal ideation and suicide attempts, which are consistently more prevalent in bipolar than in unipolar depression, as also established by other studies [39, 40].

Second, the characteristics of the clinical course and family history also differ between both illnesses. It is known that bipolar depression often occurs at earlier ages or postpartum periods, and it is more severe, recurrent, and resistant to treatment [2, 37]. As discussed previously, the main risk factor associated with bipolar disorder is the family history of the disorder. Those findings support the importance of a complete anamnesis, which should also comprehend a family "screening" for behavioral features associated with mania/hypomania.

The comprehensive clinical evaluation can be useful to distinguish bipolar and unipolar depression, aside from diagnostic criteria [37]. Nevertheless, it is necessary to elucidate that, although this symptomatology and clinical course occur more often in bipolar depression, there is no validated cutoff of risk for establishing a formal diagnosis [38]. Thus, the information presented here should be accounted for as risk factors, which must orient clinical decisions and prevent iatrogenesis. Table 5.2 summarizes characteristics associated with bipolar disorder in the context of a depressive episode.

5.7 Postpartum Depression

Postpartum depression happens in approximately 13% of women in developed countries and reaches higher prevalence in underdeveloped ones, with a global incidence of about 10%. It is associated with various concerns in the mother-infant relationship due to the increased risk of maternal suicide, compromised attachment, and infant malnutrition [41, 42]. In the literature, there is already evidence of the association between postpartum depression and an increased risk of severe maternal mental illness, such as bipolar disorder [41].

The appearance of bipolar disorder in the context of postpartum depression is complex, considering the difficulty in identifying psychiatric disorders in the postpartum period. Extreme hormonal changes during the postpartum period may contribute to the vulnerability of some women to the development of bipolar disorder. This occurs due to variables such as hormonal fluctuation, sleep deprivation, and other symptoms that precipitate difficult-to-categorize psychiatric symptoms. Clinicians should be alert to symptoms of hypomania in postpartum women for the possibility of bipolar disorder [43]. Genetic factors play a significant role in this process, as postpartum depression is associated with bipolar disorder, showing strong genetic factors among them [42, 44].

There is evidence that women with postpartum depression and thoughts of self-harm are more likely to develop bipolar disorder within a period of 7 years. It was observed that approximately 14% of patients with postpartum depression in the first month postpartum developed bipolar disorder [41]. About 20.1% of those patients showed signs of hypomania, bipolar depression, and mood episodes during pregnancy or postpartum [43].

Postpartum depression precipitating bipolar disorder is associated with a 23-fold greater risk of psychiatric hospitalizations when compared to non-postpartum women with bipolar disorder [45]. Moreover, the estimated rate of suicidal ideation in the postpartum period in women with bipolar disorder is between 5% and 14% [46]. Comprehensive assessment and evaluation are essential to enhance early identification of postpartum women with bipolar disorder to provide intervention strategies. Common screening practices in postpartum depression without investigation of symptoms of mania or hypomania can lead to incorrect diagnosis and treatment [43].

5.8 Clinical Implications

The main reason for establishing a diagnosis in medicine is to provide proper treatment to patients. That is particularly important when we are dealing with the distinction between unipolar and bipolar depression, since there are different pharmacological classes standardized for each one [47, 48]. Moreover, it is known that treating one as the other may result in ineffectiveness, morbidity-associated adverse effects, and worsening of symptomatology (or even manic switch) [27]. However, there is no risk-based instrument validated in the literature yet for such discernment [38]. Therefore, when the patient presents with a depressive episode—with associated high risk for bipolar disorder—the distinction between both diagnoses becomes blurred, possibly implying uncertainty about medical management as well.

In a depressive episode, the use of second-generation antidepressants is standard for major depressive disorder, whereas, in patients with bipolar disorder, the first choice is second-generation antipsychotics (especially quetiapine and lurasidone) [47, 48]. That said, the use of antidepressants in bipolar depressive episodes is controversial, perhaps being ineffective or even harmful in the long term for some patients [48, 49]. In a systematic review and meta-analysis of 6 clinical trials, representing 1383 patients with bipolar depression, the presence of adjunctive second-generation antidepressants to a mood stabilizer or antipsychotic was not distinct from placebo in clinical response or remission rates [50]. In addition, there was an increased risk (1.774 [1.018–3.091], $p = 0.043$) in treatment-emergent mania or hypomania after a 52-week re-evaluation (but not at the acute phase of treatment). Furthermore, the misdiagnosis of a patient with bipolar disorder may delay up to 12 years the initiation of proper treatment, implying a poorer prognosis, as the clinical progression of the disorder occurs without protective pharmacotherapy [51].

On the other hand, a patient with unipolar depression may receive treatment intended for bipolar disorder. As previously mentioned, two standard treatments for bipolar depression include the use of quetiapine or lurasidone [48]. According to the literature, quetiapine demonstrates an antidepressant effect in unipolar depression [52] but also presents important short- and long-term side effects, including weight gain and increased incidence of hypertension and cardiovascular diseases [53, 54].

Therefore, the treatment of those cases in which the patient presents with depression but is also at high risk for bipolar disorder becomes a complex decision. As suggested by some reviews, until more consistent evidence is published, the treatment should be individualized and even discussed with the patient, respecting their autonomy and in a stigma-free environment [27, 55]. Furthermore, a systematic review of 16 clinical trials involving patients at high risk of developing bipolar disorder highlights the need for more methodologically homogenous studies, specifically measuring bipolar conversion as an outcome [56].

5.9 Future Perspective

Distinguishing bipolar from unipolar disorder has significant implications for our patients, as defining this differential diagnosis can improve the prognosis of the illness [51]. Although highly important, the literature on this subject still lacks studies that establish precise clinical guidelines based on risk factors or patient symptoms [27]. Aiming to address this limitation, some studies have proposed the exploration of possible biomarkers of bipolar disorder [57, 58]. Additionally, there is growing literature approaching the differential diagnosis between unipolar and bipolar patients using machine learning techniques with neuroimaging [59], blood biomarkers [60], genetics, and clinical data [57, 58, 61]. These studies aim to build models to recognize patterns more associated with bipolar disorder that can help clinicians with more objective tools.

More studies are needed to identify risk and protective factors, as well as tools to help differentiate patients with bipolar from unipolar disorder. Early management is essential, using psychotherapy, medication, and lifestyle changes, such as ceasing substance abuse. Accurate diagnosis is important to avoid delaying treatment and to provide a better prognosis and quality of life for these patients.

References

1. Yang R, Zhao Y, Tan Z, et al. Differentiation between bipolar disorder and major depressive disorder in adolescents: from clinical to biological biomarkers. Front Hum Neurosci. 2023;17:1192544.
2. Patella AM, Jansen K, Cardoso T d A, Souza LD d M, Silva RA d, Coelho FM d C. Clinical features of differential diagnosis between unipolar and bipolar depression in a drug-free sample of young adults. J Affect Disord. 2019;243:103–7.
3. Nierenberg AA, Agustini B, Köhler-Forsberg O, Cusin C, Katz D, Sylvia LG, Peters A, Berk M. Diagnosis and treatment of bipolar disorder: a review. JAMA. 2023;330:1370–80.
4. Uchida M, Serra G, Zayas L, Kenworthy T, Faraone SV, Biederman J. Can unipolar and bipolar pediatric major depression be differentiated from each other? A systematic review of cross-sectional studies examining differences in unipolar and bipolar depression. J Affect Disord. 2015;176:1–7.
5. American Psychiatric Association (APA). DSM-5: Manual Diagnóstico e Estatístico de Transtornos Mentais. Artmed Editora; 2014.
6. American Psychiatric Association. Diagnostic and statistical manual of mental disorders: DSM-5-TR. American Psychiatric Association Publishing; 2022.
7. Geller B, Cooper TB, Chestnut EC, Anker JA, Schluchter MD. Preliminary data on the relationship between nortriptyline plasma level and response in depressed children. Am J Psychiatry. 1986;143:1283–6.
8. Faedda GL, Baldessarini RJ, Glovinsky IP, Austin NB. Pediatric bipolar disorder: phenomenology and course of illness. Bipolar Disord. 2004;6:305–13.
9. Akiskal HS, Benazzi F. Continuous distribution of atypical depressive symptoms between major depressive and bipolar II disorders: dose-response relationship with bipolar family history. Psychopathology. 2008;41:39–42.
10. Baldessarini RJ, Tondo L, Pinna M, Nuñez N, Vázquez GH. Suicidal risk factors in major affective disorders. Br J Psychiatry. 2019:1–6.
11. Johansson O, Bjärehed J, Andersson G, Carlbring P, Lundh L-G. Effectiveness of guided internet-delivered cognitive behavior therapy for depression in routine psychiatry: a randomized controlled trial. Internet Interv. 2019;17:100247.
12. Fabbri C. The role of genetics in bipolar disorder. Curr Top Behav Neurosci. 2021;48:41–60.
13. Sullivan PF, Neale MC, Kendler KS. Genetic epidemiology of major depression: review and meta-analysis. Am J Psychiatry. 2000;157:1552–62.
14. Maniglio R. Prevalence of child sexual abuse among adults and youths with bipolar disorder: a systematic review. Clin Psychol Rev. 2013;33:561–73.
15. Andreu Pascual M, Levenson JC, Merranko J, et al. The effect of traumatic events on the longitudinal course and outcomes of youth with bipolar disorder. J Affect Disord. 2020;274:126–35.
16. Jaworska-Andryszewska P, Rybakowski JK. Childhood trauma in mood disorders: neurobiological mechanisms and implications for treatment. Pharmacol Rep. 2019;71:112–20.
17. Passos IC, Vasconcelos-Moreno MP, Costa LG, Kunz M, Brietzke E, Quevedo J, Salum G, Magalhães PV, Kapczinski F, Kauer-Sant'Anna M. Inflammatory markers in post-traumatic stress disorder: a systematic review, meta-analysis, and meta-regression. Lancet Psychiatry. 2015;2:1002–12.

18. Peruzzolo TL, Pinto JV, Roza TH, et al. Inflammatory and oxidative stress markers in post-traumatic stress disorder: a systematic review and meta-analysis. Mol Psychiatry. 2022;27:3150–63.
19. Palines PA, Rabbitt AL, Pan AY, Nugent ML, Ehrman WG. Comparing mental health disorders among sex trafficked children and three groups of youth at high-risk for trafficking: a dual retrospective cohort and scoping review. Child Abuse Negl. 2020;100:104196.
20. MT MK, Cannon M, Chambers D, Conroy RM, Coughlan H, Dodd P, Healy C, O'Donnell L, Clarke MC. Childhood trauma and adult mental disorder: a systematic review and meta-analysis of longitudinal cohort studies. Acta Psychiatr Scand. 2021;143:189–205.
21. Köhler-Forsberg O, Ge F, Hauksdóttir A, et al. Adverse childhood experiences and psychological functioning among women with schizophrenia or bipolar disorder: population-based study. Br J Psychiatry. 2024;224:6–12.
22. Koenders MA, Mesman E, Giltay EJ, Elzinga BM, MHJ H. Traumatic experiences, family functioning, and mood disorder development in bipolar offspring. Br J Clin Psychol. 2020;59:277–89.
23. Aas M, Ueland T, Lagerberg TV, Melle I, Aminoff SR, Hoegh MC, Lunding SH, Laskemoen JF, Steen NE, Andreassen OA. Retrospectively assessed childhood trauma experiences are associated with illness severity in mental disorders adjusted for symptom state. Psychiatry Res. 2023;320:115045.
24. Carmassi C, Bertelloni CA, Dell'Oste V, Foghi C, Diadema E, Cordone A, Pedrinelli V, Dell'Osso L. Post-traumatic stress burden in a sample of hospitalized patients with bipolar disorder: which impact on clinical correlates and suicidal risk? J Affect Disord. 2020;262:267–72.
25. Jansen K, Cardoso TA, Fries GR, Branco JC, Silva RA, Kauer-Sant'Anna M, Kapczinski F, Magalhaes PVS. Childhood trauma, family history, and their association with mood disorders in early adulthood. Acta Psychiatr Scand. 2016;134:281–6.
26. Leverich GS, Altshuler LL, Frye MA, et al. Factors associated with suicide attempts in 648 patients with bipolar disorder in the Stanley Foundation Bipolar Network. J Clin Psychiatry. 2003;64:506–15.
27. Vieta E, Salagre E, Grande I, Carvalho AF, Fernandes BS, Berk M, Birmaher B, Tohen M, Suppes T. Early intervention in bipolar disorder. Am J Psychiatry. 2018;175:411–26.
28. McGrath JJ, Al-Hamzawi A, Alonso J, et al. Age of onset and cumulative risk of mental disorders: a cross-national analysis of population surveys from 29 countries. Lancet Psychiatry. 2023;10:668–81.
29. Levenson JC, Axelson DA, Merranko J, et al. Differences in sleep disturbances among offspring of parents with and without bipolar disorder: association with conversion to bipolar disorder. Bipolar Disord. 2015;17:836–48.
30. Hasin DS, Sarvet AL, Meyers JL, Saha TD, Ruan WJ, Stohl M, Grant BF. Epidemiology of adult DSM-5 major depressive disorder and Its specifiers in the United States. JAMA Psychiatry. 2018;75:336–46.
31. Hunt GE, Malhi GS, Lai HMX, Cleary M. Prevalence of comorbid substance use in major depressive disorder in community and clinical settings, 1990–2019: systematic review and meta-analysis. J Affect Disord. 2020;266:288–304.
32. Preuss UW, Schaefer M, Born C, Grunze H. Bipolar disorder and comorbid use of illicit substances. Medicina. 2021; https://doi.org/10.3390/medicina57111256.
33. Lalli M, Brouillette K, Kapczinski F, de Azevedo Cardoso T. Substance use as a risk factor for bipolar disorder: a systematic review. J Psychiatr Res. 2021;144:285–95.
34. Kapczinski F, Montezano BB, de Azevedo Cardoso T. Latent bipolar disorder. Lancet. 2023;401:2109.
35. Rabelo-da-Ponte FD, Marchionatti LE, Watts D, et al. Premorbid intelligence quotient and school failure as risk markers for bipolar disorder and major depressive disorder. J Psychiatr Res. 2024;169:160–5.

36. Østergaard SD, Straszek S, Petrides G, Skadhede S, Jensen SOW, Munk-Jørgensen P, Nielsen J. Risk factors for conversion from unipolar psychotic depression to bipolar disorder. Bipolar Disord. 2014;16:180–9.
37. Hirschfeld RM. Differential diagnosis of bipolar disorder and major depressive disorder. J Affect Disord. 2014;169(Suppl 1):S12–6.
38. Vöhringer PA, Perlis RH. Discriminating between bipolar disorder and major depressive disorder. Psychiatr Clin North Am. 2016;39:1–10.
39. Hantouche EG, Akiskal HS, Lancrenon S, Allilaire JF, Sechter D, Azorin JM, Bourgeois M, Fraud JP, Châtenet-Duchêne L. Systematic clinical methodology for validating bipolar-II disorder: data in mid-stream from a French national multi-site study (EPIDEP). J Affect Disord. 1998;50:163–73.
40. Hu C, Xiang Y-T, Ungvari GS, et al. Undiagnosed bipolar disorder in patients treated for major depression in China. J Affect Disord. 2012;140:181–6.
41. Chen M-H, Pan T-L, Bai Y-M, Huang K-L, Tsai S-J, Su T-P, Chen T-J, Hsu J-W. Postpartum depression and psychosis and subsequent severe mental illnesses in mothers and neurodevelopmental disorders in children: a nationwide study. J Clin Psychiatry. 2021; https://doi.org/10.4088/JCP.20m13735.
42. Zuo M, Wang Z, Li W, Chen S, Yuan Y, Yang Y, Mao Q, Liu Y. Causal effects of potential risk factors on postpartum depression: a Mendelian randomization study. Front Psych. 2023;14:1275834.
43. Freeman MP, Goldberg JF. The pursuit to recognize bipolar disorder in pregnant and postpartum women. J Clin Psychiatry. 2022; https://doi.org/10.4088/JCP.22ed14399.
44. Byrne EM, Carrillo-Roa T, Penninx BWJH, et al (2014) Applying polygenic risk scores to postpartum depression. Arch Womens Ment Health 17:519–528.
45. Sharma V, Doobay M, Baczynski C. Bipolar postpartum depression: an update and recommendations. J Affect Disord. 2017;219:105–11.
46. Batt MM, Olsavsky AK, Dardar S, St John-Larkin C, Johnson RL, Sammel MD. Course of illness and treatment updates for bipolar disorder in the perinatal period. Curr Psychiatry Rep. 2022;24:111–20.
47. Qaseem A, Owens DK, Etxeandia-Ikobaltzeta I, et al. Nonpharmacologic and pharmacologic treatments of adults in the acute phase of major depressive disorder: a living clinical guideline from the American College of Physicians. Ann Intern Med. 2023;176:239–52.
48. Levenberg K, Cordner ZA. Bipolar depression: a review of treatment options. Gen Psychiatr. 2022;35:e100760.
49. Gitlin MJ. Antidepressants in bipolar depression: an enduring controversy. Focus. 2019;17:278–83.
50. McGirr A, Vöhringer PA, Nassir Ghaemi S, Lam RW, Yatham LN. Safety and efficacy of adjunctive second-generation antidepressant therapy with A mood stabiliser or an atypical antipsychotic in acute bipolar depression: randomised systematic review and meta-analysis of A placebo-controlled trials. Focus. 2021;19:129–37.
51. Berk M, Berk L, Dodd S, Cotton S, Macneil C, Daglas R, Conus P, Bechdolf A, Moylan S, Malhi GS. Stage managing bipolar disorder. Bipolar Disord. 2014;16:471–7.
52. Maneeton N, Maneeton B, Srisurapanont M, Martin SD. Quetiapine monotherapy in acute phase for major depressive disorder: a meta-analysis of randomized, placebo-controlled trials. BMC Psychiatry. 2012;12:160.
53. Jerrell JM, McIntyre RS, Tripathi A. Childhood treatment with psychotropic medication and development of comorbid medical conditions in adolescent-onset bipolar disorder. Hum Psychopharmacol. 2011;26:451–9.
54. Pringsheim T, Gardner D, Patten SB. Adjunctive treatment with quetiapine for major depressive disorder: are the benefits of treatment worth the risks? BMJ. 2015;350:h569.
55. Ratheesh A, Cotton SM, Davey CG, Adams S, Bechdolf A, Macneil C, Berk M, McGorry PD. Ethical considerations in preventive interventions for bipolar disorder. Early Interv Psychiatry. 2017;11:104–12.

56. Saraf G, Moazen-Zadeh E, Pinto JV, Ziafat K, Torres IJ, Kesavan M, Yatham LN. Early intervention for people at high risk of developing bipolar disorder: a systematic review of clinical trials. Lancet Psychiatry. 2021;8:64–75.
57. Siegel-Ramsay JE, Bertocci MA, Wu B, Phillips ML, Strakowski SM, Almeida JRC. Distinguishing between depression in bipolar disorder and unipolar depression using magnetic resonance imaging: a systematic review. Bipolar Disord. 2022;24:474–98.
58. Phillips ML, Kupfer DJ. Bipolar disorder diagnosis: challenges and future directions. Lancet. 2013;381:1663–71.
59. Librenza-Garcia D, Kotzian BJ, Yang J, Mwangi B, Cao B, Pereira Lima LN, Bermudez MB, Boeira MV, Kapczinski F, Passos IC. The impact of machine learning techniques in the study of bipolar disorder: a systematic review. Neurosci Biobehav Rev. 2017;80:538–54.
60. Wollenhaupt-Aguiar B, Librenza-Garcia D, Bristot G, et al. Differential biomarker signatures in unipolar and bipolar depression: a machine learning approach. Aust N Z J Psychiatry. 2020;54:393–401.
61. Rabelo-da-Ponte FD, Feiten JG, Mwangi B, Barros FC, Wehrmeister FC, Menezes AM, Kapczinski F, Passos IC, Kunz M. Early identification of bipolar disorder among young adults: a 22-year community birth cohort. Acta Psychiatr Scand. 2020;142:476–85.

Chapter 6
Diagnostic Conversion from Attention-Deficit/Hyperactivity Disorder to Bipolar Disorder

Carolina Goldman Bergmann and Marina Roman Meller

6.1 Introduction

In order to prevent or delay the onset of bipolar disorder (BD), efforts have been made in research to predict and improve early identification of its signs and symptoms [1]. Some of these BD precursors are present years prior to syndrome onset [2, 3]. Among the most common subclinical symptoms preceding an initial mood episode, some of them overlap with Attention-Deficit/Hyperactivity Disorder (ADHD) symptoms, such as excessive energy, increased speech, and difficulties in the thinking process and in academic and work settings [3]. Other subclinical symptoms preceding the onset of BD include agitation, rage attacks, mood swings, irritability, distractibility, and disinhibition, which are also commonly observed in ADHD [4, 5]. Although the specificity of these prodromal BD symptoms and signs is low, it is plausible to consider ADHD symptoms, at clinical or subthreshold levels, as a possible presentation of latent bipolar disorder [1, 6].

Looking at the history of ADHD, the first description of similar features dates from 1798 by Sir Alexander Crichton. The Scottish physician described patients with impaired attention since very early in life [7]. In 1902, the British pediatrician Sir George Frederic Still described children with a "morbid defect of moral control," who were impulsive and had difficulties in controlling their own actions [8]. In 1932, German physicians Franz Kramer and Hans Pollnow described cases of children with marked motor agitation, inattention, and impulsivity, which closely aligns with the current concept of ADHD, and called it "*Hyperkinetic Disease of Infancy*" [9]. In the 1930s and 1940s, some authors proposed the association of

C. G. Bergmann
Department of Psychiatry, University of British Columbia, Vancouver, BC, Canada

M. Roman Meller (✉)
Department of Psychiatry, Federal University of São Paulo, São Paulo, SP, Brazil

T. de Azevedo Cardoso et al. (eds.), *Latent Bipolar Disorder*,
https://doi.org/10.1007/978-3-032-01297-5_6

hyperactive symptoms with brain injury, leading to the concept of "*minimal brain damage*" [10, 11]. The idea of structural brain damage was replaced by the "*minimal brain dysfunction*" hypothesis in the 1960s [10, 12]. "*Attention Deficit Disorder, with and without hyperactivity*" was incorporated in the third edition of the *Diagnostic and Statistical Manual of Mental Disorders* (*DSM-III*) in 1980 [13, 14].

Regarding the historical context of BD, the birth of the modern concept dates back to 1850 and 1854, when "*folie circulaire*" and "*folie à double forme*" were described by two French residents at La Salpetriere. Both terms referred to a cyclical disorder that encompasses both depressive and manic syndromes [15, 16]. Emil Kraepelin, a German psychiatrist and founder of modern psychiatry, later unified affective disorders into the condition called "*manic-depressive insanity*" [17]. The terminology "*insanity*" changed to "*illness*," and it was only in the third version of DSM, in 1980, that "*Bipolar Disorder*" was identified as such [13]. Due to the predominant influence of psychoanalytic theory in American psychiatry throughout the twentieth century, BD was largely disregarded as a possible diagnosis for children by the majority of authors [18]. However, the concept of children with BD regained attention with DeLong's success in treating aggressive and hyperactive youth with lithium [19, 20].

In the late twentieth century, the relationship between BD and ADHD was one of the most hotly debated topics in child psychiatry literature [21, 22]. Some researchers argued that juvenile mania differed significantly from its adult presentation. For them, BD manifests as a non-episodic illness, lacking markedly distinct episodes of mania in the child and adolescent population [23, 24]. The field was then polarized, since other authors advocated that the episodicity of "discrete episodes" is a *sine qua non* of BD [25]. Another issue revolved around the affective nature of core symptoms, with some authors arguing that severe and chronic irritability was sufficient as a cardinal symptom of mania in youth, instead of requiring signs of euphoria or elation [25–27]. Given that children with ADHD often exhibit chronic irritability, and hyperarousal symptoms overlap between ADHD and BD, the question of whether a significant number of children with BD were in fact misdiagnosed with ADHD was the subject of controversy [21].

In the 2000s, the contrasting descriptions of mania were operationalized into two distinct clinical phenotypes: a *narrow phenotype* (characterized by elevated mood or grandiosity happening in a markedly distinct episode) and a *broad phenotype* (marked by chronic, non-episodic illness, severe irritability, and hyperarousal) [28]. More than 2 decades later, there is now enough consensus that chronic irritability, despite its severity and volatility, is not sufficient for a diagnosis of BD [29]. However, questions regarding the complex relationship between ADHD and BD have continued to be an important subject in psychiatric literature. Whether ADHD is a marker of very early onset mania [30] or two facets of the same underlying process [31] remain relevant questions to this day.

In this chapter, in order to discuss the relationship between ADHD and BD, we are first going to present some aspects of ADHD, such as epidemiology, symptomatology, and clinical trajectory; how they resemble or differ from BD features; and how to make a differential diagnosis between them. Afterwards, we are going to discuss the comorbidity of ADHD and BD and finally, how ADHD symptoms can be understood as a possible presentation of latent BD.

6.2 Epidemiology of ADHD

ADHD is a disorder characterized by symptoms of inattention and hyperactivity/impulsivity. To diagnose the disorder, several symptoms must be present since childhood and persist for at least six months. These symptoms must cause impairment in two or more settings, such as home and school or work [32].

This neurodevelopmental disorder affects 5.29% of children and adolescents globally [33]. Two-thirds of children will continue to experience impairing ADHD symptoms in adulthood, either at clinical or subthreshold levels [34]. Regarding the adult population, the overall prevalence of *persistent ADHD* (with childhood onset) is 4.61%, and the prevalence of symptomatic *adult ADHD* (regardless of childhood onset) is 8.83% [35].

Males are more likely to receive an ADHD diagnosis than females. In children, the male-to-female prevalence ratio ranges from 2:1 to 4:1, while in adults this number gets closer to 1:1 [36, 37]. The prevalence is similar across different geographic regions [33]. While ADHD is one of the most common mental disorders in children, BD is described as rare in the same population [38].

ADHD is a relatively chronic disorder, with the majority of patients experiencing fluctuating symptoms from early childhood through adolescence and adulthood. Longitudinal findings from the Multimodal Treatment Study of ADHD (MTA) show that although periods of remission can be expected in most cases, 90% of children with ADHD continue to experience residual symptoms in early adulthood, and less than 10% will achieve recovery [39]. Some childhood factors affecting the persistence of ADHD into adult life include initial symptom severity, presence of comorbidities, and parental mental health problems [40]. Childhood IQ levels and household income levels are also important predictors of adult functional impairment [41].

The etiologies of ADHD point to multifactorial causes, including genetic, neurobiological, and environmental factors. Gestational and perinatal factors that occur during the development of the central nervous system, such as premature birth and perinatal hypoxia, are important risk factors for ADHD [42]. Regarding genetic factors, it is known that ADHD is highly heritable (60–70%) and reflects a polygenic condition, with 12 significant loci identified in genome-wide association studies (GWAS) [43]. Socioeconomic disadvantages such as financial difficulties are strong predictors of ADHD, and lower levels of parental involvement and the presence of adversity early in life mediate this association [44].

6.3 Clinical Trajectory of ADHD

According to National Survey of Children's Health (NSCH) data, the average age of ADHD diagnosis is 6 years, ranging from 4 years in severe forms to 7 years in mild presentations of the disorder [45]. A recent systematic review in European children showed that the median age of onset of ADHD symptoms ranged from 2.25 years to 7.5 years, highlighting that symptoms can be present very early in life [46].

For diagnosis, the current version of the DSM requires that several symptoms be present before the age of 12 [32]. According to the predominant symptoms at the time of diagnosis, patients can be classified into three presentations: inattentive, hyperactive/impulsive or combined [32]. However, due to its heterotypic trajectory, ADHD symptoms often change over time within individuals across their lifespan [47].

In preschool age, the most common ADHD symptom is hyperactivity, which peaks before declining during the rest of childhood [48]. On the other hand, as the children confront school demands, symptoms of inattention gradually increase and become more important [49]. It is important to note that children with ADHD might be able to remain focused when performing specific tasks, such as watching television, playing video games, and other pleasure activities [50].

The domain of inattention becomes detrimental, especially in social contexts during both adolescence and adulthood [51]. During adolescence, hyperactivity wanes and impulsivity peaks, exacerbating the tendency to make risky decisions that is common in this age range even in healthy adolescents [52, 53]. Hyperactivity during adolescence may manifest as fidgetiness or inner feelings of jitteriness, restlessness, and impatience [32]. In adults, besides inattention, hyperactivity may manifest as extreme restlessness, and impulsivity can remain problematic [32].

More recent literature shows that the functional impairments associated with ADHD across the lifespan cannot be solely attributed to the core symptoms of inattention and hyperactivity/impulsivity [54]. Emotion regulation deficits (ERDs), also named as emotional dysregulation/impulsiveness/lability, are consistently observed in patients with ADHD [55]. These deficits are present across the lifespan, affecting children, adolescents, and adults with ADHD [56], and are associated with significant functional impairments [57]. Moreover, ERD during childhood is associated with the persistence of ADHD symptomatology after four years [58]. Recent theories highlight ERD as a central component of ADHD, with executive dysfunction and motivational difficulties accounting for most, if not all, symptoms of the disorder [57].

6.4 Differential Diagnosis Between ADHD and BD

Attention-deficit/hyperactivity disorder (ADHD) and episodes of mania/hypomania exhibit numerous overlapping symptoms, including excessive or rapid speech, hyperactivity, racing thoughts, inappropriate behavior, lack of inhibition, irritability, emotional dysregulation, distractibility, and impulsivity [59]. Other features, although not overlapping, can still be difficult to distinguish, such as the ones regarding sleep ("decreased need" in BD versus "difficulties in sleep" in ADHD), cognition ("flight of ideas" in BD versus impaired sustained attention in ADHD), energy/volition ("excessive involvement in pleasurable activities with high potential for painful consequences" in BD versus impulsivity and hyperfocus in ADHD), and functional and/or social impairments [21, 32]. These phenomenological similarities may result in diagnostic ambiguity between BD and ADHD, and may also lead to a failure to diagnose one disorder when both are present [60].

The clinical distinction between these conditions is further complicated by the fact that not only do they frequently co-occur with each other, but also they are both highly comorbid with other disorders, such as oppositional defiant disorder (ODD) and conduct disorder (CD) [21, 31]. Given that aggression and behavioral disinhibition are present in ODD and CD, but also are associated with bipolarity, the diagnostic challenge and clinical decision-making gain an additional layer of complexity [31]. Moreover, the challenge of differential diagnosis is exacerbated by inter-episode cognitive deficits and functional impairments, and the presence of hypomanic episodes in BD type II, where the state-like features of BD and the trait-like nature of ADHD must be carefully considered [61].

To conduct a differential diagnosis, it is crucial to clarify whether the symptoms denote a consistent pattern within the individual, persisting chronically, or if they denote a distinct episode [32, 62]. In the case of ADHD, symptoms typically manifest continuously prior to the age of 12, with some degree of variability and developmental changes [32, 63]. On the other hand, during the acute phase of BD, symptoms manifest within a circumscribed period, during the mood episode [32].

Mood instability in BD is often triggered by various factors such as limit setting, sleep deprivation, hypoglycemia, dehydration, heat, or emotional overstimulation. Tantrums in BD can endure for longer than one hour, and individuals may harbor anger, hold grudges, and become unforgiving. In contrast, mood dysregulation in ADHD typically arises from difficulties with tasks (such as learning), demands on sustained attention, or other frustrating situations, lasting approximately 20–30 minutes, with the individual often forgetting the reason for their distress after calming down [64].

Moreover, individuals with ADHD may demonstrate heightened and more frequent agitation, energy levels, pressured speech, impulsivity, distractibility, irritability, mood dysregulation, and engagement in risky behaviors compared to the general population, potentially resulting in a misdiagnosis of BD [59, 60].

In Table 6.1, several symptoms potentially manifesting in both disorders are delineated, along with the distinctions in their presentation within each respective disorder.

Table 6.1 Presentation of symptoms in ADHD and BD—key differences

Differential diagnosis	Bipolar disorder (BD)	Attention deficit hyperactivity disorder (ADHD)
Age of onset	Adolescence/young adulthood	The average age of diagnosis is 6 years old
Gender	Male = female	Male > female
Course	Episodic	Persistent
Trajectory	Symptoms manifest during discrete episodes. Episodes have a minimum duration of one week (mania), four days (hypomania), or two weeks (depression). During the episode, symptoms are present most of the day, nearly every day throughout this specific period. In between mood episodes, the patient is euthymic but can maintain cognitive and functional impairment.	Despite variability in symptom manifestation and intensity over the lifespan, they are frequently and continuously present. Symptoms often have a heterotypic trajectory, in which the clinical presentation changes over time within individuals across their lifespan.
Mood symptoms	In a (hypo)manic episode, an abnormal, elevated, expansive, or irritable mood is present for a specific period of time. This mood is persistently altered, or there is mood dysregulation over several days and is different or more intense than the individual's usual pattern.	Emotional dysregulation is frequent. Episodes of intense irritation or disproportionality in response to a frustrating situation may occur. A trigger for mood dysregulation is often present. Throughout the day, the mood of a person with ADHD may vary, presenting episodes of intense irritability, intense sadness, and intense joy; however, it returns to a baseline mood after a short period of time.
Increased energy levels	A distinct period of abnormally and persistently increased energy. Increased goal-directed activity (whether socially, at work or school, or sexually).	Individuals may want to do several tasks at the same time or spend several hours focused on a specific activity (hyperfocus). People with ADHD may experience hyperfocus and also have a poor sense of time. This characteristic is continuously present.
Psychomotor agitation	Presence of psychomotor agitation (e.g., purposeless activity not directed towards goals).	Long-standing presence of chronic agitation/hyperactivity manifested as difficulty in remaining still, needing to frequently move hands or feet, or squirming in the chair. May have difficulty staying seated or waiting in line or for an activity.
Inflated self-esteem or grandiosity	Inflated self-esteem or grandiosity is characteristic of mania or hypomania. The individual clearly believes in this feeling persistently during the mood episode.	It is not a common symptom in ADHD, but transient episodes of increased self-esteem are sometimes observed. It is important to note that children with ADHD may attempt clearly dangerous acts more frequently than children of the same age, but these acts occur more frequently over development and not sporadically as in manic/hypomanic episodes.

(continued)

Table 6.1 (continued)

Sleep disturbance	Reduced need for sleep without feeling tired. The individual sleeps a few hours, has difficulties getting to sleep, wakes up several times, or wakes up hours earlier than usual but continues to feel rested or full of energy during the day.	Insomnia or other sleep disorders are common in ADHD. Patients usually feel tired if they present insomnia. It is common for individuals with ADHD to procrastinate going to bed even when they are feeling tired (sleep resistance).
Speech	Faster, more pressured, louder, and more difficult to interrupt than usual. Individuals may speak intrusively or without regard for others' communication desires. Speech may contain jokes, theatricality, and excessive gestures.	As a reflection of their hyperactivity and impulsivity, individuals with ADHD may speak excessively, make jokes at inappropriate times, or interrupt others while they speak.
Inattention	Attention is diverted very easily by insignificant or irrelevant external stimuli.	In ADHD, symptoms of inattention manifest as failing to follow instructions through the end, failing to finish work or school activities, wandering off, having difficulty in remaining focused, having trouble being organized, and losing things.
Engagement in risky behaviors	Excessive involvement in activities with high potential for painful consequences is usually secondary to increased self-esteem and grandiosity.	Involvement in activities with high potential for painful consequences occurs impulsively and frequently over the lifespan.
Suicidality	Can have suicidal ideas/behavior, especially in depressive and mixed episodes.	Rare suicidal ideation or behavior.
Hypersexuality	Common during (hypo)manic episodes.	Rare.
Thought	Flight of ideas, or the subjective experience of accelerated thoughts.	Individuals diagnosed with ADHD may experience a chronic sense of accelerated thought processes, distinct from episodic occurrences.
Psychotic symptoms	Can present with psychotic symptoms during an acute phase of a mood episode	No psychotic symptoms.

6.5 Comorbidity Between ADHD and BD

The co-occurrence of ADHD and BD has been extensively studied [65, 66]. To make a comorbid ADHD and bipolar disorder diagnosis, the criteria for both disorders must be present. According to the International Society for Bipolar Disorders Task Force, it is important to not "double-count" overlapping diagnostic items (e.g., hyperactivity in ADHD and increase of energy in BD) when making comorbid diagnoses [29].

Substantial heterogeneity of comorbidity rates in children is found in the literature. In clinical samples, high rates of comorbidity were found in previous studies. In 1996, a follow-up study with children and adolescents with ADHD found that 11% met criteria for BD at baseline and an additional 12% met criteria for BD during the four-year follow-up, with rates significantly higher than controls [67, 68]. Another study found even more expressive values, showing rates of ADHD up to 85% in children with pediatric BD and 22% of pediatric BD in children with ADHD, pointing to a bidirectional overlap between the two entities [69].

In a multisite NIMH study with 348 youth aged 7–17 years with BD type I, II, and not otherwise specified (NOS), ADHD was reported in 59.8% of subjects, ranging from 43.4% in the BD type II group to 62.1% in the BD-NOS group [70, 71].

Children with ADHD and comorbid BD had higher rates of psychopathology, hospitalization, and psychosocial impairment than children with ADHD alone. They also had a very severe symptomatic picture of ADHD [68] and higher family rates of aggression and psychiatric disorders [72].

Regarding this co-occurrence in adults, in a cohort of 1000 patients with BD, 14.7% of male and 5.8% of female patients also had ADHD, with an overall lifetime prevalence of 9.5%. Those who presented with the comorbidity had shorter periods of wellness and were more frequently depressed [73]. In a smaller study with 100 adults with BD in remission, a lifetime rate of co-occurrence with ADHD of 18% was found and a current rate of 10% [74]. In adults with BD, the presence of ADHD comorbidity was associated with a significantly earlier onset of mood disorder, a higher number of mood episodes, higher impulsivity, and more suicidal history than adults with BD without ADHD [74, 75].

A recent systematic review and meta-analysis of 71 studies with 646,766 participants found that about one in thirteen adults with ADHD were also diagnosed with BD (7.95%) and one in six adults with BD had ADHD (17.11%) [61].

A possible explanation for this comorbidity involves shared genetic effects, given findings of family-based studies [61]. When studying first-degree relatives of children with ADHD, some authors proposed that comorbid ADHD-BD represents a distinct familial subtype from other forms of ADHD [30, 76]. Moreover, two meta-analyses found a significantly higher prevalence of ADHD in relatives of probands with BD and higher rates of BD in relatives of probands with ADHD, compared with relatives of controls [58, 61].

A GWAS study revealed a substantial and significant genetic correlation between ADHD and BD, indicative of a genetic overlap between the two disorders [77]. Furthermore, this study also supports the idea that ADHD comorbid with BD represents an early-onset subtype of bipolar illness, with distinct genetic mechanisms implicated in early and later forms of BD [77]. However, a recent meta-analysis with GWAS studies found only a small significant genetic correlation [78]. Thus, authors suggested that the observed rates of cross-transmission of ADHD and BD in family studies may be attributable to rare variants, the effect of environmental risk factors, and gene-environment interactions [78].

6.6 Treatment of the Comorbidity

The primary goal in treating comorbid BD and ADHD should always be mood stabilization [79, 80]. Mood stabilization with mood stabilizers and/or antipsychotics acts as a protective factor against mood destabilization and allows for a reassessment of ADHD symptom severity and treatment. However, guidance on subsequent ADHD treatment is limited due to insufficient data.

During acute mood episodes, especially mania or hypomania, treating ADHD is not recommended [79]. However, mood stabilizers typically do not address the specific symptoms of ADHD [81]. Many patients report residual ADHD symptoms, such as difficulty concentrating, memory issues, irritability, and mood dysregulation, even when euthymic [81–83].

Thus, after mood re-stabilization, specific treatment for ADHD may be prescribed [80] since untreated ADHD is linked to a worsened course of bipolar disorder in individuals with comorbid BD-ADHD, along with an increased burden of other psychiatric comorbidities [73].

The first-line treatment for ADHD, according to various guidelines, consists of stimulant medication such as methylphenidate (MPH) and amphetamines (AMP), followed by atomoxetine (ATX) and guanfacine XR (only for children and adolescents) as second-line treatment [80, 84]. As a third line of treatment, bupropion, clonidine, imipramine, and modafinil may be considered [80].

Following mood stabilization, stimulants have demonstrated both safety and efficacy in patients with BD [80]. When comparing stimulants, there is no evidence of superior tolerability or efficacy. There is evidence from double-blind, placebo-controlled trials that euthymic youth with BD and ADHD benefit from concomitant treatment with methylphenidate [85].

In the youth population with comorbid BD-ADHD, after stabilizing mood, it is suggested that MPH or mixed-salt amphetamine be considered as first-line treatments for ADHD, followed by guanfacine as second-line and ATX as third-line options [86].

The risk of manic switch when initiating a stimulant or ATX, although small when the patient is using a mood stabilizer, should be carefully monitored [80, 84]. When the patient has a clear diagnosis of ADHD, but the diagnosis of BD is only suspected, ADHD can be treated first. However, the clinician should be vigilant regarding the presence of mood symptoms [81].

A recent Swedish study found no association between MPH use and manic switch in patients concurrently using mood stabilizers. Associating MPH with mood stabilizers decreased the risk of new manic episodes. In contrast, patients treated solely with MPH experienced a sixfold to sevenfold rise in manic episodes during the first three months of therapy [87]. Additionally, another study showed that children with ADHD treated with MPH had lower rates of developing a first episode of BD compared to those who did not receive treatment [88]. Lisdexamfetamine was studied as an adjunctive treatment in patients with treatment-resistant bipolar depression. This stimulant has also been shown to be safe and effective in treating comorbid ADHD-BD [83]. Long-acting stimulants appear to be less associated with manic switches and have a lower risk of abuse compared to short-acting ones. Extended-release methylphenidate (MPH-ER) MPH-ER (extended-release) has demonstrated efficacy in controlling emotional dysregulation in patients with comorbid ADHD-BD [82].

In case a patient experiences an acute manic or hypomanic episode during treatment with stimulant/ATX, the medication should be discontinued, and BD treatment prioritized. When the patient's mood is stabilized again, the stimulant/ATX can be restarted—it is important to start at a low dose and gradually increase it [80, 81]. In summary, the treatment of comorbid ADHD-BD should be hierarchical, prioritizing mood stabilization and adding bupropion, a stimulant, or ATX afterward.

6.7 ADHD Symptoms as a Clinical Presentation of Latent BD

The prodromal phase of BD has garnered increasing attention in recent research. BD prodrome includes *precursor symptoms* (affective symptoms preceding BD onset), as well as *clinical risk factors* (non-affective psychopathology). Additionally, it involves other psychiatric diagnoses and functional impairments [89, 90]. Prodromal symptoms typically manifest insidiously, may display episodicity during childhood, and frequently emerge over two years before BD onset (27.1 ± 23.1 months; range = 4.6–130.0 months) [91].

Although endophenotypes do not represent prodromes, they can aid in the early detection of individuals at risk for specific disorders. Evidence supports deficits in executive function and sustained attention—biological traits closely linked to ADHD—as potential endophenotypes of BD [92].

Among the clinical risk factors, ADHD and impulsivity emerge as reliable predictors for BD in community and outpatient samples [89]. Previous literature has strongly suggested that ADHD symptoms may represent a prodromal or early manifestation of BD in certain at-risk individuals, implying that ADHD, whether clinical or subsyndromal, could represent a latent presentation of bipolar disorder [69].

Regarding precursor symptoms, in bipolar disorder offspring cohorts, subthreshold manic/hypomanic symptoms emerge as the most robust predictors of imminent BD diagnosis [4]. Compared to community offspring, children of parents with BD are at higher risk of many psychiatric disorders, including ADHD (30.7% compared with 18.1%) [4, 93]. Moreover, among BD offspring, the majority of those who later experience manic or hypomanic episodes previously received a psychiatric diagnosis such as ADHD [4, 93, 94].

Recent research highlights that prodromal symptoms reported in over 50% of youth who later developed BD type I showed overlapping symptoms with ADHD, including irritability (61.5%), increased energy/activity (50%), school/work impairment (65.4%), and inattention (51.9%) [5]. A recent meta-analysis also identifies common prodromal symptoms that overlap with ADHD phenomenology, such as excessive energy (68%), talkativeness (60%), academic or work difficulties (56%), and sleep issues (54%) [91]. Despite the absence of pathognomonic symptoms of bipolar disorder, the prolonged duration of the initial prodrome shows that there is an ample window of intervention if symptoms and individuals are identified early [91].

In a 6-year follow-up prospective study, authors investigated the rate, risk, and predictors of switching from ADHD to BD type I. To qualify as a "switcher," the children had to meet criteria for a manic or mixed episode, with cardinal symptoms of elated mood and/or grandiosity to avoid misdiagnosis due to symptom overlap with ADHD. The cumulative risk of switching was 28.5%, significantly higher than the 2% switching rate observed in healthy controls. Significant predictors of switching included more severe baseline scores on the Children's Global Assessment Scale (CGAS), paternal recurrent major depressive disorder (MDD), and lower stimulant use. Family history of BD in first-degree relatives, antidepressant use, psychosocial measures, and life events were not predictive of switching from ADHD to BD [95]. In another study, ADHD youth were followed prospectively into adulthood; the authors found that a CBCL score >= 180 in deficient emotional self-regulation was associated with manic switching [58].

Furthermore, adolescents with ADHD who also receive a diagnosis of CD, ODD, anxiety disorders, or substance use disorder (SUD) face significantly increased odds of developing BD later on [96–98].

ADHD was also associated with a significantly higher risk of switches from unipolar MDD to BD. In subjects with ADHD, switches from unipolar MDD to BD were predicted by baseline comorbid CD, school behavior problems, and a positive family history of parental mood disorder [99]. Similarly, in a longitudinal sample of ADHD youth, the presence of these subthreshold BD symptoms and deficits in emotional regulation at baseline significantly increased the risk for switching from unipolar MDD to BD in later adolescence and young adulthood. Such findings emphasize the clinical relevance of subsyndromal forms of BD in children with ADHD and comorbid MDD, as they substantially elevate the risk for bipolar switches [100].

In the adult sample of patients with MDD, it was found that individuals with ADHD reported higher rates of adverse responses to previous antidepressant treatment compared to those without ADHD. Specifically, antidepressant use was associated with (hypo)manic switches, mood lability, and irritability. Moreover, the most common (hypo)manic symptoms in individuals with ADHD were emotional/mood lability and distractibility, followed by impulsivity, talkativeness/pressured speech, and racing thoughts. Mixed features during the current depressive episode were more prevalent in patients with comorbid ADHD compared to the remaining sample [101].

6.8 Conclusion

An ADHD diagnosis or subsyndromal symptoms often precede the onset of the first mood episode in individuals with BD. The prolonged duration of the clinical presentation before a BD diagnosis provides clinicians with an opportunity for early intervention and proactive management. Early intervention is associated with better prognosis and should always be a goal. Further research could enhance our understanding of the association between ADHD symptomatology and the subsequent onset of mood episodes, shedding light on potential neurodevelopmental aspects of both disorders along with possible implications for pathogenesis and intervention strategies.

Clinical Tips

- Given the symptom overlap and shared comorbidities between Attention Deficit Hyperactivity Disorder (ADHD) and Bipolar Disorder (BD), a careful clinical approach is crucial for accurate differential diagnosis.
- While ADHD typically exhibits a chronic heterotypic trajectory and is prevalent among children, BD follows an episodic course of symptoms and is comparatively rare in the same demographic.
- Individuals with ADHD face a higher risk of developing BD than the general population, and vice versa, underscoring the potential coexistence of both disorders as comorbidities, thereby complicating diagnostic assessments.
- Prioritizing mood stabilization is paramount in the management of comorbid ADHD and BD.
- Treatment for ADHD should be avoided during acute mood episodes.
- Following mood stabilization, initiation of stimulant therapy is advisable.
- Long-acting stimulant formulations are typically preferred over short-acting due to their enhanced safety profile.
- The prodromal phase of BD frequently emerges years before the onset of BD itself.
- ADHD diagnosis or subsyndromal symptoms frequently precede the onset of an initial mood episode in individuals with BD, potentially serving as a prodromal or early manifestation of BD.

References

1. Geoffroy PA, Leboyer M, Scott J. Predicting bipolar disorder: what can we learn from prospective cohort studies? L'Encéphale. 2015;41(1):10–6.
2. Faedda GL, Marangoni C, Serra G, Salvatore P, Sani G, Vázquez GH, et al. Precursors of bipolar disorders: a systematic literature review of prospective studies. J Clin Psychiatry. 2015;76(5):614–24.
3. Rabelo-da-Ponte FD, Feiten JG, Mwangi B, Barros FC, Wehrmeister FC, Menezes AM, et al. Early identification of bipolar disorder among young adults—a 22-year community birth cohort. Acta Psychiatr Scand. 2020;142(6):476–85.

4. Axelson D, Goldstein B, Goldstein T, Monk K, Yu H, Hickey MB, et al. Diagnostic precursors to bipolar disorder in offspring of parents with bipolar disorder: a longitudinal study. Am J Psychiatry. 2015;172(7):638–46.
5. Correll CU, Hauser M, Penzner JB, Auther AM, Kafantaris V, Saito E, et al. Type and duration of subsyndromal symptoms in youth with bipolar I disorder prior to their first manic episode. Bipolar Disord. 2014;16(5):478–92.
6. Skjelstad DV, Malt UF, Holte A. Symptoms and signs of the initial prodrome of bipolar disorder: a systematic review. J Affect Disord. 2010;126(1–2):1–13.
7. Crichton A. An inquiry into the nature and origin of mental derangement. Comprehending a concise system of the physiology and pathology of the human mind.... London: T. Cadell, Junior, and W. Davies; 1798.
8. Still GF. Some abnormal psychical conditions in children. Lancet. 1902;
9. Kramer F, Pollnow H. Über eine hyperkinetische Erkrankung im Kindesalter. Eur Neurol. 1932;82(1–2):1–20.
10. Ross DM, Ross SA. Hyperactivity: research, theory, and action. New York: Wiley; 1976.
11. Kessler JW. History of minimal brain dysfunctions. In: Rie H, Rie L, editors. Handbook of minimal brain dysfunctions: a critical view. New York: Wiley, 1980. p. 18–52.
12. Clements SD. Minimal brain dysfunction in children: terminology and identification: phase one of a three-phase project. Washington (DC): US Department of Health, Education and Welfare; 1966.
13. American Psychiatric Association. Diagnostic and statistical manual of mental disorders. DSM IV. Washington, DC: American Psychiatric Association Press; 1980.
14. Lange KW, Reichl S, Lange KM, Tucha L, Tucha O. The history of attention deficit hyperactivity disorder. Atten Defic Hyperact Disord. 2010;2(4):241–55.
15. Falret J. Leçons cliniques de mé decine mentale. 10e Con Suite Marche Mal. Ment. Paris: JB Bailliere; 1854. p. 225–63.
16. Pichot P. The birth of the bipolar disorder. Eur Psychiatry. 1995;10(1):1–10.
17. Angst J, Sellaro R. Historical perspectives and natural history of bipolar disorder. Biol Psychiatry. 2000;48(6):445–57.
18. Glovinsky I. A brief history of childhood-onset bipolar disorder through 1980. Child Adolesc Psychiatr Clin N Am. 2002;11(3):443–60. vii
19. DeLong G, Nieman G. Lithium-induced behavior changes in children with symptoms suggesting manic-depressive illness. Psychopharmacol Bull. 1983;19(2):258–65.
20. DeLong R. Lithium treatment and bipolar disorders in childhood. N C Med J. 1990;51(4):152–4.
21. Giedd JN. Bipolar disorder and attention-deficit/hyperactivity disorder in children and adolescents. J Clin Psychiatry. 2000;61(Suppl 9):31–4.
22. Carlson GA, Glovinsky I. The concept of bipolar disorder in children: a history of the bipolar controversy. Child Adolesc Psychiatr Clin N Am. 2009;18(2):257–71. vii
23. Geller B, Sun K, Zimerman B, Luby J, Frazier J, Williams M. Complex and rapid-cycling in bipolar children and adolescents: a preliminary study. J Affect Disord. 1995;34(4):259–68.
24. Geller B, Luby J. Child and adolescent bipolar disorder: a review of the past 10 years. J Am Acad Child Adolesc Psychiatry. 1997;
25. Wozniak J, Biederman J, Kiely K, Ablon JS, Faraone SV, Mundy E, et al. Mania-like symptoms suggestive of childhood-onset bipolar disorder in clinically referred children. J Am Acad Child Adolesc Psychiatry. 1995;34(7):867–76.
26. Biederman J, Klein RG, Pine DS, Klein DF. Resolved: mania is mistaken for ADHD in prepubertal children. J Am Acad Child Adolesc Psychiatry. 1998;37(10):1091–6. discussion 6–9
27. Carlson GA. Juvenile mania versus ADHD. J Am Acad Child Adolesc Psychiatry. 1999;38(4):353–4.
28. Leibenluft E, Charney DS, Towbin KE, Bhangoo RK, Pine DS. Defining clinical phenotypes of juvenile mania. Am J Psychiatry. 2003;160(3):430–7.

29. Goldstein BI, Birmaher B, Carlson GA, DelBello MP, Findling RL, Fristad M, et al. The International society for bipolar disorders task force report on pediatric bipolar disorder: knowledge to date and directions for future research. Bipolar Disord. 2017;19(7):524–43.
30. Faraone SV, Biederman J, Wozniak J, Mundy E, Mennin D, O'Donnell D. Is comorbidity with ADHD a marker for juvenile-onset mania? J Am Acad Child Adolesc Psychiatry. 1997;36(8):1046–55.
31. Zepf FD. Attention deficit-hyperactivity disorder and early-onset bipolar disorder: two facets of one entity? Dialogues Clin Neurosci. 2009;11(1):63–72.
32. American Psychiatric Association. Diagnostic and statistical manual of mental disorders. 5th ed., text rev. ed. Washington (DC): American Psychiatric Publishing; 2022.
33. Posner J, Polanczyk GV, Sonuga-Barke E. Attention-deficit hyperactivity disorder. Lancet. 2020;395(10222):450–62.
34. Faraone SV, Biederman J, Mick E. The age-dependent decline of attention deficit hyperactivity disorder: a meta-analysis of follow-up studies. Psychol Med. 2006;36(2):159–65.
35. Song P, Zha M, Yang Q, Zhang Y, Li X, Rudan I. The prevalence of adult attention-deficit hyperactivity disorder: a global systematic review and meta-analysis. J Glob Health. 2021;11:04009.
36. Ramtekkar UP, Reiersen AM, Todorov AA, Todd RD. Sex and age differences in attention-deficit/hyperactivity disorder symptoms and diagnoses: implications for DSM-V and ICD-11. J Am Acad Child Adolesc Psychiatry. 2010;49(3):217–28.e1–3.
37. Bitsko RH. Mental health surveillance among children—United States, 2013–2019. MMWR Suppl. 2022;71
38. Merikangas KR, Nakamura EF, Kessler RC. Epidemiology of mental disorders in children and adolescents. Dialogues Clin Neurosci. 2009;11(1):7–20.
39. Sibley MH, Arnold LE, Swanson JM, Hechtman LT, Kennedy TM, Owens E, et al. Variable patterns of remission from ADHD in the multimodal treatment study of ADHD. Am J Psychiatry. 2022;179(2):142–51.
40. Roy A, Hechtman L, Arnold LE, Sibley MH, Molina BS, Swanson JM, et al. Childhood factors affecting persistence and desistence of attention-deficit/hyperactivity disorder symptoms in adulthood: results from the MTA. J Am Acad Child Adolesc Psychiatry. 2016;55(11):937–44.e4.
41. Roy A, Hechtman L, Arnold LE, Swanson JM, BSG M, Sibley MH, et al. Childhood predictors of adult functional outcomes in the multimodal treatment study of attention-deficit/hyperactivity disorder (MTA). J Am Acad Child Adolesc Psychiatry. 2017;56(8):687–95.e7.
42. Núñez-Jaramillo L, Herrera-Solís A, Herrera-Morales WV. ADHD: reviewing the causes and evaluating solutions. J Pers Med. 2021;11(3)
43. Demontis D, Walters RK, Martin J, Mattheisen M, Als TD, Agerbo E, et al. Discovery of the first genome-wide significant risk loci for attention deficit/hyperactivity disorder. Nat Genet. 2019;51(1):63–75.
44. Russell AE, Ford T, Russell G. Socioeconomic associations with ADHD: findings from a mediation analysis. PLoS One. 2015;10(6):e0128248.
45. Visser SN, Danielson ML, Bitsko RH, Holbrook JR, Kogan MD, Ghandour RM, et al. Trends in the parent-report of health care provider-diagnosed and medicated attention-deficit/hyperactivity disorder: United States, 2003–2011. J Am Acad Child Adolesc Psychiatry. 2014;53(1):34–46.e2.
46. Rocco I, Corso B, Bonati M, Minicuci N. Time of onset and/or diagnosis of ADHD in European children: a systematic review. BMC Psychiatry. 2021;21(1):575.
47. Epstein JN, Loren RE. Changes in the definition of ADHD in DSM-5: subtle but important. Neuropsychiatry (London). 2013;3(5):455–8.
48. Olson SL. Developmental perspectives. In: Sandberg S, editor. Hyperactivity disorders of childhood. Cambridge: Cambridge University Press; 1996. p. 242–89.

49. Hart EL, Lahey BB, Loeber R, Applegate B, Frick PJ. Developmental change in attention-deficit hyperactivity disorder in boys: a four-year longitudinal study. J Abnorm Child Psychol. 1995;23(6):729–49.
50. de Freitas de Sousa A, Coimbra IM, Castanho JM, Polanczyk GV, Rohde LA. Attention deficit hyperactivity disorder. In: Rey JM, Martin A, editors. JM Rey's IACAPAP e-Textbook of Child and Adolescent Mental Health. Portuguese ed. F. Dias Silva, editor. Geneva: International Association for Child and Adolescent Psychiatry and Allied Professions; 2020.
51. Kumperscak HG. ADHD through different developmental stages. In: Gregoric H, editor. Attention deficit hyperactivity disorder in children and adolescents. Rijeka: InTech; 2013. p. 3–19. https://doi.org/10.5772/53963.
52. Martel MM, Levinson CA, Langer JK, Nigg JT. A network analysis of developmental change in ADHD symptom structure from preschool to adulthood. Clin Psychol Sci. 2016;4(6):988–1001.
53. Dekkers TJ, de Water E, Scheres A. Impulsive and risky decision-making in adolescents with attention-deficit/hyperactivity disorder (ADHD): the need for a developmental perspective. Curr Opin Psychol. 2022;(44):330–6.
54. Szuromi B, Bitter I, Czobor P. Functional impairment in adults positively screened for attention-deficit hyperactivity disorder: the role of symptom presentation and executive functioning. Compr Psychiatry. 2013;54(7):974–81.
55. Graziano PA, Garcia A. Attention-deficit hyperactivity disorder and children's emotion dysregulation: a meta-analysis. Clin Psychol Rev. 2016;46:106–23.
56. Christiansen H, Hirsch O, Albrecht B, Chavanon ML. Attention-deficit/hyperactivity disorder (ADHD) and emotion regulation over the life span. Curr Psychiatry Rep. 2019;21(3):17.
57. Barkley RA, Fischer M. The unique contribution of emotional impulsiveness to impairment in major life activities in hyperactive children as adults. J Am Acad Child Adolesc Psychiatry. 2010;49(5):503–13.
58. Biederman J, Spencer TJ, Petty C, Hyder LL, O'Connor KB, Surman CB, et al. Longitudinal course of deficient emotional self-regulation CBCL profile in youth with ADHD: prospective controlled study. Neuropsychiatr Dis Treat. 2012;8:267–76.
59. Zaravinos-Tsakos F, Kolaitis G. Disentangling pediatric bipolar disorder and attention deficit-hyperactivity disorder: a neuropsychological approach. Psychiatriki. 2020;31(4):332–40.
60. Salvi V, Ribuoli E, Servasi M, Orsolini L, Volpe U. ADHD and bipolar disorder in adulthood: clinical and treatment implications. Medicina (Kaunas). 2021;57(5)
61. Schiweck C, Arteaga-Henriquez G, Aichholzer M, Edwin Thanarajah S, Vargas-Cáceres S, Matura S, et al. Comorbidity of ADHD and adult bipolar disorder: a systematic review and meta-analysis. Neurosci Biobehav Rev. 2021;124:100–23.
62. Youngstrom EA, Arnold LE, Frazier TW. Bipolar and ADHD comorbidity: both artifact and outgrowth of shared mechanisms. Clin Psychol (New York). 2010;17(4):350–9.
63. Kooij SJ, Bejerot S, Blackwell A, Caci H, Casas-Brugué M, Carpentier PJ, et al. European consensus statement on diagnosis and treatment of adult ADHD: the European network adult ADHD. BMC Psychiatry. 2010;10:67.
64. Marangoni C, De Chiara L, Faedda GL. Bipolar disorder and ADHD: comorbidity and diagnostic distinctions. Curr Psychiatry Rep. 2015;17(8):604.
65. Fu-I L. Bipolar disorder in childhood and adolescence. Braz J Psychiatry. 2004;26(Suppl 3):22–6.
66. Spencer TJ. ADHD and comorbidity in childhood. J Clin Psychiatry. 2006;67(Suppl 8):27–31.
67. Biederman J, Faraone S, Mick E, Wozniak J, Chen L, Ouellette C, et al. Attention-deficit hyperactivity disorder and juvenile mania: an overlooked comorbidity? J Am Acad Child Adolesc Psychiatry. 1996;35(8):997–1008.
68. Biederman J, Faraone S, Milberger S, Guite J, Mick E, Chen L, et al. A prospective 4-year follow-up study of attention-deficit hyperactivity and related disorders. Arch Gen Psychiatry. 1996;53(5):437–46.

69. Singh MK, MP DB, Kowatch RA, Strakowski SM. Co-occurrence of bipolar and attention-deficit hyperactivity disorders in children. Bipolar Disord. 2006;8(6):710–20.
70. Birmaher B, Axelson D, Goldstein B, Strober M, Gill MK, Hunt J, et al. Four-year longitudinal course of children and adolescents with bipolar spectrum disorders: the course and outcome of bipolar youth (COBY) study. Am J Psychiatry. 2009;166(7):795–804.
71. Scheffer RE. Concurrent ADHD and bipolar disorder. Curr Psychiatry Rep. 2007;9(5):415–9.
72. Pliszka SR. Comorbidity of attention-deficit/hyperactivity disorder with psychiatric disorder: an overview. J Clin Psychiatry. 1998;59(Suppl 7):50–8.
73. Nierenberg AA, Miyahara S, Spencer T, Wisniewski SR, Otto MW, Simon N, et al. Clinical and diagnostic implications of lifetime attention-deficit/hyperactivity disorder comorbidity in adults with bipolar disorder: data from the first 1000 STEP-BD participants. Biol Psychiatry. 2005;57(11):1467–73.
74. Bernardi S, Cortese S, Solanto M, Hollander E, Pallanti S. Bipolar disorder and comorbid attention deficit hyperactivity disorder. A distinct clinical phenotype? Clinical characteristics and temperamental traits. World J Biol Psychiatry. 2010;11(4):656–66.
75. Harmanci H, Çam Çelikel F, Etikan İ. Comorbidity of adult attention deficit and hyperactivity disorder in bipolar and unipolar patients. Noro Psikiyatr Ars. 2016;53(3):257–62.
76. Biederman J, Faraone SV, Petty C, Martelon M, Woodworth KY, Wozniak J. Further evidence that pediatric-onset bipolar disorder comorbid with ADHD represents a distinct subtype: results from a large controlled family study. J Psychiatr Res. 2013;47(1):15–22.
77. van Hulzen KJE, Scholz CJ, Franke B, Ripke S, Klein M, McQuillin A, et al. Genetic overlap between attention-deficit/hyperactivity disorder and bipolar disorder: evidence from genome-wide association study meta-analysis. Biol Psychiatry. 2017;82(9):634–41.
78. plee0@mgh.harvard.edu C-DGotPGCEa, Consortium C-DGotPG. Genomic relationships, novel loci, and pleiotropic mechanisms across eight psychiatric disorders. Cell. 2019;179(7):1469–82.e11.
79. Bond DJ, Hadjipavlou G, Lam RW, RS MI, Beaulieu S, Schaffer A, et al. The Canadian network for mood and anxiety treatments (CANMAT) task force recommendations for the management of patients with mood disorders and comorbid attention-deficit/hyperactivity disorder. Ann Clin Psychiatry. 2012;24(1):23–37.
80. CADDRA–Canadian A. Resource alliance: Canadian ADHD practice guidelines. Toronto ON; 2020.
81. Asherson P, Young AH, Eich-Höchli D, Moran P, Porsdal V, Deberdt W. Differential diagnosis, comorbidity, and treatment of attention-deficit/hyperactivity disorder in relation to bipolar disorder or borderline personality disorder in adults. Curr Med Res Opin. 2014;30(8):1657–72.
82. Perugi G, Pallucchini A, Rizzato S, Pinzone V, De Rossi P. Current and emerging pharmacotherapy for the treatment of adult attention deficit hyperactivity disorder (ADHD). Expert Opin Pharmacother. 2019;20(12):1457–70.
83. Brus MJ, Solanto MV, Goldberg JF. Adult ADHD vs. bipolar disorder in the DSM-5 era: a challenging differentiation for clinicians. J Psychiatr Pract. 2014;20(6):428–37.
84. National Institute for Health and Care Excellence (NICE). Attention deficit hyperactivity disorder: diagnosis and management. London: NICE; 2018.
85. Findling RL, Short EJ, NK MN, Demeter CA, Stansbrey RJ, Gracious BL, et al. Methylphenidate in the treatment of children and adolescents with bipolar disorder and attention-deficit/hyperactivity disorder. J Am Acad Child Adolesc Psychiatry. 2007;46(11):1445–53.
86. Schneck CD, Chang KD, Singh MK, MP DB, Miklowitz DJ. A pharmacologic algorithm for youth who are at high risk for bipolar disorder. J Child Adolesc Psychopharmacol. 2017;27(9):796–805.
87. Viktorin A, Rydén E, Thase ME, Chang Z, Lundholm C, D'Onofrio BM, et al. The risk of treatment-emergent mania with methylphenidate in bipolar disorder. Am J Psychiatry. 2017;174(4):341–8.

88. Wang LJ, Shyu YC, Yuan SS, Yang CJ, Yang KC, Lee TL, et al. Attention-deficit hyperactivity disorder, its pharmacotherapy, and the risk of developing bipolar disorder: a nationwide population-based study in Taiwan. J Psychiatr Res. 2016;72:6–14.
89. Faedda GL, Serra G, Marangoni C, Salvatore P, Sani G, Vázquez GH, et al. Clinical risk factors for bipolar disorders: a systematic review of prospective studies. J Affect Disord. 2014;168:314–21.
90. Conroy S, Francis M, Hulvershorn LA. Identifying and treating the prodromal phases of bipolar disorder and schizophrenia. Curr Treat Options Psychiatry. 2018;5(1):113–28.
91. Van Meter AR, Burke C, Youngstrom EA, Faedda GL, Correll CU. The bipolar prodrome: meta-analysis of symptom prevalence prior to initial or recurrent mood episodes. J Am Acad Child Adolesc Psychiatry. 2016;55(7):543–55.
92. Luby JL, Navsaria N. Pediatric bipolar disorder: evidence for prodromal states and early markers. J Child Psychol Psychiatry. 2010;51(4):459–71.
93. Nurnberger JI, McInnis M, Reich W, Kastelic E, Wilcox HC, Glowinski A, et al. A high-risk study of bipolar disorder. Childhood clinical phenotypes as precursors of major mood disorders. Arch Gen Psychiatry. 2011;68(10):1012–20.
94. Sparks GM, Axelson DA, Yu H, Ha W, Ballester J, Diler RS, et al. Disruptive mood dysregulation disorder and chronic irritability in youth at familial risk for bipolar disorder. J Am Acad Child Adolesc Psychiatry. 2014;53(4):408–16.
95. Tillman R, Geller B. Controlled study of switching from attention-deficit/hyperactivity disorder to a prepubertal and early adolescent bipolar I disorder phenotype during 6-year prospective follow-up: rate, risk, and predictors. Dev Psychopathol. 2006;18(4):1037–53.
96. Chen MH, Su TP, Chen YS, Hsu JW, Huang KL, Chang WH, et al. Higher risk of developing mood disorders among adolescents with comorbidity of attention deficit hyperactivity disorder and disruptive behavior disorder: a nationwide prospective study. J Psychiatr Res. 2013;47(8):1019–23.
97. Jerrell JM, RS MI, Park YM. Correlates of incident bipolar disorder in children and adolescents diagnosed with attention-deficit/hyperactivity disorder. J Clin Psychiatry. 2014;75(11):e1278–83.
98. Koolwijk I, Stein DS, Chan E, Powell C, Driscoll K, Barbaresi WJ. "Complex" attention-deficit hyperactivity disorder, more norm than exception? Diagnoses and comorbidities in a developmental clinic. J Dev Behav Pediatr. 2014;35(9):591–7.
99. Biederman J, Petty CR, Byrne D, Wong P, Wozniak J, Faraone SV. Risk for switch from unipolar to bipolar disorder in youth with ADHD: a long term prospective controlled study. J Affect Disord. 2009;119(1–3):16–21.
100. Biederman J, Wozniak J, Tarko L, Serra G, Hernandez M, McDermott K, et al. Re-examining the risk for switch from unipolar to bipolar major depressive disorder in youth with ADHD: a long term prospective longitudinal controlled study. J Affect Disord. 2014;152–154:347–51.
101. Vannucchi G, Medda P, Pallucchini A, Bertelli M, Angst J, Azorin JM, et al. The relationship between attention deficit hyperactivity disorder, bipolarity and mixed features in major depressive patients: evidence from the BRIDGE-II-Mix Study. J Affect Disord. 2019;246:346–54.

Chapter 7
Autism Spectrum Disorder and Latent Bipolar Disorder

Mirela Paiva Vasconcelos-Moreno, Jairo Vinícius Pinto, Cintia Vasquez Cruz Heidemann, Ingrid Souza-Melo, and Flavio Kapczinski

7.1 Autism Spectrum Disorder and Latent Bipolar Disorder

Bipolar disorder (BD) is a highly heritable condition, with twin studies estimating its heritability between 60% and 90%, emphasizing the role of genetics in its etiology [1, 2]. Family studies have shown that the risk of developing BD is up to 7.9 times higher in first-degree relatives of individuals with the condition than those without a family history [3, 4]. As a result, children of individuals with BD are an identifiable at-risk group whose mental health should be closely monitored from an early age [5].

In this context, prospective studies have shown that individuals at familial risk follow a sequence in the development of BD. This sequence begins in childhood

M. P. Vasconcelos-Moreno (✉)
Laboratory of Molecular Psychiatry, Hospital de Clínicas de Porto Alegre (HCPA), Porto Alegre, Brazil

Universidade Federal do Rio Grande do Sul, School of Medicine, Graduate Program in Psychiatry and Behavioral Sciences, Department of Psychiatry, Porto Alegre, RS, Brazil

Instituto Nacional de Ciência e Tecnologia Translacional em Medicina (INCT-TM), Porto Alegre, RS, Brazil

J. V. Pinto
Laboratory of Molecular Psychiatry, Hospital de Clínicas de Porto Alegre (HCPA), Porto Alegre, Brazil

Universidade Federal do Rio Grande do Sul, School of Medicine, Graduate Program in Psychiatry and Behavioral Sciences, Department of Psychiatry, Porto Alegre, RS, Brazil

University Hospital, Universidade Federal de Santa Catarina (HU-UFSC), Florianópolis, SC, Brazil

C. V. C. Heidemann
Laboratory of Molecular Psychiatry, Hospital de Clínicas de Porto Alegre (HCPA), Porto Alegre, Brazil

T. de Azevedo Cardoso et al. (eds.), *Latent Bipolar Disorder*,
https://doi.org/10.1007/978-3-032-01297-5_7

with symptoms of anxiety, sleep disturbances, and sometimes neurodevelopmental disorders. As these individuals reach adolescence, they exhibit the first signs of mood disturbances, including their first depressive episodes and suicidal behaviors. In adulthood, the manic and hypomanic episodes finally emerge [6, 7].

Consequently, young persons with a familial predisposition and exhibiting nonspecific symptoms but who have not yet developed hypomania or mania may demonstrate a latent form of BD [8].

Understanding who these high-risk individuals are, their psychopathological manifestations, and their healthcare needs allows for the planning of preventive strategies [5]. Early interventions in bipolar disorder are crucial, as they are more effective than those implemented in later stages and contribute to preventing unfavorable long-term outcomes [9, 10]. However, early diagnosis remains challenging for clinicians, given that approximately half of patients present depression as their initial mood episode, often during adolescence [7, 11]. Furthermore, prodromal symptoms preceding the first manic episode are nonspecific, including anxiety, sleep disturbances, and subthreshold hypomanic symptoms [6, 12, 13]. Consequently, patients with a latent BD are frequently misdiagnosed as having unipolar depression or anxiety disorders [7].

Although BD is classified as a mood disorder and diagnosis typically occurs in early adulthood, longitudinal studies indicate that neurodevelopmental disorders, such as attention-deficit/hyperactivity disorder (ADHD) and learning disorders, may play a role in the trajectory of BD onset in individuals with a family risk [6]. Interestingly, BD is highly prevalent in individuals with autism spectrum disorder (ASD), another neurodevelopmental condition. Data shows a significant overlap in the prevalence of BD among those with ASD [14]. Therefore, other conditions related to neurodevelopment, such as ASD, should be explored both as a comorbidity and as a differential diagnosis for latent BD [15].

ASD is characterized by a heterogeneous array of neurodevelopmental symptoms that manifest early in childhood and affect individuals across the lifespan [16]. Similar to BD, ASD also exhibits a significant heritability ranging from 64% to 91% [17]. The severity of ASD and the manifestation of its symptoms can vary widely among individuals. Therefore, a thorough and individualized assessment is essential for an accurate diagnosis. Early diagnoses are often made in individuals with more severe symptoms and evident neurodevelopmental delays [18]. However, in some cases, such as those with ASD Level I, diagnosis may not occur until adulthood despite the presence of clinical impairments [19]. In adolescents or adults with undiagnosed ASD co-occurring with latent BD, diagnostic and therapeutic

I. Souza-Melo
Laboratory of Molecular Psychiatry, Hospital de Clínicas de Porto Alegre (HCPA), Porto Alegre, Brazil

Universidade Federal do Rio Grande do Sul, School of Medicine, Graduate Program in Psychiatry and Behavioral Sciences, Department of Psychiatry, Porto Alegre, RS, Brazil

F. Kapczinski
Psychiatry Department, Federal University of Rio Grande do Sul, Porto Alegre, Rio Grande do Sul, Brazil

challenges are particularly significant. Unspecific shared symptoms, such as mood dysregulation, impulsivity, and social skills deficits, complicate the diagnostic process and increase the risk of misdiagnosis [14, 20, 21].

The main goal of this chapter is to explore the clinical characteristics, diagnostic criteria, genetic factors, differential diagnosis, and treatment considerations of ASD in the context of latent BD. The focus is on improving the identification of ASD, especially in individuals with latent BD who may not have a prior diagnosis. The discussion mainly addresses adolescents and adults with ASD requiring minimal support (ASD level 1 of support).

7.2 Epidemiology and Comorbidity of Autism Spectrum Disorder and Bipolar Disorder

Recent epidemiological data indicates a notable increase in the prevalence of ASD, with estimates suggesting that around 1 in 36 children in the United States may be affected [22]. ASD exhibits a male-to-female prevalence ratio of approximately 4:1, reflecting potential differences in diagnostic patterns and gender-specific presentations [23]. The observed rise in prevalence is attributed to enhanced diagnostic practices, broader diagnostic criteria, and increased public and clinical awareness [23]. BD, in turn, exhibits a global prevalence of approximately 1–2% in the general population, with significant variations across studies and populations [24]. Gender distribution in BD is relatively balanced, though some studies suggest a slightly higher incidence in females, particularly for bipolar II disorder [24]. Both ASD and BD are highly heritable, as cited above, with substantial evidence indicating a strong genetic predisposition for both conditions [1, 25].

Historically, emotional and behavioral problems in individuals with ASD have often been attributed solely to ASD itself [26]. However, recent studies suggest these symptoms may warrant additional diagnoses, such as BD [27]. Currently, the majority of patients with ASD receive at least one comorbid psychiatric diagnosis, frequently with delays or under-recognition due to the complexities of the condition [28]. BD is a common comorbid psychiatric disorder in this population, along with ADHD, anxiety disorders, and depression [14, 29]. Additionally, clinical evidence indicates that relatives of individuals with ASD have a significantly higher prevalence of affective disorders, suggesting a potential familial or genetic link between these conditions [30].

More recent cohort studies point out that the presence of BD in first-degree relatives is a significant and consistent risk factor for ASD [31]. A population-based study demonstrated that individuals with ASD have a heightened risk of developing BD, schizophrenia, and other non-affective psychotic disorders compared to age- and sex-matched individuals without ASD from the general population [32]. In another cohort study, individuals with ASD by age 30 exhibited a cumulative incidence of BD at 7.3%, depression at 54.1%, and anxiety at 50.0%, while control subjects had respective incidences of 0.9%, 28.9%, and 22.2% [33].

The largest cohort study on this topic followed 700,000 children for 11 years, and although it reported lower comorbidity rates of BD and ASD (0.6% of patients diagnosed with ASD by age 16 also met the criteria for BD by the study's end), this rate was six times higher than in the control group (0.1%) [34]. Overall, the estimated prevalence of BD in individuals with ASD ranges from 5% to 8%, significantly higher than the approximately 2% found in the general population [14]. Rosenberg et al. found that 5.2% of the 4343 patients with ASD up to 18 years old, evaluated from a national online registry, received a comorbid diagnosis of BD [29]. Both studies identified higher rates of BD in patients with greater intellectual abilities, which can be associated with a more typical disease course, better communication of emotions, and a presumed higher risk of developing depressive episodes [14, 29].

There is considerable variability in studies examining the comorbidity of BD and ASD, particularly in evaluating autistic traits among patients with BD [35]. High reported prevalence of autistic traits in patients with BD (42.7–56.9%) may reflect an artificial co-occurrence due to ASD's heterogeneous nature and differing evaluation methods [36–38]. Limitations include the reliance on screening questionnaires, which are inadequate for a definitive ASD diagnosis, and the atypical, nonspecific presentation of BD in patients with ASD, which complicates accurate diagnosis [35].

When examining the overlap between ASD and BD, it is crucial to address the comorbid conditions frequently observed in both disorders. ASD and BD are associated with an increased risk of developing other psychiatric disorders. Up to 79% of individuals with ASD meet criteria for at least one psychiatric disorder during their lifetime, including ADHD (28%), anxiety disorders (20%), sleep-wake disorders (13%), depressive disorders (11%), obsessive-compulsive disorder (OCD) (9%), and BD (5%) [39]. Individuals with BD, in turn, often have comorbid conditions such as ADHD, anxiety disorders, OCD, and substance use disorder [24]. The presence of substance use disorder in both ASD and BD can complicate diagnosis by masking symptom presentation, may exacerbate mood dysregulation, impair social functioning, and complicate the management of both conditions [19, 24, 28, 40]. Moreover, behaviors associated with ASD and BD can overlap with traits found in personality disorders, such as borderline or schizotypal personalities [39, 41]. This overlap presents challenges for identifying comorbidities and distinguishing between these conditions in differential diagnosis.

7.3 The Clinical Manifestations and Diagnosis of Autism in Adults

7.3.1 Clinical Manifestations in Adults

ASD is characterized by two core symptom clusters: (1) deficits in social interaction and social communication and (2) repetitive patterns of behaviors, interests, or activities that are atypical or excessive for the age and sociocultural context [16].

Symptoms typically manifest during developmental stages, often observed in early childhood, though full manifestation may be delayed until social demands surpass the individual's adaptive capacities. These deficits are apparent across various contexts, though they may fluctuate with environmental influences and can result in significant functional impairments in multiple domains, such as personal, familial, social, educational, and occupational spheres [16]. The severity of ASD symptoms, along with cognitive and linguistic abilities, varies widely among affected individuals, necessitating a spectrum of support levels [42].

The clinical presentation of ASD level 1 of support in adolescentes and adults is highly heterogeneous. The core features of ASD typically emerge in childhood, but therapeutic interventions, compensatory strategies, and supportive environments can mitigate symptoms, complicating diagnosis in adults [19]. Besides, individuals with ASD may consciously or unconsciously camouflage or mask their symptoms; it involves concealing or suppressing autistic traits to meet societal norms [43]. This concealment of symptoms can make it challenging to recognize the clinical manifestation and address ASD diagnosis in adult populations.

According to DSM-5-TR, nonverbal communication in individuals with ASD is often marked by an absence, reduction, or atypical use of gestures, eye contact, and facial expressions. Even those who acquire functional gestures, exhibit fluent speech, and maintain relatively good eye contact may display a narrower repertoire of nonverbal behaviors compared to typical peers and often exhibit inadequate integration of eye contact, gestures, posture, prosody, and facial expressions [16, 44–46]. This disintegration can impair social communication and become more pronounced under stress [47]. In adults with fluent language, difficulties in aligning nonverbal communication with verbal speech may result in interactions characterized by "strange," rigid, or exaggerated body language [16].

Individuals who do not exhibit language or cognitive impairments may still display subtle communication deficits [45, 48]. Their communication tends to be one-sided, focusing on naming, narrating, or categorizing rather than engaging in reciprocal dialogue, sharing emotions, or expressing ideas [16, 49].

Deficits in understanding, maintaining, and developing relationships should be evaluated in the context of age, gender, and cultural norms [16]. Individuals may express a strong desire to form friendships without a full or realistic understanding of the requirements and dynamics of these relationships, potentially leading to unbalanced interactions or relationships based solely on shared special interests [16, 50].

Restricted and repetitive interests should be evaluated in relation to the individual's age, functional abilities, therapeutic interventions, and available supports [16]. Manifestations of restricted behavioral patterns may include excessive adherence to routines, resistance to minor changes, adherence to rules, rigidity in thought processes, or ritualistic verbal or non-verbal behaviors [16]. Interests are typically characterized by abnormal focus and intensity [51]. Certain routines may be associated with hyper- or hyporeactivity to sensory stimuli and can present as extreme responses to specific auditory or tactile inputs, excessive smelling or touching of objects, or a marked lack of response to pain, temperature extremes, or other sensory experiences [16]. Extreme reactions or ritualistic behaviors related to the taste, smell, texture, or appearance of food, as well as severe dietary restrictions, are frequently observed [52, 53].

A clear association exists between increased stereotypies and lower intelligence quotient, younger age, and greater severity of symptoms in individuals with ASD [54]. Significant impairment in social, occupational, or other key areas of functioning must be evident [16]. Even when possessing above-average intelligence and experiencing fewer psychosocial impairments, individuals with ASD often struggle with independent functioning [19, 55, 56]. They may remain socially naive and vulnerable [19], find it challenging to manage practical demands without support, and are more susceptible to anxiety and depression [57, 58]. Due to their rigidity and difficulties with novelty, planning, organizing, and adapting to change can adversely affect their academic, professional, and interpersonal relationships [16].

Individuals with average or high intelligence often exhibit a disparate profile of abilities [55, 59]. There is typically a notable gap between functional adaptive skills and intellectual capabilities [60]. Commonly observed deficits include impaired theory of mind (difficulty understanding others' perspectives), executive function impairments, and challenges with central coherence (difficulty grasping the broader context or seeing the whole situation, with a tendency to focus excessively on details) [61–64]. Impairments in social cognition will be explored in more detail in the following section.

Women with ASD often demonstrate more effective reciprocal conversation skills, are more likely to share interests, and integrate verbal and non-verbal behaviors more adeptly [65, 66]. Nevertheless, they may report that maintaining adherence to social conventions can be mentally exhausting [65].

It is important to note that ASD is not a degenerative disorder; rather, learning and adaptive strategies typically continue to develop throughout the lifespan [16]. ASD can present with a wide range of intellectual abilities, from intellectual disability to high intelligence [67, 68]. Individuals with elevated intellectual abilities may demonstrate distinct intensities and heightened sensitivities, which can contribute to issues such as perfectionism, rumination, and increased anxiety [67, 69]. These characteristics may predispose individuals to anxiety and depression, complicating diagnostic challenges [70].

7.3.2 Social Cognition

Social cognition encompasses the cognitive processes of perceiving, interpreting, and responding to social information, including recognizing and understanding others' emotions, intentions, and social norms. It is essential for effective social interaction and navigating complex social environments involving both neural and behavioral components [71]. Green in 2008 proposed five key aspects of social cognition, including (1) theory of mind (involves attributing mental states to oneself and others); (2) social perception (ability to identify social context and rules, e.g., perception of the nature of relationships between people); (3) social knowledge (internalized understanding of social rules and expectations); (4) attributional bias (how people typically infer the causes of particular positive and negative events); and (5) emotional processing (refers broadly to perceiving and using emotions) [72].

Individuals with ASD present persistent difficulties in social communication and social cognition [16, 73]. The identification of the deficit in the theory of mind was one of the first findings in the study of social cognition in ASD, and it is the most studied cognitive function in ASD, with robust evidence of significant deficits [62, 74]. Theory of mind is a key element in applying social skills in contexts involving interpersonal contact, and it is one of the skills that should be examined when ASD is suspected [19, 62]. Additionally, individuals with ASD often struggle with interpreting nonverbal cues and social signals, which can result in misunderstandings and difficulties in forming meaningful connections [73]. These impairments in social cognition contribute to the broader challenges that individuals with ASD face in achieving social maturity and maintaining peer relationships [73, 75]. These impairments are correlated with increased rates of social isolation, reduced employment opportunities, heightened anxiety and depression, and a higher risk of suicide [76]. Impaired social cognition is a major driver of poor psychosocial functioning in ASD [75].

7.3.3 Diagnosis of Autism in Adults

There are two core symptom clusters in ASD, as cited above: (1) deficits in social interaction and social communication and (2) repetitive patterns of behaviors, interests, or activities that are atypical or excessive for the age and sociocultural context [16]. The DSM-5-TR stipulates that for an ASD diagnosis, an individual must exhibit at least three symptoms from Criterion A, which includes persistent challenges in reciprocal social communication and social interaction. Additionally, at least two symptoms from Criterion B are required, characterized by restricted and repetitive patterns of behavior, interests, or activities. These symptoms should be evident from the early developmental stages and cause considerable impairment in daily functioning, as outlined in Criteria C and D [16]. Conversely, the ICD-11, in its eleventh edition, does not specify a minimum number of symptoms for diagnosis. Nevertheless, it requires the presence of symptoms from both core groups: persistent deficits in initiating and sustaining social communication and reciprocal social interactions, and persistent restricted, repetitive, and inflexible patterns of behavior, interests, or activities. Furthermore, ICD-11 states that the onset of the disorder occurs during the developmental period, and the symptoms result in significant impairment in functioning [42].

Table 7.1 summarizes the DSM-5-TR and ICD-11 criteria for ASD.

The UK National Institute for Health and Care Excellence (NICE) guidelines recommend assessing adults for autism if they show signs of the condition and meet at least one of these criteria: difficulties with employment or education, challenges

Table 7.1 DSM-5-TR and ICD-11 criteria for autism spectrum disorder

DSM-5-TR—Autism spectrum disorder		ICD-11—Autism spectrum disorder
A.	Persistent deficits in social communication and social interaction across multiple contexts, manifested by *all of the following* (currently or by history):	Persistent deficits in social communication and social interactions that are outside the expected range of typical functioning given the individual's age and level of intellectual development. Manifestations may include limitations in the following:
1.	Deficits in social-emotional reciprocity Abnormal social approach and failure of typical back-and-forth conversation. Reduced sharing of interests, emotions, or affect. Failure to initiate or respond to social interactions.	Understanding and use of language in social contexts Ability to initiate and sustain reciprocal social conversations. Mutual sharing of interests. Ability to imagine and respond to the feelings, emotions and attitudes of others.
2.	Deficits in nonverbal communicative behaviors used for social interaction Poorly integrated verbal and nonverbal communication. Abnormalities in eye contact and body language, lack of facial expressions Deficits in understanding and use of gestures.	Understanding/interest the verbal or non-verbal social communications of others. Inappropriate responses to the verbal or non-verbal social communications. Integration of spoken language with typical complimentary non-verbal cues. Non-verbal behaviors may be reduced in frequency or intensity.
3.	Deficits in developing, maintaining, and understanding relationships Difficulties adjusting behavior to suit various social contexts. Difficulties in sharing imaginative play or in making friends. Absence of interest in peers.	Social awareness, leading to behavior that is not appropriately modulated according to the social context. Ability to make and sustain typical peer relationships.
B.	Restricted, repetitive patterns of behavior, interests, or activities, as manifested by *at least two of the following* (currently or by history):	Persistent restricted, repetitive, and inflexible patterns of behavior, interests, or activities that are clearly atypical or excessive for the individual's age and sociocultural context. These may include:

(continued)

Table 7.1 (continued)

DSM-5-TR—Autism spectrum disorder		ICD-11—Autism spectrum disorder
1.	Stereotyped or repetitive motor movements, use of objects, or speech Simple motor stereotypies. Lining up toys or flipping objects. Echolalia, idiosyncratic phrases.	Repetitive and stereotyped motor movements, Whole body movements, atypical gait, unusual posturing Unusual hand or finger movements Excessive and persistent ritualized behavior with no apparent external purpose.
2.	Insistence on sameness, inflexible adherence to routines, or ritualized patterns of verbal or nonverbal behavior Extreme distress at small changes, difficulties with transitions. Rigid thinking patterns, greeting rituals, need to take same route or eat same food every day.	Excessive adherence to rules Inflexible adherence to particular routines. Lack of adaptability to new experiences and circumstances, with associated distress
3.	Highly restricted, fixated interests that are abnormal in intensity or focus Strong attachment to or preoccupation with unusual objects. Excessively circumscribed or perseverative interests.	Persistent preoccupation with one or more special interests or parts of objects. Persistent preoccupation with specific types of stimuli. Unusually strong attachment to particular objects.
4.	Hyper/hyporeactivity or unusual interest in sensory input. Hypereativity or hyporeactivity to sensory input. Unusual interest in sensory aspects of the environment.	Lifelong excessive and persistent hypersensitivity or hyposensitivity to sensory stimuli Unusual interest in a sensory stimulus
C.	Symptoms must be present in the early developmental period *Symptoms but may not become fully manifest until social demands exceed limited capacities or may be masked by learned strategies in later life.*	Onset occurs during the developmental period, typically in early childhood, *Characteristic symptoms may not become fully manifest until later, when social demands exceed limited capacities.*
D.	Symptoms cause clinically significant impairment in social, occupational, or other important areas of current functioning.	Symptoms result in significant impairment in personal, family, social, educational, occupational or other important areas of functioning. *Some individuals with ASD can function adequately in many contexts through exceptional effort, such that their deficits may not be apparent to others. A diagnosis of ASD is still appropriate in such cases.*

(continued)

Table 7.1 (continued)

DSM-5-TR—Autism spectrum disorder		ICD-11—Autism spectrum disorder
E.	These disturbances are not better explained by intellectual developmental disorder (intellectual disability) or global developmental delay. *Intellectual developmental disorder and autism spectrum disorder frequently co-occur; to make comorbid diagnoses of autism spectrum disorder and intellectual developmental disorder, social communication should be below that expected for general developmental level.*	–
	Specifiers:	
	With or without accompanying intellectual impairment With or without accompanying language impairment Associated with a known genetic or other medical condition or environmental factor Associated with a neurodevelopmental, mental, or behavioral problem With catatonia ---	Co-occurring disorder of intellectual development Degree of functional language impairment --- --- --- With or without loss of previously acquired skills
	Specify current severity based on social communication impairments and restricted, repetitive patterns of behavior Requiring very substantial support Requiring substantial support Requiring support	–

DSM-5-TR: Diagnostic and Statistical Manual of Mental Disorders, Fifth Edition, Text Revision; ICD-11: International Classification of Diseases 11th Revision

in social relationships, interaction with mental health or learning disability services, or a history of neurodevelopmental or mental health disorders [19, 77].

7.3.4 Diagnostic Assessment Scales and Clinical Rating Scales

The diagnosis of autism spectrum disorder (ASD) is primarily clinical and should involve multiple sources of information rather than relying on a single questionnaire or observation tool [16]. However, standardized diagnostic and screening instruments like the Autism Diagnostic Observation Schedule (ADOS) and the Autism Diagnostic Interview-Revised (ADI-R) are considered the gold standard and are highly reliable for complementarily diagnosing ASD in adults [78]. Additional tools include the Social Responsiveness Scale (SRS-2), which is frequently used for screening autism symptoms and is recognized as effective for identifying ASD in adults, and the Autism Spectrum Quotient (AQ-50), which has demonstrated satisfactory psychometric properties in adults without cognitive impairments [79, 80].

7.3.5 Symptoms Overlap Between ASD and BD

ASD and BD clearly have different core symptoms: BD is characterized by mood episodes, whereas ASD is primarily marked by deficits in social communication and the presence of repetitive behaviors [16]. Besides, there are overlapping symptoms between ASD and BD, leading to varying clinical presentations and underlying mechanisms. Mood dysregulation in BD is characterized by clear episodic swings between depressive and manic states, influenced by stress, life events, and sleep disturbances [81]. In contrast, ASD involves persistent symptoms and heightened sensitivity to environmental stimuli and routine changes, which can lead to mood swings that may mimic or obscure affective disorders [19, 82]. Emotional instability in ASD often arises from difficulties in emotional recognition and expression, while in BD, it is more pronounced during mood episodes [32]. Additionally, irritability, impulsivity, and aggressive behaviors are common to both disorders but may present differently, complicating differential diagnoses [14]. Individuals with ASD may exhibit heightened irritability, which can be triggered by sensory overload, changes in routine, or difficulties in communication and social interactions [15]. Individuals with ASD often experience difficulties with sleep initiation and maintenance, which can exacerbate emotional dysregulation [83].

ASD and BD can involve impairments in social skills and social cognition [73, 84]. Deficits in social cognition in bipolar disorder can impact individuals both during mood episodes and in periods of remission, but mood dysregulation may further exacerbate these social impairments [84, 85]. A review of 29 studies revealed moderate deficits in social cognition among individuals with BD, with observed variations across specific domains, including theory of mind, emotion recognition, and social judgment [84].

ASD and BD are associated with deficits in executive functioning, including impaired performance in planning, organizing, decision-making, inhibitory control, set-shifting, verbal fluency, working memory, and problem-solving [86, 87]. These shared cognitive impairments may contribute to difficulties in adaptive functioning observed in both conditions [86, 87]. Sensory sensitivities are another overlapping feature. Individuals with ASD frequently experience sensory sensitivities to light, sound, touch, or taste [88]. Similarly, individuals with BD may exhibit heightened sensitivity to sensory stimuli during manic or depressive episodes [89]. Figure 7.1 provides an overview of the primary similarities and differences between the two disorders.

Diagnostic overshadowing in ASD occurs when coexisting conditions or preconceived notions about ASD stereotypes obscure the recognition of its symptoms, resulting in delayed or inaccurate diagnoses [90]. Symptom overlap may cause misdiagnosis. It may be challenging to differentiate what these overlapping symptoms represent: a single disorder with a broader presentation, the co-occurrence of both ASD and BD (comorbidity), or the presence of another condition altogether. Challenges also include evolving presentations over time and ASD symptoms like social withdrawal (difficulty expressing emotions can be obscured by depressive

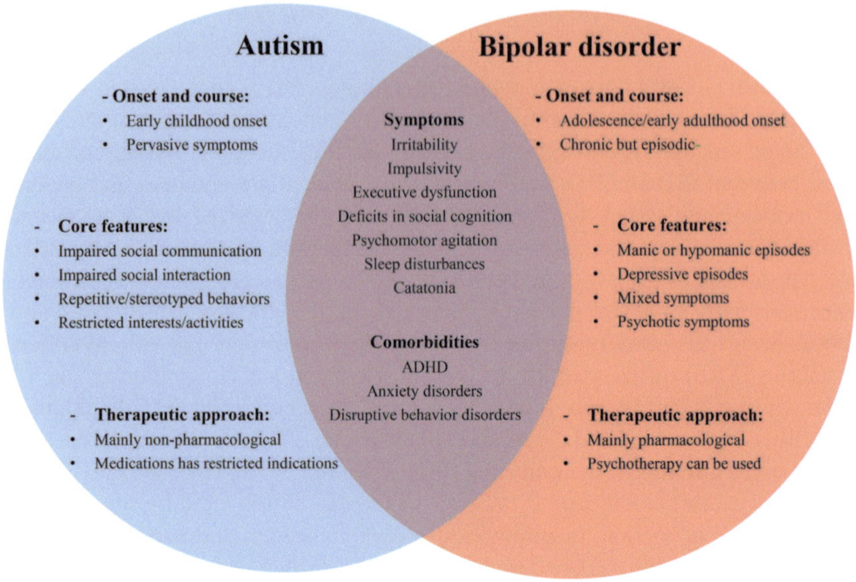

Fig. 7.1 Symptoms overlap between bipolar disorder and autism spectrum disorder. This figure illustrates the distinct and overlapping symptoms associated with bipolar disorder and autism spectrum disorder. Bipolar disorder's core symptoms include manic and depressive episodes, while the core symptoms of autism spectrum disorder feature social communication challenges, repetitive behaviors, and restricted interests. The overlapping area represents symptoms that may be present in both conditions, such as irritability, impulsivity, psychomotor agitation, executive dysfunction, difficulties with social interaction, and shared comorbidities. ADHD attention deficit hyperactivity disorder

symptoms) [14]. In the context of latent bipolar disorder, diagnosis may be further complicated because prodromal symptoms are nonspecific.

7.4 Genetic Factors and Heritability

The etiology of ASD remains incompletely understood; however, the role of genetics in the condition has been progressively established. In 1977, Folstein and Rutter published a pioneering twin study on ASD that unequivocally demonstrated a predominant genetic influence [91]. Recent meta-analyses, as previously cited, showed substantial heritability in ASD estimates of 64–91% [17]. Rare variants with large effect sizes and common gene variants with smaller effects contribute to the risk of ASD [92]. Genetic alterations may include (1) single gene mutations, (2) large structural genomic alterations (such as deletions or duplications), (3) smaller copy number variants (CNVs), and other polygenic conditions susceptible to environmental and epigenetic influences [93–95]. Despite the high degree of locus heterogeneity, recent studies have underscored the involvement of genes in two main domains: synaptic structure/function and chromatin modification [96–102].

BD, in turn, also is highly heritable and shows genetic overlap with other psychiatric diseases [3, 103, 104]. For instance, research using the GeneAnalytics program revealed 23 genes shared among ASD, BD, and schizophrenia [104]. These genes participate in nine biological super pathways, prominently including circadian entrainment. Also, they impact dopamine and serotonin regulation and signal transduction pathways, influencing mood, behavior, and physical activity levels [104]. Ardesch and colleagues recently pointed to common expression patterns of risk genes associated with major psychiatric disorders (schizophrenia, BD, ASD, and major depressive disorder) [103]. This study converges on specific cortical regions, suggesting a common vulnerability of the cortex to transcriptional dysregulation across these disorders. These findings support the hypothesis that psychiatric disorders share genetic mechanisms and may suggest a foundational etiological connection between these neuropsychiatric disorders [103, 104].

7.5 Differential Diagnosis for Autism Spectrum Disorder

The list of differential diagnoses for ASD is extensive and varies depending on the individual's age and required level of support. For instance, in preschoolers, other neurodevelopmental disorders such as global developmental delay and language delays may manifest with communicative challenges that need to be distinguished from those of ASD, which involve more significant impairments in nonverbal communication, in addition to impairments in socio-emotional reciprocity and social interaction [105]. In young children, ADHD emerges as a salient differential diagnosis, both for overactivity and for social difficulties in peer interactions at this age [23]. Within this age group, clinicians must also distinguish ASD from selective mutism, characterized by the lack of spoken communication in particular settings such as in school, which engenders subsequent challenges in social interaction. Throughout the preschool period, neurological diseases such as epileptic syndromes, genetic diseases, and other general pediatric conditions that involve alterations in sleep and eating patterns will also be significant differential diagnoses [23].

In school-age children, neurodevelopmental conditions such as intellectual disability, ADHD, and communication disorders persist as relevant differential diagnoses for ASD due to difficulties in interacting with peers and their impact on academic performance. Nevertheless, at this stage of life, other psychiatric disorders become more common and thus warrant consideration as relevant differential diagnoses [23]. For instance, in early-onset obsessive-compulsive disorder, particularly when accompanied by tic disorders, the compulsive rituals may resemble the restricted and repetitive behaviors of ASD; moreover, in children, obsessions may not be as well described or verbalized as in the adult population, and the degree of insight regarding the symptoms is often limited. Other mental health conditions that may also be mistaken are social anxiety disorder, due to its difficulties in social interaction with peers, and disruptive behavior disorders, due to irritability [23].

Throughout adolescence, many of the conditions present in childhood continue to be critical differential diagnoses; however, other diagnoses, such as schizophrenia and schizotypal disorder, become more prevalent in this age group. Specific characteristics of these conditions, such as social withdrawal, impairments in social cognition, and unusual behaviors, may resemble those of ASD [19, 23]. Within this age group, mood disorders, particularly latent BD, may also be a challenge when differentiating from ASD due to overlapping symptoms like irritability, mood instability, social isolation, and difficulties in peer relationships [19, 23].

By persisting from early childhood through late adolescence, these differential diagnoses continue to be pertinent in adulthood; however, certain conditions, such as schizophrenia, BD, and major depressive disorder, become more pronounced. Concurrently, in this adult population, other differential diagnoses emerge, including personality disorders [19, 105]. A critical point to emphasize in distinguishing ASD from other conditions with similar symptomatology is the precocious manifestation of ASD, typically in the initial years of life. Despite the possibility that these manifestations may elude detection during childhood or may not engender substantial impairment due to many factors, their presence is imperative early on [105]. This fact helps to differentiate ASD from other psychiatric disorders whose symptoms typically start later in life, such as schizophrenia and BD; even though these conditions may have their prodromal symptoms during adolescence, the hallmark episodes that characterize the disorders (i.e., mania or psychotic episode) commonly emerge in early adulthood. It is also noteworthy that a considerable portion of the differential diagnoses for ASD are also co-occurring conditions; these include intellectual disability, ADHD, anxiety disorders, mood disorders, and OCD, among others [19].

ASD and latent bipolar disorder may co-occur and also be a differential diagnosis, given their shared symptoms such as irritability, impulsivity, anxiety, and social skills deficits that can be due to their core features or secondary to other shared psychiatric comorbidities. These symptoms may arise from their intrinsic features or other coexisting psychiatric conditions [15, 40, 106]. In addition, it is noteworthy that impairments in social cognition are present in individuals with a familial predisposition to BD [107]. Those individuals diagnosed with BD who have higher autistic traits frequently experience an earlier onset of the disorder and a greater prevalence of anxiety disorders relative to individuals with fewer autistic traits [36]. Consequently, within clinical settings, a suspicion of ASD should be considered in individuals previously diagnosed with BD when substantial social cognitive impairments are detected or when there is resistance to standard therapeutic interventions. On the other hand, when a patient with ASD exhibits episodic irritability or agitation in conjunction with other affective or neurovegetative symptoms, BD should be considered [19].

7.6 Interventions for Bipolar Disorder and Autism Spectrum Disorder

Interventions for BD and Autism Spectrum Disorder ASD differ markedly in their approaches. For BD, pharmacotherapy is a crucial aspect of treatment, with medications used to stabilize acute mood swings and prevent future episodes. Psychotherapeutic approaches complement pharmacological treatment, especially during certain phases of the disorder [108]. Conversely, the management of ASD primarily involves psychological interventions, focusing on behavioral and developmental strategies [23]. While pharmacological treatments for ASD are limited to addressing specific symptoms such as irritability, they do not target the core features of the disorder [109].

The management of BD involves a range of interventions aimed at addressing acute episodes, maintaining euthymic states, and preventing relapses. While non-pharmacological strategies are utilized, pharmacotherapy remains the cornerstone of treatment across all phases of BD, encompassing medications such as lithium, anticonvulsants, and antipsychotics [108]. Despite the critical role of pharmacotherapy, adjunctive psychosocial interventions may be employed to manage depressive symptoms during the maintenance phase and to improve the patient's overall quality of life [108]. Psychoeducation combined with medication is considered a first-line approach for the maintenance phase, while cognitive-behavioral therapy and family-focused therapy are recommended as second-line treatments for maintenance and depressive episodes. Currently, there is no evidence supporting the effectiveness of non-pharmacological interventions for manic episodes [108].

The management of ASD, as previously mentioned, is primarily centered on non-pharmacological approaches, in contrast to the treatment of BD [23]. For preschool-aged children, early intervention is crucial to enhance communication and social interaction with family members and peers. Various protocols are utilized, many derived from applied behavior analysis practices. However, the most evidence-supported programs integrate behavioral strategies with developmental approaches within the child's everyday activities, known as "naturalistic developmental behavioral interventions." [23] Additionally, specific parental training methods are employed to address irritability and challenging behaviors [109].

Behavioral strategies may be employed in school-aged children and adolescents to enhance communication abilities and social skills training [23]. As the individuals transition into adulthood, the focus of interventions shifts from the core features of ASD to addressing associated symptoms and coexisting conditions, as well as promoting autonomy and independence [19]. For older children, adolescents, and adults, cognitive-behavioral therapy is indicated for the treatment of comorbidities, particularly anxiety disorders [23].

The use of pharmacotherapy in the management of ASD has very restricted indications. Pharmacological interventions are not recommended for the core features of ASD, namely, impairments in social interaction and communication, as well as restricted and repetitive patterns of behavior; these characteristics of ASD are always addressed through psychological approaches [23]. The use of medications is reserved for addressing irritability in persons with ASD, and this is typically considered after trying non-pharmacological strategies. In such scenarios, the primary pharmacological agents employed are risperidone and aripiprazole [109]. When behavioral interventions fail to yield improvements, melatonin may be indicated for sleep disturbances [110].

The administration of other medication classes is only recommended for individuals diagnosed with ASD when concurrent psychiatric conditions are identified. For example, psychostimulants might be prescribed in the presence of ADHD, antidepressants for OCD, anxiety, or depression, and lithium or other mood stabilizers for comorbid BD. In cases where a latent BD is suspected in a patient with a prior autism diagnosis, it is prudent to evaluate the potential risks and prescribe medication only after trying behavioral interventions, notwithstanding if there are plans to use risperidone or aripiprazole for irritability [23]. Notably, there is no evidence to support the initiation of pharmacological treatment aimed at preventing the onset of a full-blown BD in patients at risk of developing such a condition [5].

7.7 Conclusion

This chapter offers an in-depth analysis of ASD and examines its associations with BD, focusing on the symptomatic overlaps between these disorders. It underscores how these overlaps and frequent comorbidities can complicate diagnostic processes and impede timely treatment. Identifying overlapping symptoms is crucial for clinicians, especially when dealing with latent or less apparent bipolar cases, which adds an additional layer of complexity. Furthermore, clinicians should consider the possibility of ASD in individuals with a prior diagnosis of BD, particularly when significant deficits in social cognition and daily functioning are evident, when patients show resistance to standard therapeutic interventions, and in cases with a history of multiple psychiatric diagnoses.

References

1. Craddock N, Sklar P. Genetics of bipolar disorder. Lancet. 2013;381(9878):1654–62.
2. Smoller JW, Finn CT. Family, twin, and adoption studies of bipolar disorder. Am J Med Genet C Semin Med Genet. 2003;123C(1):48–58.
3. O'Connell KS, Coombes BJ. Genetic contributions to bipolar disorder: current status and future directions. Psychol Med. 2021;51(13):2156–67.
4. Song J, Bergen SE, Kuja-Halkola R, Larsson H, Landén M, Lichtenstein P. Bipolar disorder and its relation to major psychiatric disorders: a family-based study in the Swedish population. Bipolar Disord. 2015;17(2):184–93.

5. Saraf G, Moazen-Zadeh E, Pinto JV, Ziafat K, Torres IJ, Kesavan M, et al. Early intervention for people at high risk of developing bipolar disorder: a systematic review of clinical trials. Lancet Psychiatry. 2021;8(1):64–75.
6. Duffy A, Goodday S, Keown-Stoneman C, Grof P. The emergent course of bipolar disorder: observations over two decades from the Canadian high-risk offspring cohort. Am J Psychiatry. 2019;176(9):720–9.
7. Thapar A, Eyre O, Patel V, Brent D. Depression in young people. Lancet. 2022;400(10352):617–31.
8. Gitlin MJ. Diagnosing latent bipolar disorder: a clinical dilemma. Bipolar Disord. 2018;20(4):300–2.
9. Goi PD, Vianna-Sulzbach M, Silveira L, Grande I, Chendo I, Sodré LA, et al. Treatment delay is associated with more episodes and more severe illness staging progression in patients with bipolar disorder. Psychiatry Res. 2015;227(2–3):372–3.
10. Pinto JV, Kauer-Sant'Anna M, Yatham LN. What impact does bipolar disorder staging have on the use of pharmacotherapy? Expert Opin Pharmacother. 2021;22(12):1513–6.
11. Pinto JV, Saraf G, Kozicky J, Beaulieu S, Sharma V, Parikh SV, et al. Remission and recurrence in bipolar disorder: the data from health outcomes and patient evaluations in bipolar disorder (HOPE-BD) study. J Affect Disord. 2020;268:150–7.
12. Andrade-González N, Álvarez-Cadenas L, Saiz-Ruiz J, Lahera G. Initial and relapse prodromes in adult patients with episodes of bipolar disorder: a systematic review. Eur Psychiatry. 2020;63(1):e12.
13. Duffy A, Horrocks J, Doucette S, Keown-Stoneman C, McCloskey S, Grof P. The developmental trajectory of bipolar disorder. Br J Psychiatry. 2014;204(2):122–8.
14. Dunalska A, Rzeszutek M, Dębowska Z, Bryńska A. Comorbidity of bipolar disorder and autism spectrum disorder—review paper. Psychiatr Pol. 2021;55(6):1421–31.
15. Oakley B, Loth E, Murphy DG. Autism and mood disorders. Int Rev Psychiatry. 2021;33(3):280–99.
16. American Psychiatric Association. Diagnostic and statistical manual of mental disorders [Internet]. DSM-5-TR. American Psychiatric Association Publishing; 2022. [cited 2024 Aug 29]. Available from: https://psychiatryonline.org/doi/book/10.1176/appi.books.9780890425787.
17. Tick B, Bolton P, Happé F, Rutter M, Rijsdijk F. Heritability of autism spectrum disorders: a meta-analysis of twin studies. J Child Psychol Psychiatry. 2016;57(5):585–95.
18. Mandell DS, Novak MM, Zubritsky CD. Factors associated with age of diagnosis among children with autism spectrum disorders. Pediatrics. 2005;116(6):1480–6.
19. Lai MC, Baron-Cohen S. Identifying the lost generation of adults with autism spectrum conditions. Lancet Psychiatry. 2015;2(11):1013–27.
20. Borue X, Mazefsky C, Rooks BT, Strober M, Keller MB, Hower H, et al. Longitudinal course of bipolar disorder in youth with high-functioning autism spectrum disorder. J Am Acad Child Adolesc Psychiatry. 2016;55(12):1064–1072.e6.
21. Vannucchi G, Masi G, Toni C, Dell'Osso L, Erfurth A, Perugi G. Bipolar disorder in adults with Asperger's syndrome: a systematic review. J Affect Disord. 2014;168:151–60.
22. Maenner MJ, Warren Z, Williams AR, Amoakohene E, Bakian AV, Bilder DA, et al. Prevalence and characteristics of autism spectrum disorder among children aged 8 years — autism and developmental disabilities monitoring network, 11 sites, United States, 2020. MMWR Surveill Summ. 2023;72(2):1–14.
23. Lord C, Brugha TS, Charman T, Cusack J, Dumas G, Frazier T, et al. Autism spectrum disorder. Nat Rev Dis Primer. 2020;6(1):5.
24. Merikangas KR, Jin R, He JP, Kessler RC, Lee S, Sampson NA, et al. Prevalence and correlates of bipolar spectrum disorder in the world mental health survey initiative. Arch Gen Psychiatry. 2011;68(3):241.
25. Sandin S, Lichtenstein P, Kuja-Halkola R, Larsson H, Hultman CM, Reichenberg A. The familial risk of autism. JAMA. 2014;311(17):1770.

26. Lainhart JE. Psychiatric problems in individuals with autism, their parents and siblings. Int Rev Psychiatry. 1999;11(4):278–98.
27. Skokauskas N, Gallagher L. Psychosis, affective disorders and anxiety in autistic spectrum disorder: prevalence and nosological considerations. Psychopathology. 2010;43(1):8–16.
28. Simonoff E, Pickles A, Charman T, Chandler S, Loucas T, Baird G. Psychiatric disorders in children with autism spectrum disorders: prevalence, comorbidity, and associated factors in a population-derived sample. J Am Acad Child Adolesc Psychiatry. 2008;47(8):921–9.
29. Rosenberg RE, Kaufmann WE, Law JK, Law PA. Parent report of community psychiatric comorbid diagnoses in autism spectrum disorders. Autism Res Treat. 2011;2011:1–10.
30. De Long R, Nohna C. Psychiatric family history and neurological disease in autistic spectrum disorders. Dev Med Child Neurol. 1994;36(5):441–8.
31. Sullivan PF, Magnusson C, Reichenberg A, Boman M, Dalman C, Davidson M, et al. Family history of schizophrenia and bipolar disorder as risk factors for autism. Arch Gen Psychiatry [Internet]. 2012 [cited 2024 Aug 29];69(11). Available from: http://archpsyc.jamanetwork.com/article.aspx?doi=10.1001/archgenpsychiatry.2012.730.
32. Selten JP, Lundberg M, Rai D, Magnusson C. Risks for nonaffective psychotic disorder and bipolar disorder in young people with autism spectrum disorder: a population-based study. JAMA Psychiatry. 2015;72(5):483.
33. Kirsch AC, Huebner ARS, Mehta SQ, Howie FR, Weaver AL, Myers SM, et al. Association of comorbid mood and anxiety disorders with autism spectrum disorder. JAMA Pediatr. 2020;174(1):63.
34. Wozniak J, Biederman J, Faraone SV, Frazier J, Kim J, Millstein R, et al. Mania in children with pervasive developmental disorder revisited. J Am Acad Child Adolesc Psychiatry. 1997;36(11):1552–9.
35. Skokauskas N, Frodl T. Overlap between autism spectrum disorder and bipolar affective disorder. Psychopathology. 2015;48(4):209–16.
36. Dell'Osso L, Carpita B, Bertelloni CA, Diadema E, Barberi FM, Gesi C, et al. Subthreshold autism spectrum in bipolar disorder: prevalence and clinical correlates. Psychiatry Res. 2019;281:112605.
37. Pine DS, Guyer AE, Goldwin M, Towbin KA, Leibenluft E. Autism spectrum disorder scale scores in pediatric mood and anxiety disorders. J Am Acad Child Adolesc Psychiatry. 2008;47(6):652–61.
38. Abu-Akel A, Clark J, Perry A, Wood SJ, Forty L, Craddock N, et al. Autistic and schizotypal traits and global functioning in bipolar I disorder. J Affect Disord. 2017;207:268–75.
39. Lai MC, Kassee C, Besney R, Bonato S, Hull L, Mandy W, et al. Prevalence of co-occurring mental health diagnoses in the autism population: a systematic review and meta-analysis. Lancet Psychiatry. 2019;6(10):819–29.
40. Pehlivanidis A, Papanikolaou K, Mantas V, Kalantzi E, Korobili K, Xenaki LA, et al. Lifetime co-occurring psychiatric disorders in newly diagnosed adults with attention deficit hyperactivity disorder (ADHD) or/and autism spectrum disorder (ASD). BMC Psychiatry. 2020;20(1):423.
41. Dell'Osso L, Cremone IM, Nardi B, Tognini V, Castellani L, Perrone P, et al. Comorbidity and overlaps between autism spectrum and borderline personality disorder: state of the art. Brain Sci. 2023;13(6):862.
42. World Health Organization. Clinical descriptions and diagnostic requirements for ICD-11 mental, behavioural and neurodevelopmental disorders. [Internet]. 2024. 852 p. Available from: https://www.who.int/publications/i/item/9789240077263.
43. Cook J, Hull L, Crane L, Mandy W. Camouflaging in autism: a systematic review. Clin Psychol Rev. 2021;89:102080.
44. Åsberg Johnels J, Hovey D, Zürcher N, Hippolyte L, Lemonnier E, Gillberg C, et al. Autism and emotional face-viewing. Autism Res. 2017;10(5):901–10.
45. Vogindroukas I, Stankova M, Chelas EN, Proedrou A. Language and speech characteristics in autism. Neuropsychiatr Dis Treat. 2022;18:2367–77.

46. Roy M, Strate P. Autism spectrum disorders in adulthood. Dtsch Ärztebl Int [Internet]. 2023 [cited 2024 Aug 29]; Available from: https://www.aerzteblatt.de/10.3238/arztebl.m2022.0379.
47. Drmic IE, Szatmari P, Volkmar F. Life course health development in autism spectrum disorders. In: Halfon N, Forrest CB, Lerner RM, Faustman EM, editors. Handbook of life course health development [Internet]. Cham: Springer; 2018. [cited 2024 Aug 29]. Available from: http://www.ncbi.nlm.nih.gov/books/NBK543697/.
48. Mirkovic B, Gérardin P. Asperger's syndrome: what to consider? L'Encéphale. 2019;45(2):169–74.
49. Baird G, Norbury CF. Social (pragmatic) communication disorders and autism spectrum disorder. Arch Dis Child. 2016;101(8):745–51.
50. Mazurek MO. Loneliness, friendship, and well-being in adults with autism spectrum disorders. Autism. 2014;18(3):223–32.
51. Uljarević M, Cooper MN, Bebbington K, Glasson EJ, Maybery MT, Varcin K, et al. Deconstructing the repetitive behaviour phenotype in autism spectrum disorder through a large population-based analysis. J Child Psychol Psychiatry. 2020;61(9):1030–42.
52. Dovey TM, Kumari V, Blissett J. Eating behaviour, behavioural problems and sensory profiles of children with avoidant/restrictive food intake disorder (ARFID), autistic spectrum disorders or picky eating: same or different? Eur Psychiatry. 2019;61:56–62.
53. Baraskewich J, Von Ranson KM, McCrimmon A, McMorris CA. Feeding and eating problems in children and adolescents with autism: a scoping review. Autism. 2021;25(6):1505–19.
54. Melo C, Ruano L, Jorge J, Pinto Ribeiro T, Oliveira G, Azevedo L, et al. Prevalence and determinants of motor stereotypies in autism spectrum disorder: a systematic review and meta-analysis. Autism. 2020;24(3):569–90.
55. Farley MA, McMahon WM, Fombonne E, Jenson WR, Miller J, Gardner M, et al. Twenty-year outcome for individuals with autism and average or near-average cognitive abilities. Autism Res. 2009;2(2):109–18.
56. Alvares GA, Bebbington K, Cleary D, Evans K, Glasson EJ, Maybery MT, et al. The misnomer of 'high functioning autism': intelligence is an imprecise predictor of functional abilities at diagnosis. Autism. 2020;24(1):221–32.
57. Frank F, Jablotschkin M, Arthen T, Riedel A, Fangmeier T, Hölzel LP, et al. Education and employment status of adults with autism spectrum disorders in Germany—a cross-sectional-survey. BMC Psychiatry. 2018;18(1):75.
58. Crawley D, Zhang L, Jones EJH, Ahmad J, Oakley B, San José Cáceres A, et al. Modeling flexible behavior in childhood to adulthood shows age-dependent learning mechanisms and less optimal learning in autism in each age group. Ramus F, editor. PLOS Biol. 2020;18(10):e3000908.
59. Geurts HM, Pol SE, Lobbestael J, Simons CJP. Executive functioning in 60+ autistic males: the discrepancy between experienced challenges and cognitive performance. J Autism Dev Disord. 2020;50(4):1380–90.
60. Torske T, Nærland T, Øie MG, Stenberg N, Andreassen OA. Metacognitive aspects of executive function are highly associated with social functioning on parent-rated measures in children with autism spectrum disorder. Front Behav Neurosci. 2018;11:258.
61. Brewer N, Young RL, Barnett E. Erratum to: Measuring theory of mind in adults with autism spectrum disorder. J Autism Dev Disord. 2017;47(7):1942–3.
62. Kimhi Y, Mirsky Y, Bauminger-Zviely N. The role of theory of mind, executive functions, and central coherence in reading comprehension for children with ASD and typical development. J Autism Dev Disord [Internet]. 2024 [cited 2024 Aug 29]. Available from: https://link.springer.com/10.1007/s10803-024-06272-y.
63. Braconnier ML, Siper PM. Neuropsychological assessment in autism spectrum disorder. Curr Psychiatry Rep. 2021;23(10):63.
64. Happé F, Frith U. The weak coherence account: detail-focused cognitive style in autism spectrum disorders. J Autism Dev Disord. 2006;36(1):5–25.

65. Cruz S, Zubizarreta SCP, Costa AD, Araújo R, Martinho J, Tubío-Fungueiriño M, et al. Is there a bias towards males in the diagnosis of autism? A systematic review and meta-analysis. Neuropsychol Rev [Internet]. 2024 [cited 2024 Aug 29]. Available from: https://link.springer.com/10.1007/s11065-023-09630-2.
66. Lai MC, Baron-Cohen S, Buxbaum JD. Understanding autism in the light of sex/gender. Mol Autism. 2015;6(1):24.
67. Karpinski RI, Kinase Kolb AM, Tetreault NA, Borowski TB. High intelligence: a risk factor for psychological and physiological overexcitabilities. Intelligence. 2018;66:8–23.
68. Srivastava AK, Schwartz CE. Intellectual disability and autism spectrum disorders: causal genes and molecular mechanisms. Neurosci Biobehav Rev. 2014;46:161–74.
69. Boschi A, Planche P, Hemimou C, Demily C, Vaivre-Douret L. From high intellectual potential to Asperger syndrome: evidence for differences and a fundamental overlap—a systematic review. Front Psychol [Internet]. 2016 [cited 2024 Aug 29];7. Available from: http://journal.frontiersin.org/article/10.3389/fpsyg.2016.01605/full.
70. Nolen-Hoeksema S. The role of rumination in depressive disorders and mixed anxiety/depressive symptoms. J Abnorm Psychol. 2000;109(3):504–11.
71. Eisenberg N, Miller PA. The relation of empathy to prosocial and related behaviors. Psychol Bull. 1987;101(1):91–119.
72. Green MF, Penn DL, Bentall R, Carpenter WT, Gaebel W, Gur RC, et al. Social cognition in schizophrenia: an NIMH workshop on definitions, assessment, and research opportunities. Schizophr Bull. 2008;34(6):1211–20.
73. Fernandes JM, Cajão R, Lopes R, Jerónimo R, Barahona-Corrêa JB. Social cognition in schizophrenia and autism spectrum disorders: a systematic review and meta-analysis of direct comparisons. Front Psych. 2018;9:504.
74. Baron-Cohen S, Leslie AM, Frith U. Does the autistic child have a "theory of mind" ? Cognition. 1985;21(1):37–46.
75. Bishop-Fitzpatrick L, Mazefsky CA, Eack SM, Minshew NJ. Correlates of social functioning in autism spectrum disorder: the role of social cognition. Res Autism Spectr Disord. 2017;35:25–34.
76. Cassidy S, Au-Yeung S, Robertson A, Cogger-Ward H, Richards G, Allison C, et al. Autism and autistic traits in those who died by suicide in England. Br J Psychiatry. 2022;221(5):683–91.
77. National Collaborating Centre for Mental Health (UK). Autism: recognition, referral, diagnosis and management of adults on the autism spectrum [Internet]. Leicester: British Psychological Society; 2012. [cited 2024 Aug 29]. (National Institute for Health and Clinical Excellence: Guidance). Available from: http://www.ncbi.nlm.nih.gov/books/NBK299070/.
78. Frigaux A, Evrard R, Lighezzolo-Alnot J. L'ADI-R et l'ADOS face au diagnostic différentiel des troubles du spectre autistique : intérêts, limites et ouvertures. L'Encéphale. 2019;45(5):441–8.
79. Takei R, Matsuo J, Takahashi H, Uchiyama T, Kunugi H, Kamio Y. Verification of the utility of the social responsiveness scale for adults in non-clinical and clinical adult populations in Japan. BMC Psychiatry. 2014;14(1):302.
80. Woodbury-Smith MR, Robinson J, Wheelwright S, Baron-Cohen S. Screening adults for Asperger syndrome using the AQ: a preliminary study of its diagnostic validity in clinical practice. J Autism Dev Disord. 2005;35(3):331–5.
81. Stratta P, Tempesta D, Bonanni RL, De Cataldo S, Rossi A. Emotional reactivity in bipolar depressed patients: emotional reactivity in bipolar depression. J Clin Psychol. 2014;70(9):860–5.
82. Richman KA, Bidshahri R. Autism, theory of mind, and the reactive attitudes. Bioethics. 2018;32(1):43–9.
83. Wiggs L, Stores G. Sleep patterns and sleep disorders in children with autistic spectrum disorders: insights using parent report and actigraphy. Dev Med Child Neurol. 2004;46(6):372–80.

84. Gillissie ES, Lui LMW, Ceban F, Miskowiak K, Gok S, Cao B, et al. Deficits of social cognition in bipolar disorder: systematic review and meta-analysis. Bipolar Disord. 2022;24(2):137–48.
85. Hoertnagl CM, Hofer A. Social cognition in serious mental illness. Curr Opin Psychiatry. 2014;27(3):197–202.
86. Dickinson T, Becerra R, Coombes J. Executive functioning deficits among adults with Bipolar Disorder (types I and II): a systematic review and meta-analysis. J Affect Disord. 2017;218:407–27.
87. Diamond A. Executive functions. Annu Rev Psychol. 2013;64(1):135–68.
88. Nimbley E, Golds L, Sharpe H, Gillespie-Smith K, Duffy F. Sensory processing and eating behaviours in autism: a systematic review. Eur Eat Disord Rev. 2022;30(5):538–59.
89. Parker G, Paterson A, Romano M, Graham R. Altered sensory phenomena experienced in bipolar disorder. Am J Psychiatry. 2017;174(12):1146–50.
90. Gupta N, Gupta M. Diagnostic overshadowing in high-functioning autism: mirtazapine, buspirone, and modified Cognitive Behavioral Therapy (CBT) as treatment options. Cureus [Internet]. 2023 [cited 2024 Aug 30]. Available from: https://www.cureus.com/articles/156324-diagnostic-overshadowing-in-high-functioning-autism-mirtazapine-buspirone-and-modified-cognitive-behavioral-therapy-cbt-as-treatment-options.
91. Folstein S, Rutter M. Infantile autism: a genetic study of 21 twin pairs. J Child Psychol Psychiatry. 1977;18(4):297–321.
92. Thapar A, Rutter M. Genetic advances in autism. J Autism Dev Disord. 2021;51(12):4321–32.
93. Genovese A, Butler MG. Clinical assessment, genetics, and treatment approaches in autism spectrum disorder (ASD). Int J Mol Sci. 2020;21(13):4726.
94. Heil KM, Schaaf CP. The genetics of autism spectrum disorders—a guide for clinicians. Curr Psychiatry Rep. 2013;15(1):334.
95. Roberts JL, Hovanes K, Dasouki M, Manzardo AM, Butler MG. Chromosomal microarray analysis of consecutive individuals with autism spectrum disorders or learning disability presenting for genetic services. Gene. 2014;535(1):70–8.
96. The DDD Study, Homozygosity Mapping Collaborative for Autism, UK10K Consortium, The Autism Sequencing Consortium, De Rubeis S, He X, et al. Synaptic, transcriptional and chromatin genes disrupted in autism. Nature. 2014;515(7526):209–15.
97. Iossifov I, O'Roak BJ, Sanders SJ, Ronemus M, Krumm N, Levy D, et al. The contribution of de novo coding mutations to autism spectrum disorder. Nature. 2014;515(7526):216–21.
98. Manoli DS, State MW. Autism spectrum disorder genetics and the search for pathological mechanisms. Am J Psychiatry. 2021;178(1):30–8.
99. O'Roak BJ, Deriziotis P, Lee C, Vives L, Schwartz JJ, Girirajan S, et al. Exome sequencing in sporadic autism spectrum disorders identifies severe de novo mutations. Nat Genet. 2011;43(6):585–9.
100. O'Roak BJ, Vives L, Girirajan S, Karakoc E, Krumm N, Coe BP, et al. Sporadic autism exomes reveal a highly interconnected protein network of de novo mutations. Nature. 2012;485(7397):246–50.
101. Sanders SJ, Ercan-Sencicek AG, Hus V, Luo R, Murtha MT, Moreno-De-Luca D, et al. Multiple recurrent de novo CNVs, including duplications of the 7q11.23 Williams syndrome region, are strongly associated with autism. Neuron. 2011;70(5):863–85.
102. Zoghbi HY. Postnatal neurodevelopmental disorders: meeting at the synapse? Science. 2003;302(5646):826–30.
103. Ardesch DJ, Libedinsky I, Scholtens LH, Wei Y, Van Den Heuvel MP. Convergence of brain transcriptomic and neuroimaging patterns in schizophrenia, bipolar disorder, autism spectrum disorder, and major depressive disorder. Biol Psychiatry Cogn Neurosci Neuroimaging. 2023;8(6):630–9.
104. Khanzada N, Butler M, Manzardo A. GeneAnalytics pathway analysis and genetic overlap among autism spectrum disorder, bipolar disorder and schizophrenia. Int J Mol Sci. 2017;18(3):527.

105. American Psychiatric Association. Diagnostic and statistical manual of mental disorders [Internet]. Fifth ed. American Psychiatric Association; 2013. [cited 2024 Aug 29]. Available from: https://psychiatryonline.org/doi/book/10.1176/appi.books.9780890425596.
106. Varcin KJ, Herniman SE, Lin A, Chen Y, Perry Y, Pugh C, et al. Occurrence of psychosis and bipolar disorder in adults with autism: a systematic review and meta-analysis. Neurosci Biobehav Rev. 2022;134:104543.
107. Bora E, Özerdem A. Social cognition in first-degree relatives of patients with bipolar disorder: a meta-analysis. Eur Neuropsychopharmacol. 2017;27(4):293–300.
108. Yatham LN, Kennedy SH, Parikh SV, Schaffer A, Bond DJ, Frey BN, et al. Canadian Network for Mood and Anxiety Treatments (CANMAT) and International Society for Bipolar Disorders (ISBD) 2018 guidelines for the management of patients with bipolar disorder. Bipolar Disord. 2018;20(2):97–170.
109. Choi H, Kim JH, Yang HS, Kim JY, Cortese S, Smith L, et al. Pharmacological and non-pharmacological interventions for irritability in autism spectrum disorder: a systematic review and meta-analysis with the GRADE assessment. Mol Autism. 2024;15(1):7.
110. Williams Buckley A, Hirtz D, Oskoui M, Armstrong MJ, Batra A, Bridgemohan C, et al. Practice guideline: treatment for insomnia and disrupted sleep behavior in children and adolescents with autism spectrum disorder: report of the Guideline Development, Dissemination, and Implementation Subcommittee of the American Academy of Neurology. Neurology. 2020;94(9):392–404.

Chapter 8
Women's Mental Health and the Latent Stage in Bipolar Disorder

Divya Prasad, Vanessa Gnielka, and Luisa Caropreso

8.1 Background

Bipolar disorder (BD) is a multifaceted psychiatric condition characterized by mood instability. Research shows that the disorder is more common in female patients [24], who are more likely to experience rapid cycling [9] and to present more psychiatric comorbidities than men [3]. Bipolar disorder typically arises in women between the ages of 15 and 23, often starting with depressive episodes rather than manic or hypomanic episodes [64]. Thus, BD frequently emerges in women during critical reproductive periods. BD recognition and treatment remain challenging, particularly in those initially diagnosed with major depressive disorder (MDD) [117]. In this chapter, we aim to review the BD diagnosis and treatment in women, examining the factors associated with new onset of BD and diagnostic conversion, with a focus on the perinatal period, the menopause transition, and its interaction with premenstrual dysphoric disorder (PMDD).

D. Prasad
Warneford Hospital, Warneford Ln, Oxford, UK

Department of Psychiatry, University of Oxford, Oxford, UK

V. Gnielka
Post Graduate Program in Psychiatry and Behavioral Sciences, Department of Psychiatry, School of Medicine, Universidade Federal do Rio Grande do Sul (UFRGS), Porto Alegre, RS, Brazil

Mood Disorders Clinic, McMaster University, Hamilton, ON, Canada

L. Caropreso (✉)
Women's Health Concerns Clinic, Department of Psychiatry and Behavioural Neurosciences, McMaster University, Hamilton, ON, Canada
e-mail: caroprel@mcmaster.ca

T. de Azevedo Cardoso et al. (eds.), *Latent Bipolar Disorder*,
https://doi.org/10.1007/978-3-032-01297-5_8

8.2 Bipolar Disorder in the Perinatal Period

Pregnancy and childbirth are significant triggers for mood episodes [37, 38]. Affective episodes during the perinatal period, which includes pregnancy and up to one year postpartum, can either be a recurrence of a previous psychiatric condition or the first episode in a person's lifetime.

While up to one in four women experience depression during the perinatal period [107], close to a quarter (22.6%) of women with a positive screening for perinatal depression receive a diagnosis of BD if further assessed [150]. However, BD remains underdiagnosed and misdiagnosed in this population [117].

Multiple factors contribute to the development of BD during the perinatal period [69], including those of a psychological, neurobiological, and immunological nature. Hormonal fluctuations during pregnancy, along with a significant decrease in gonadal steroids after childbirth, can potentially trigger mood instability. Additionally, sleep deprivation and disruptions in biological rhythms during late pregnancy, labor, and breastfeeding can exacerbate these symptoms [69, 150].

The accurate diagnosis of perinatal BD is essential, as women with this condition are at a significantly greater risk of severe outcomes. For instance, in the first 3 months postpartum, women with BD are 37 times more likely to be admitted to a psychiatric facility than at any other time in their lives, with a particularly elevated risk of postpartum psychosis (PPP). While the risk of PPP in the general population is 1–2 per 1000 deliveries [142], approximately 1 in 5 women with BD may experience PPP [89, 104, 146].

8.2.1 Factors Associated with Diagnostic Conversion and New-Onset BD in the Perinatal Period

While it is estimated that 2–3% of the general population is affected by bipolar spectrum disorders [85], a recent study reported that the pooled prevalence of bipolar spectrum mood episodes increases to 20.1% during the perinatal period [83]. Interestingly, in this study, only 2.6% of the study group had a diagnosis of BD before pregnancy. Although this research utilized the Mood Disorders Questionnaire instead of a formal diagnostic assessment, which could have resulted in an overestimate, the results raise the question of how many women struggled with undiagnosed BD prior to pregnancy and how many experienced a new onset of BD during the peripartum period. Together, these findings highlight the importance of heightened clinical vigilance for BD during the perinatal period.

Growing evidence indicates that psychiatric disorders with first onset in the postpartum period are strong predictors of latent BD. This finding is particularly relevant for PPP, as research suggests that it is a distinct nosological entity within the bipolar disorder spectrum [8]. For example, a cross-sectional study of patients with a first major depressive episode (MDE) revealed that those experiencing their first depressive episode postpartum presented elevated clinical traits that potentially indicated BD, such as atypical depressive symptoms [4]. Additionally, a retrospective study revealed that approximately 1 in 3 women with BD experienced their first lifetime occurrence of the disorder surrounding childbirth. In the same study, more than half of the women with BD who experienced postpartum affective psychosis had no prior psychiatric history [27].

Similarly, an investigation of polygenic risk scores in women with first-onset PPP demonstrated that, compared with controls, the genetic vulnerability to BD was similar in women who experienced PPP and those with BD [28]. A cohort study revealed that approximately 14% of women who had their first psychiatric contact within the first month after delivery developed BD within 15 years, which was a threefold greater risk than those with initial psychiatric contact at other times within the first postpartum year. Additionally, the risk of conversion to BD was greater among women who had inpatient admissions and among women with a paternal history of BD than among women with a family history of other psychiatric diagnoses or women with parents without psychiatric conditions [90].

The perinatal period is also a time of higher rates of diagnostic conversion from MDD to BD. A prospective study assessing the diagnostic conversion rate from MDD to BD during pregnancy and up to 12 months postpartum revealed that 6 out of 92 women (6.5%) experienced a diagnostic change from MDD to BD within the first 6 months postpartum, with all but one conversion occurring in the first 3 months after delivery and 50% occurring in the first month. In this study, the only statistically significant risk factor for diagnostic conversion was a family history of BD, which was present in approximately 67% of women who experienced diagnostic conversion compared with 22% of women who did not [116]. Similarly, a prospective study investigated symptoms of mania/hypomania during pregnancy and up to 3 months postpartum among women with a self-reported lifetime history of MDD (n = 107) and reported that 34.6% of participants had scores above the cutoff for mania/hypomania in the Altman Self-Rated Mania Scale (ASRM) [57]. These findings show that the perinatal period is crucial for assessing BD [73, 74].

Several studies have screened for symptoms of mania/hypomania in perinatal women with depressive symptoms. One study with a sample of 10,000 participants screened women for postpartum depression (PPD) and conducted diagnostic assessments via the Structured Clinical Interview for the DSM (SCID) on those who screened positive on the EPDS [150]. Among the women who scored ≥10 on the Edinburgh Postnatal Depression Scale (EPDS), 22.6% were found to have BD. When considering women who scored ≥13, 26.7% met the diagnostic criteria for BD. Similar results were reported in a pilot study with 342 participants, where among patients with a positive screening for depression on the EPDS, 21.4% also screened positive for BD on the Mood Disorder Questionnaire (MDQ) [86].

Furthermore, higher rates of BD were found in studies conducted in tertiary centers. One study assessed 56 women referred to a specialty clinic with a diagnosis of PPD. The participants were interviewed via the SCID, the Highs scale, and the MDQ. The study revealed that 54% of patients with PPD had bipolar spectrum disorder [115]. Similarly, a recent cross-sectional study screened 61 women with high-risk pregnancies via the EPDS, MDQ, and SCID. The results indicated that among the participants who met the criteria for a current depressive episode, 50% also met the diagnostic criteria for BD [109].

It should also be considered that elation and transient, low-grade hypomanic symptoms, referred to as "postpartum highs"—the hypomanic equivalent of the "postpartum blues"—are also common. A systematic review of the nosological status of the highs identified studies from several countries showing that 9.6–49.1% of women have hypomanic symptoms in the postpartum period. Although some studies have reported an association between postpartum highs and later PPD [46], no definite conclusions can be drawn regarding the association between postpartum highs and BD due to the methodological limitations of the available studies [120].

8.2.2 *Investigating BD During the Perinatal Period: Screening Tools and Frequency of Assessment*

As demonstrated in the studies described above, screening for perinatal depression without concurrent screening for BD can lead to the misrecognition of PPD as unipolar depression instead of bipolar [47].

In support of this finding, the American College of Obstetricians and Gynecologists (ACOG) has recently updated its guidelines on perinatal mental health screening, which now includes the recommendation to screen for BD, especially before starting medications for anxiety or depression [94]. This recommendation aligns with the CANMAT guidelines, which recommends that every woman with perinatal depressive symptoms should be screened for BD. Both guidelines also recommend screening for common co-occurring mental conditions, such as anxiety disorders and obsessive–compulsive disorder (OCD).

Among several validated screening tools for BD, the MDQ has been studied the most in the perinatal population [40, 113]. The MDQ is a 15-item self-report scale that assesses the lifetime prevalence of (hypo)manic symptoms. Originally, the threshold for a positive screening was the presence of seven or more symptoms in question one, a positive answer to question two (symptoms occurring at the same time), and symptoms causing moderate to severe impairment (question three) [51]. Revised scoring systems have been tested and have shown improved sensitivity while maintaining high specificity. Importantly, a positive screening does not substitute for a formal diagnostic investigation [20, 156].

When traditional scoring is used in pregnant women, the MDQ has a sensitivity of 39% and a specificity of 91%, whereas the revised scoring of 7 or more positive symptoms without supplementary questions has a sensitivity of 89% and a specificity of 84% [40]. More recently, Masters et al. [82] reported that 18.8% of participants screened positive for BD via the revised scoring of the MDQ in a sample of 574 perinatal women versus 8.7% via the original scoring method.

Considering that more than half of the patients with affective episodes in the postpartum period have symptom onset before childbirth [57, 150], the ACOG recommends screening for BD once per pregnancy. Nevertheless, Sharma et al. [117] suggested continuing screening until 3 months postpartum, especially in women with subthreshold scores on the MDQ.

8.2.3 Course of Illness

Across the mood disorder spectrum, perinatal episodes tend to occur within the first 4 weeks postpartum, with manic and psychotic presentations appearing earlier than depression [25]. Some studies propose that manic episodes occur more often during pregnancy or following childbirth than during other stages of life [44]. Thus, it is conceivable that bipolar perinatal depression is more likely to be mixed [117]. Other features associated with bipolar rather than unipolar depression are atypical depressive symptoms, psychotic features, and agitation [4, 58, 114]. Furthermore, patients with bipolar perinatal depression often have comorbid psychiatric diagnoses, particularly anxiety disorders and OCD [117].

A first onset of depression during the postpartum period and a younger age at illness onset are suggestive of bipolarity. Interestingly, among women with BD, those who began experiencing BD alongside PPD may have more favorable outcomes [49], with fewer lifetime depressive episodes and fewer suicide attempts [135]. This may be because an onset during reproductive years represents a later onset, whereas an earlier onset predicts a more severe illness course. Another hypothesis is that several mechanisms during childbirth may lower the threshold for BD onset, which may not develop otherwise [47].

With respect to manic episodes, when investigators compared postpartum manic episodes with other life periods, it was found that postpartum manic episodes were more likely to be mixed, with a higher frequency of depressive symptoms. These included excessive guilt, perplexity, and less 'classic' manic symptoms [49].

8.2.3.1 Risk of Relapse

Studies consistently show that the risk of a mood episode in women with BD peaks in the postpartum period. In a meta-analysis, Weseloo et al. [146] reported an overall relapse risk of 35% postpartum, with a significant difference between patients who continued pharmacotherapy and patients not treated with pharmacotherapy (23% versus 66%, respectively). The risk of recurrence during pregnancy has greater variability across studies, depending on the population assessed and study design, where higher relapse rates are observed in studies including patients with BD type II [44]. A recent cross-sectional study including 436 women with BD type I revealed a sixfold greater probability of episodes after delivery than during pregnancy (30.1% vs 5.2%), notably peaking in the early postpartum period (<4 weeks). In contrast, a prospective cohort study of women with BDs I and II [145] reported that the overall risk of experiencing at least one mood episode during pregnancy was 71%, with 85% among women who discontinued mood stabilizer medication. Although there is a higher episode risk following live births, women who experience perinatal losses are also at risk for relapse, where approximately 1 in 4 women experience a bipolar mood episode after an induced abortion [26, 44].

Women with a history of perinatal bipolar affective episodes face an even greater risk of recurrence in subsequent deliveries [44, 146]. Di Florio et al. [27] examined clinical predictors of perinatal recurrence in 887 multiparous women with lifetime BD or schizoaffective disorder (bipolar type), revealing that 55% of women with BD who experienced episodes of affective psychosis or depression during pregnancy or after childbirth experienced a recurrence in the subsequent perinatal period.

Those with a history of PPP are at the highest risk of experiencing another severe postpartum episode; the risk of experiencing a manic/psychotic episode after a subsequent delivery is nearly one in two. Interestingly, women with a history of non-psychotic perinatal depression face a slightly greater risk of any form of perinatal recurrence than those with a history of postpartum affective psychosis [27].

The authors also reported that the absence of mood episodes during or after their initial pregnancy does not ensure that they will not face perinatal illness in subsequent pregnancies, as approximately one-third of women may encounter some form of perinatal episode during a second pregnancy, even if they do not experience any illness following their first pregnancy [27].

8.2.4 Treatment Recommendations

In patients with a high suspicion of bipolar diathesis, antidepressant medications should be used with caution because of the risk of inducing mood instability and mixed symptoms [1, 43, 115]. Therapeutic challenges are further complicated in the perinatal period, given that a relapse or new onset of mood episodes in this period could interfere with fetal and child development, affecting parenting ability and bonding, potentially leading to drastic outcomes, including suicide and infanticide [5, 12, 98]. As such, when latent BD is presumed, psychoeducation concerning the course of illness and identification of symptoms is critical.

Women who are of childbearing age and are diagnosed with BD should receive contraceptive counseling to reduce the risk of unplanned pregnancies. Some anticonvulsants, such as carbamazepine, lamotrigine, and topiramate, can reduce the effectiveness of oral contraceptives. Similarly, some contraceptives might affect the efficacy of lamotrigine. Owing to its high teratogenic potential, valproate is contraindicated in women of childbearing potential, and where alternative treatments are ineffective, contraception during treatment should be ensured, and the risks discussed with the patient [48, 50].

For patients on pharmacotherapy or with an indication to start on medications, a risk–benefit analysis concerning the risks of medications versus the risks of untreated mental illness across conception, pregnancy, postpartum, and lactation is indicated. This should be a shared decision-making process between the patient and her healthcare provider, ideally involving the partner [36, 48, 77].

For patients planning to conceive, preconception counseling should be promoted. Given the risk of relapse faced by women with perinatal BD, pharmacotherapy continuation during pregnancy is highly recommended [144, 146]. Ideally, patients should be receiving monotherapy at the lowest effective dose. When opting to discontinue medications, this should be performed gradually, and medication changes should ideally be made before pregnancy. Whenever possible, patients who are not in treatment before pregnancy should start medications only after the first trimester and prioritize psychosocial measures to decrease the risk of teratogenicity. Patients with BD who are not on medications during pregnancy should be encouraged to start maintenance treatment as soon as possible after delivery and continue with close monitoring for early detection of mood episodes or psychotic symptoms [153].

8.2.4.1 BD Treatment in Pregnancy

There is a paucity of studies investigating the effectiveness of medications for managing BD in the perinatal period. Therefore, pharmacological management should follow the treatment hierarchies for BD guidelines in the general population, considering the risks related to each medication [117]. As of 2015, the FDA has replaced the risk categories with the Pregnancy and Lactation Labeling Rule (PLLR), which provides updated information for risks. Updated information on the effects of individual psychotropic drugs on fetal and infant health during pregnancy is available in databases such as the UK Teratology Information Service (https://uktis.org) and the FDA List of Pregnancy Exposure Registries (LPER; https://www.fda.gov/consumers/womens-health-topics/pregnancy-exposure-registries). Preference should be given to medications that have been effective in the past and could be effective in preventing both polarities [118, 119].

A recent systematic review confirmed the teratogenic risks of valproate and carbamazepine, finding no statistically significant increased risk for lamotrigine [14]. Scandinavian register-based studies revealed no meaningful associations of neurodevelopmental associations with pregnancy exposure to lamotrigine or carbamazepine monotherapy for seizure disorders [11, 21], whereas a significant risk was found for valproate, as previously demonstrated.

Lithium is the medication that has been studied the most for the prevention of perinatal mood episodes [77]. The risk of heart defects associated with lithium use during the period of organogenesis may be lower than previously thought, although the difference is still statistically significant [97]. Therefore, if a patient is stable on lithium, it could be used in pregnancy at the lowest effective dose, with careful monitoring of the therapeutic response and serum lithium levels [147, 148]. Lithium serum concentrations decrease during pregnancy due to increased plasma volume and glomerular filtration. Thus, the dose usually needs to be increased to maintain effective serum concentrations. Supplementation with 5 mg of folate may reduce the risk of congenital heart disease [54], and screening via fetal echocardiography at 16–18 weeks gestation is recommended. To mitigate the risk of adverse neonatal outcomes associated with elevated lithium levels, it is recommended to hold the lithium dose at labor onset or for 24–48 hours before a planned delivery. After childbirth, the lithium dose should be decreased to the prepregnancy dose [19, 35, 118, 119, 147, 148].

A recent birth cohort study of 3.4 million children did not find a significantly increased risk of developmental disorders associated with antipsychotic exposure in the perinatal period, with the potential exception of aripiprazole, which requires replication [131]. Another large study revealed no significant risk for congenital malformations with antipsychotic exposure during pregnancy, apart from a small increased risk for risperidone [55].

8.2.4.2 BD Treatment During Lactation

Breastfeeding provides many benefits to the mother and the infant and should not be discouraged [108], unless in cases of mania or psychosis [137]. However, the sleep deprivation associated with breastfeeding can trigger mood episodes and PPP. If the woman decides to breastfeed, the patient and her family should be oriented to protect the patient's sleep as a measure of utmost importance. Strategies such as having the patient's partner bottle-feed at night may be recommended [153].

Deciding whether to use psychotropic medication in breastfeeding mothers should involve a thorough risk–benefit analysis. Selecting the appropriate medication should rely on safety information to reduce infant exposure and potential side effects [118, 119]. Updated information on medication safety during lactation can be found in the FDA LPER and the LactMed database (https://www.ncbi.nlm.nih.gov/books/NBK501922/).

Although breastfeeding is usually not recommended for women on lithium, many professionals do not consider it an absolute contraindication. Breastfeeding while taking lithium monotherapy can be deemed appropriate in cases of healthy full-term infants, as long as the mother adheres to monitoring recommendations, with the involvement of a pediatrician [56].

Second-generation antipsychotics, except for clozapine, are considered relatively safe breastfeeding choices [141]. While risperidone, olanzapine, and quetiapine have the most available information on exposure risk during lactation, a systematic review recommended olanzapine and quetiapine as preferred options [95].

Finally, a systematic review on anticonvulsants during lactation revealed that very low infant drug levels are associated with carbamazepine and valproate, whereas higher levels are reported for lamotrigine. Adverse reactions in infants were considered rare. According to the review, the use of these medications by lactating women was not associated with poorer developmental outcomes in their offspring, according to prospective long-term follow-up studies [139].

8.2.4.3 Postpartum Psychosis

PPP is a psychiatric emergency requiring psychiatric admission and early initiation of pharmacotherapy. Although there is limited research available on the treatment of PPP, the evidence supports the use of antipsychotics, lithium, and electroconvulsive therapy (ECT) for acute management [59]. Bergink et al. [7] developed a stepwise treatment algorithm for the treatment of PPP. The first step was lorazepam at bedtime for 3 days; if there was no response, the next step would be adding an antipsychotic on day 4; if there was no response after 2 weeks, the third step was adding lithium. Nonrespondents would have an indication for ECT, although 98.4% of the women in this study achieved remission within the first three steps. After symptom remission, benzodiazepines and antipsychotics were discontinued, and lithium was continued for 9 months (or antipsychotics were given if the treatment response was without lithium). Given the high risk of recurrence, prophylactic treatment should be started immediately after delivery, with lithium having the most substantial level of evidence for relapse prevention [6].

8.3 Premenstrual Dysphoric Disorder and Bipolar Disorder

Female reproductive life events are frequently linked to physical and psychological adversities [155]. Two to five percent of women are affected by premenstrual dysphoric disorder (PMDD), which is the most severe manifestation of premenstrual syndrome (PMS) [32]. According to the Diagnostic and Statistical Manual of Mental Disorders, Fifth Edition (DSM-5), this condition manifests through both psychological and physical symptoms, as shown in Box 8.1. In most menstrual cycles, at least five symptoms are present in the final week before menses [2]. They typically improve within a few days after the onset of menses and become minimal or absent in the week following menstruation. Notably, characterization of the disorder requires that the patient experiences clinically negative impacts on work, school, interpersonal relationships, or social activities.

Box 8.1: Symptoms of PMDD According to the DSM-5

- Marked affective lability
- Excessive irritability/anger/interpersonal conflicts
- Depressed mood, feelings of hopelessness, or self-deprecating thoughts
- Higher anxiety, or internal tension
- Lack of interest in usual activities
- Subjective perception of decrease in concentration
- Lethargy, easy fatigability, or marked lack of energy
- Marked change in appetite: Overeating or specific food cravings
- Changes in sleep quality: Hypersomnia or insomnia
- A sense of being overwhelmed or out of control
- Physical symptoms: Breast tenderness or swelling, joint or muscle pain, a sensation of "bloating," or weight gain

Studies have evaluated the interaction between BD and PMDD and have shown that women who present with PMDD are at a greater risk of developing BD [71, 121]. The opposite is also true: patients with BD are more likely to report PMDD than the general population is [23, 70, 121, 133, 134]. Thus, there appears to be bidirectional vulnerability between PMDD and BD, such that individuals with either disorder are more prone to experiencing symptoms of the other.

The diagnosis and clinical management of comorbid BD/PMDD can be challenging. The first step in diagnosing comorbid PMDD is to stabilize the underlying BD, followed by at least 2 months of prospective mood charting [153]. These criteria are necessary to distinguish PMDD from a premenstrual exacerbation (PME) of mood disorders. In contrast to PMDD, PME of mood disorders presents as a premenstrual aggravation of an ongoing mood episode and can affect approximately 60% of women with mood disorders [67]. A comprehensive review revealed that while menstrual cycle-related mood changes were highly prevalent among women with BD (64–68%), only 15–27% of the sample presented a history of PMDD, which highlights the importance of a proper diagnosis [133, 134].

According to a recent meta-analysis [106], the pooled prevalence of PMDD is estimated to be 3.2%, with the rate climbing to 7.7% when provisional diagnoses are considered (i.e., diagnosis not confirmed throughout 2 months of prospective mood charting). In the context of comorbidity with BD, the rates of PMDD appear to be markedly higher [33, 41, 42, 133, 134]. For example, a systematic review reported that 15–27% of women with BD met the criteria for PMDD [133, 134]. Consistent with this research, Frey et al. [41, 42] reported that among a sample of 52 women with mood disorders, close to half met a provisional diagnosis of PMDD. These findings indicate that women with mood disorders, particularly BD, may be more vulnerable to hormonal fluctuations [111]. In parallel, Wittchen [151] reported that 10% of women with PMDD met the criteria for BD.

8.3.1 Factors Associated with PMDD and BD Comorbidity

As described in Table 8.1, studies have identified specific features associated with comorbid PMDD and BD. For example, an earlier age of BD onset is linked to comorbid BD and PMDD in females [99, 122–125]. Additionally, females with premenstrual mood worsening seem to have a shorter time to relapse into a subsyndromal or syndromal episode of BD [29, 30] and to exhibit more severe depressive and manic symptoms [72, 124, 125]. These findings indicate that PMDD could be a marker for a more recurrent and symptomatic course of illness in women with BD. Moreover, it suggests that hormonal sensitivity may lead to chronic and persistent mood instability, even without a full-blown illness episode [29, 30].

Slyepchenko et al. [122, 123] also reported that women with PMDD and BD had a higher risk of rapid cycling, hypomanic, and depressive episodes in the past year, as well as a higher lifetime incidence of depressive episodes. Importantly, females with comorbid PMDD and BD appear to be at greater risk for comorbid psychiatric conditions such as generalized anxiety disorder (GAD), posttraumatic stress disorder (PTSD), panic disorder, bulimia nervosa, attention deficit hyperactivity disorder (ADHD), OCD, and body dysmorphia [72, 122, 123].

Table 8.1 Factors associated with PMDD and BD comorbidity

Illness onset	Earlier onset of bipolar illness Reduced time between BD onset and age of menarche
Illness course and symptoms	Increased rates of rapid cycling Increased number and severity of hypo/manic and depressive episodes Increased depressive and anxious symptoms throughout the menstrual cycle Increased psychiatric comorbidities, including anxiety disorders, PTSD, OCD, eating disorders, substance abuse, and ADHD Greater likelihood of seasonality Greater disruption in biological rhythms Impaired social functioning Greater severity of mood symptoms during the perinatal period and during use of oral contraceptives
Clinical correlates	Greater likelihood of inflammatory or autoimmune disease
Family history	Greater likelihood of familial mental disorders

Research also suggests that comorbid BD and PMDD are associated with an earlier age of menarche and a shorter interval between menarche and BD onset [72, 122, 123]. These individuals are at greater risk of severe mood symptoms when oral contraceptives are used, indicating vulnerability to hormonal changes [122, 123]. This is supported by findings that individuals with BD and PMDD are more likely to experience mood symptoms during reproductive milestones (e.g., pregnancy, postpartum, and menopause). For example, a study of 158 women with BD type I or BD type II revealed that 77% experienced mood worsening during the perimenstrual, postnatal, or menopausal periods, which was linked to a poorer BD course [101, 102].

With respect to the greater symptomatic burden of BD/PMDD comorbidity, studies have reported increased rates of anxious and somatic symptoms and greater sleep and biological rhythm disruptions in these individuals [31, 132]. Interestingly, a recent study by Liang et al. [72] that assessed 262 women with BD revealed that patients with comorbid BD/PMDD were more likely to have a family history of mental disorders and inflammatory or autoimmune diseases.

Furthermore, Syan et al. [132] reported functional differences associated with BD/PMDD in premotor and frontal cortical areas, as well as the hippocampus. The author hypothesized that the altered connectivity observed in BD/PMDD patients could reflect efforts to manage the stress response or potentially an abnormality that could make these individuals susceptible to later episodes. Structural differences also emerged in the parietal, temporal, frontal, and caudate areas, suggesting a distinct neurobiological phenotype for patients with BD/PMDD vs. patients with BD.

8.3.2 Treatment Recommendations

Studies on the treatment of PMDD in patients with BD represent a significant research gap and an unmet clinical need for these comorbid conditions. While no randomized, placebo-controlled trials have been conducted on the treatment of PMDD comorbid with BD, some clinical recommendations can be made.

First, stabilizing bipolar symptoms and optimizing medication dosages are critical. This is necessary to ensure that the symptoms arise from the premenstrual phase alone, not from inadequately treated BD [126]. Once BD is stabilized, there must be at least 2 months of prospective daily monitoring of symptoms [153]. There are several tools available for prospective mood charting [41, 42, 84].

For a confirmed diagnosis of comorbid PMDD, measures such as sleep hygiene, physical activity, and a healthy diet can help relieve menstrual symptoms [143]. Moreover, there is some evidence that cognitive behavioral therapy (CBT) can help relieve mood and anxiety symptoms in PMDD but is not effective in treating physical symptoms [16, 62, 66].

Dietary supplements have also been shown to provide symptom relief in PMDD. There is evidence for 600 mg of elemental calcium twice daily [138], and up to 100 mg of vitamin B6 daily may also be considered, although there is some concern for peripheral neuropathy at higher doses [10, 63, 152]. Vitex agnus castus, a phytotherapeutic compound, has also been proven to be well tolerated and effective in alleviating PMDD symptoms [17]. Importantly, none of these compounds have been tested in individuals with comorbid BD and PMDD.

Selective serotonin reuptake inhibitors (SSRIs), either continuously or taken during the luteal phase, are considered first-line treatments for PMDD [52, 105, 112]. However, when there is a comorbid diagnosis of BD, the use of SSRIs raises significant safety concerns due to the increased risk of a manic switch [34, 45]. Thus, antidepressants should be restricted to patients with severe PMDD who are unresponsive to hormonal treatments [126].

Oral contraceptives with shortened or no hormone-free intervals are also considered among the most effective therapeutic options for severe PMS and PMDD [76, 112, 154]. The combination of drospirenone and ethinyl estradiol seems particularly effective [75, 76]. However, other risks and benefits associated with hormonal therapies must always be considered before these agents are prescribed. Two case studies address comorbid PMDD and BD treatment with the use of adjunctive hormonal contraceptives, with promising results [39, 126].

Finally, severe treatment-resistant PMDD may have an indication for more invasive treatments, such as the use of GnRH analogs combined with estrogen and progesterone therapies or even surgical interventions [78, 96].

8.4 Bipolar Disorder in the Menopause Transition

Perimenopause, or menopause transition (MT), is a dynamic process that begins with changes in the menstrual cycle and ends during the final menstrual period. It typically starts when women are in their mid-to-late 40s and can last 4–7 years [140]. This transition is characterized by clinical and hormonal changes, including changes in menstrual cycle length, flow, and regularity [130]. Decreased ovarian function and dysregulation of the hypothalamus–pituitary–gonadal (HPG) axis lead to various physical symptoms in middle-aged women, such as hot flashes, night sweats, and genitourinary symptoms [93]. Additionally, women in the menopausal transition may experience symptoms that overlap with depression, including sleep disturbances, cognitive difficulties, fatigue, and low libido [60, 127]. Moreover, the physical changes associated with the menopausal transition and the aging process can reduce the quality of life of women [103, 128].

Despite the widespread belief that perimenopause is universally experienced as a very distressing event and linked to severe mental health outcomes, evidence to support these claims has often not been subject to rigorous scientific review [15]. Women with a previous history of MDD may be at greater risk of recurrence during the MT [13], and several factors can predict the risk for depressive symptoms during this period (Table 8.2; [15]). Although the data concerning the impact of menopause on BD are an underrepresented research topic, preliminary evidence suggests that the menopause transition may affect the course of BD and the severity of the disease [81, 101, 102]. A post hoc analysis of the prospective Systematic Treatment Enhancement Program for Bipolar Disorder (STEP-BD) study revealed that women experience higher rates of depressive episodes, but not manic episodes, during perimenopause [79].

Menopause symptoms might be directly associated with mood changes. A recent study revealed that greater hot flash severity and sleep disturbance were significantly correlated with symptoms of depression, anxiety, and stress in patients with BD [100]. Moreover, studies have shown that patients with BD who experience menopause-related mood symptoms are more likely to present comorbid anxiety disorders, rapid cycling, and mixed mood features [101–103]. These patients also presented tendencies toward higher rates of previous self-harm and suicide attempts, in addition to an earlier age of onset for both first depressive and manic/hypomanic episodes [101, 102].

8.4.1 Factors Associated with Diagnostic Conversion and First-Onset BD During the Menopause Transition

Research on the diagnostic conversion of MDD to BD during perimenopause is scarce. Chen et al. [18] analyzed a Taiwanese health research database with over 50,273 middle-aged women (40–60 years) with major depression. They divided

Table 8.2 Factors associated with increased risk of depressive symptoms in the menopausal transition

Menopause-related risk factors	*Psychosocial risk factors*
Early menopause	History of depression
Long menopause transition	Adverse childhood events
Sleep disruption	Stressful life events
Nocturnal vasomotor symptoms	Financial difficulties
Mood sensitivity to sex steroid fluctuation	Lack of social support
Lifestyle factors	*Psychological factors*
High BMI	Negative beliefs related to menopause/aging
Sedentarism	Neuroticism
Smoking	

patients on the basis of whether they had symptomatic MT (n = 21,120) or not (n = 29,153). Individuals who went on to develop BD during follow-up were documented. Even after adjusting for demographic and psychiatric characteristics, the results revealed that middle-aged women who had both depression and symptomatic MT had a greater incidence of diagnostic conversion to BD (7.3% vs. 6.6%, $p = 0.003$) than did individuals with major depression only.

Using the same database as Chen et al. [18], an earlier study by Hu et al. [53] assessed the risk of psychiatric disorders in women following symptomatic menopausal transition. The results revealed that the incidence of BD (HR = 1.69, 95% confidence interval [CI] = 1.01–2.80) was greater among women with symptomatic menopausal transition than among age-matched asymptomatic women. Additionally, the incidence of new-onset BD following the initial diagnosis of symptomatic MT remained significantly greater, even over longer-term follow-up periods of 1–5 years and then five or more years.

Kim et al. [65] recently utilized a South Korean nationwide database of medical records to assess postmenopausal women aged 40 years or older and followed them to observe new-onset cases. The authors reported that women who received hormone therapy (HT) had an increased risk of BD, with an association between prolonged exposure and increased BD risk. Additionally, the authors reported that women who experienced menopause at the age of 45 years or older and women who had breastfed for one year or more presented a lower risk of BD. The absence of control for confounding variables, such as psychiatric comorbidities other than mood disorders, psychosocial factors, and adverse life events, affects the validity of the study.

Together, these findings suggest that a symptomatic menopause transition may be associated with a higher incidence of diagnostic conversion to BD, as well as new-onset BD [18, 53]. Furthermore, the incidence of BD may be influenced not only by the duration of estrogen exposure but also by the type (endogenous vs. exogenous) and the timing of exposure to estrogen [65]. Nevertheless, further research is needed on diagnostic conversion and first-onset BD during perimenopause and its associations with hormones and other predisposing factors [91].

8.4.2 Treatment Recommendations

The evidence for menopause treatments in the BD population is scarce; thus, patients should be treated as at other life stages [153]. Clinicians should be aware of a possible increased risk for relapse in perimenopausal women with a previous history of mood disorders. While it should not be assumed that psychological distress during the MT is attributed solely to hormonal changes, special consideration should be given to treating modifiable risk factors, such as severe vasomotor symptoms (VMS) and sleep problems [15].

Vasomotor symptoms have been associated with the onset of depressive symptoms, in part because nocturnal symptoms interfere with sleep [61]. Some evidence suggests that estrogen therapy (ET) could be effective in the management of unipolar depression in perimenopausal but not postmenopausal women [88, 110, 129]. Furthermore, it has been suggested that ET may augment the antidepressant response in middle-aged women [87]. However, a meta-analysis that included both perimenopausal and postmenopausal women revealed that bioidentical estrogen had no benefit on depression [149]. Despite the mixed results, some organizations recommend considering the use of HT to treat concurrent depressive symptoms in patients with VMS. Importantly, HT is not approved by regulatory agencies in the United States or Europe for the treatment of mood disturbances [15, 92]. With respect to the use of HT in perimenopausal women with BD, while one study indicated that HT could be protective against worsening mood symptoms [37, 38], other findings suggest that HT neither worsens nor stabilizes mood in this population [79, 80].

Many nonhormonal medications with applications in psychiatry have been found to significantly decrease VMS in menopausal women and are recommended by the North American Menopause Society for those who are not good candidates for HT ([136]; Table 8.3). Interestingly, gabapentin is considered a third-line adjunctive treatment for BD and has been shown to decrease anxiety symptoms in patients with BD [153]. As drowsiness is a potential side effect of gabapentin, it could be considered a strategy for the management of sleep disturbances associated with VMS [92].

Finally, CBT is well established as a treatment for VMS [136], in addition to being a first-line treatment for MDD [68] and a second-line treatment for the depressive and maintenance phases of BD [153]. However, there is a lack of data regarding CBT protocols for patients with BD experiencing menopausal symptoms [22].

Table 8.3 Psychotropic medications suggested as nonhormonal treatments for vasomotor symptoms

SSRIs	*Suggested dosing range*
Paroxetine	10–25 mg/day
Citalopram	10–20 mg/day
Escitalopram	10–20 mg/day
SNRIs	
Desvenlafaxine	100–150 mg/day
Venlafaxine	37.5–150 mg/day
Gabapentinoids	
Gabapentin	900–2400 mg/day

Adapted from NAMS [136]
SNRIs serotonin-norepinephrine reuptake inhibitors, *SSRIs* selective serotonin reuptake inhibitors

8.5 Conclusion

This chapter highlights that pregnancy and childbirth are potent triggers for mood episodes. Moreover, psychiatric disorders with first onset in the perinatal period are strong predictors of BD. The evolving understanding of perinatal BD reflects an urgent call for comprehensive mental health screening during and after pregnancy, when offspring may face additional psychological and social consequences if maternal psychopathology is neglected or poorly managed.

Similarly, women who experience severe premenstrual disturbances should also be monitored, particularly in the case of PMDD, given a heightened vulnerability to BD. Moreover, studies emphasize a more severe course of illness in individuals who suffer from comorbid BD/PMDD. Further work is needed to elucidate shared risk factors, clinical features, and the efficacy of treatments targeted specifically toward BD/PMDD.

Finally, the interplay between BD and the menopause transition underscores the need for integrated, individualized treatment approaches. Despite advances, significant gaps remain in research and clinical practice, particularly regarding managing BD during key reproductive transitions. Future research should continue to explore these intersections, with an emphasis on developing evidence-based treatments that address the unique needs of women across different reproductive stages. Ultimately, improving the recognition and treatment of BD holds promise for enhancing the quality of life for women, their families, and society at large.

Clinical Considerations

- Psychiatric disorders with first onset in the postpartum period are strong predictors of latent bipolar disorder.
- Screening for perinatal depression without concurrent screening for BD can lead to the misrecognition of perinatal depression as unipolar instead of bipolar.
- The first 3 months postpartum seem to be a critical period for diagnostic conversion from MDD to BD.

- It is critical to stabilize bipolar symptoms to diagnose PMDD in women with BD and assess mood with the aid of prospective mood charting to ensure that the symptoms arise from the premenstrual phase alone and not from inadequately treated BD.
- There appears to be a bidirectional vulnerability between PMDD and BD, such that individuals with either disorder are more prone to experiencing the other.
- Clinicians should be aware of a possible increased risk for relapse in perimenopausal women with a previous history of mood disorders.
- A symptomatic menopause transition may be associated with a higher incidence of diagnostic conversion to bipolar disorder, as well as new-onset bipolar disorder.

In perimenopausal women with BD, special consideration should be given to treating modifiable risk factors for depression, such as severe vasomotor symptoms and sleep problems.

References

1. Akiskal HS, Benazzi F, Perugi G, et al. Agitated unipolar depression re-conceptualized as a depressive mixed state: implications for the antidepressant-suicide controversy. J Affect Disord. 2005;85:245–58.
2. American Psychiatric Association. Desk reference to the diagnostic criteria from DSM-5. Washington, DC: American Psychiatric Publishing; 2013.
3. Arnold LM. Gender differences in bipolar disorder. Psychiatr Clin North Am. 2003;26:595–620. https://doi.org/10.1016/s0193-953x(03)00036-4.
4. Azorin J, Angst J, Gamma A, Bowden CL, Perugi G, Vieta E, et al. Identifying features of bipolarity in patients with first episode postpartum depression: findings from the international BRIDGE study. J Affect Disord. 2012;136:710–5.
5. Balazs J, Benazzi F, Rihmer Z, et al. The close link between suicide attempts and mixed (bipolar) depression: implications for suicide prevention. J Affect Disord. 2006;91:133–8.
6. Bergink V, Bouvy PF, Vervoort JS, et al. Prevention of postpartum psychosis and mania in women at high risk. Am J Psychiatry. 2012;169:609–15.
7. Bergink V, Burgerhout KM, Koorengevel KM, et al. Treatment of psychosis and mania in the postpartum period. Am J Psychiatry. 2015;172:115–23.
8. Bergink V, Rasgon N, Wisner KL. Postpartum psychosis: madness, mania, and melancholia in motherhood. Am J Psychiatry. 2016;173(12):1179–88. https://doi.org/10.1176/appi.ajp.2016.16040454.
9. Berk M, Dodd S. Review: rapid cycling bipolar disorder associated with female gender and bipolar type II subgroup. Evid Based Ment Health. 2004;7:91. https://doi.org/10.1136/ebmh.7.3.91.
10. Biggs WS, Demuth RH. Premenstrual syndrome and premenstrual dysphoric disorder. Am Fam Physician. 2011;84:918–24.
11. Bjørk MH, Zoega H, Leinonen MK, Cohen JM, Dreier JW, Furu K, et al. Association of prenatal exposure to antiseizure medication with risk of autism and intellectual disability. JAMA Neurol. 2022;79:672–81. https://doi.org/10.1001/jamaneurol.2022.1269.
12. Boukakiou R, Glangeaud-Freudenthal NMC, Falissard B, et al. Impact of a prenatal episode and diagnosis in women with serious mental illnesses on neonatal complications (prematurity, low birth weight, and hospitalization in neonatal intensive care units). Arch Womens Ment Health. 2018. https://doi.org/10.1007/s00737-018-0915-1.

13. Bromberger JT, Kravitz HM, Chang YF, Cyranowski JM, Brown C, Matthews KA. Major depression during and after the menopausal transition: study of women's health across the nation (SWAN). Psychol Med. 2011;41:1879–88. https://doi.org/10.1017/S003329171100016X.
14. Bromley R, Adab N, Bluett-Duncan M, Clayton-Smith J, Christensen J, Edwards K, Greenhalgh J, Hill RA, Jackson CF, Khanom S, McGinty RN, Tudur Smith C, Pulman J, Marson AG. Monotherapy treatment of epilepsy in pregnancy: congenital malformation outcomes in the child. Cochrane Database Syst Rev. 2023;8. https://doi.org/10.1002/14651858.CD010224.pub3.
15. Brown L, Hunter MS, Chen R, et al. Promoting good mental health over the menopause transition. Lancet (London, England). 2024;403(10430):969–83. https://doi.org/10.1016/S0140-6736(23)02801-5.
16. Busse JW, Montori VM, Krasnik C, Patelis-Siotis I, Guyatt GH. Psychological intervention for premenstrual syndrome: a meta-analysis of randomized controlled trials. Psychother Psychosom. 2009;78:6–15. https://doi.org/10.1159/000162296.
17. Cerqueira RO, Frey BN, Leclerc E, Brietzke E. Vitex agnus castus for premenstrual syndrome and premenstrual dysphoric disorder: a systematic review. Arch Womens Ment Health. 2017;20:713–9. https://doi.org/10.1007/s00737-017-0791-0.
18. Chen VCH, Shen CC, Chen TT, et al. Symptomatic menopausal transition and the risk of developing bipolar disorder in women with major depression: a nationwide longitudinal study. J Affect Disord. 2017;223:74–9.
19. Clark CT, Wisner KL. Treatment of peripartum bipolar disorder. Obstet Gynecol Clin N Am. 2018;45:403–17. https://doi.org/10.1016/j.ogc.2018.05.002.
20. Clark CT, Sit DK, Driscoll K, Eng HF, Confer AL, Luther JF, Wisniewski SR, Wisner KL. Does screening with the MDQ and EPDS improve identification of bipolar disorder in an obstetrical sample? Depress Anxiety. 2015;32:518–26. https://doi.org/10.1002/da.22373.
21. Cohen JM, Alvestad S, Cesta CE, Bjørk MH, Leinonen MK, Nørgaard M, Einarsdóttir K, Engeland A, Gissler M, Karlstad Ø, Klungsøyr K, Odsbu I, Reutfors J, Selmer RM, Tomson T, Ulrichsen SP, Zoega H, Furu K. Comparative safety of antiseizure medication monotherapy for major malformations. Ann Neurol. 2023;93:551–62. https://doi.org/10.1002/ana.26561.
22. Conklin D, Carpenter JS, Whitney MS, DeLozier S, Ogede DO, Bazella C, McVoy M, Sajatovic M. Narrative analyses: cognitive behavior group therapy for women with menopause and bipolar or major depressive disorders. Womens Health Rep (New Rochelle). 2021;2:430–42. https://doi.org/10.1089/whr.2021.0025.
23. de Carvalho RR, Dias RS, Freire RC, et al. Premenstrual dysphoric disorder and psychiatric comorbidities: a systematic review. Rev Bras Psiquiatr. 2018;40(2):188–97. https://doi.org/10.1590/1516-4446-2017-2397.
24. Dell'Osso B, Cafaro R, Ketter TA. Has bipolar disorder become a predominantly female gender related condition? Analysis of recently published large sample studies. Int J Bipolar Disord. 2021;9:3. https://doi.org/10.1186/s40345-020-00207-z.
25. Di Florio A, Forty L, Gordon-Smith K, Heron J, Jones L, Craddock N, Jones I. Perinatal episodes across the mood disorder spectrum. JAMA Psychiatry. 2013;70:168–75.
26. Di Florio A, Jones L, Forty L, Gordon-Smith K, Craddock N, Jones I. Bipolar disorder, miscarriage, and termination. Bipolar Disord. 2015;17:102–5. Available from: http://resolver.scholarsportal.info.libaccess.lib.mcmaster.ca/resolve/13985647/v17i0001/102_bdmat.xml.
27. Di Florio A, Gordon-Smith K, Forty L, Kosorok MR, Fraser C, Perry A, Bethell A, Craddock N, Jones L, Jones I. Stratification of the risk of bipolar disorder recurrences in pregnancy and postpartum. Br J Psychiatry. 2018;213:542–7. https://doi.org/10.1192/bjp.2018.92.
28. Di Florio A, Mei Kay Yang J, Crawford K, et al. Post-partum psychosis and its association with bipolar disorder in the UK: a case-control study using polygenic risk scores. Lancet Psychiatry. 2021;8(12):1045–52. https://doi.org/10.1016/S2215-0366(21)00253-4.
29. Dias RS, Freire RC, Fernandes FM, et al. Premenstrual mood symptoms as a predictor of time to relapse in women with bipolar disorder. Rev Bras Psiquiatr. 2011a;33(4):372–5.

30. Dias RS, Lafer B, Russo C, Del Debbio A, Nierenberg AA, Sachs GS, Joffe H. Longitudinal follow-up of bipolar disorder in women with premenstrual exacerbation: findings from STEP-BD. Am J Psychiatry. 2011b;168:386–94. https://doi.org/10.1176/appi.ajp.2010.09121816.
31. El Dahr Y, de Azevedo CT, Syan SK, et al. Investigating biological rhythms disruptions across the menstrual cycle in women with comorbid bipolar disorder and premenstrual dysphoric disorder. Arch Womens Ment Health. 2022;25(2):345–53. https://doi.org/10.1007/s00737-022-01220-0.
32. Epperson CN, Steiner M, Hartlage SA, Eriksson E, Schmidt PJ, Jones I, Yonkers KA. Premenstrual dysphoric disorder: evidence for a new category for DSM-5. Am J Psychiatry. 2012;169:465–75. https://doi.org/10.1176/appi.ajp.2012.11081302.
33. Fornaro M, Perugi G. Prevalence and clinical features associated with bipolar disorder-polycystic ovary syndrome comorbidity: a systematic review. J Affect Disord. 2020;263:97–104.
34. Fornaro M, Anastasia A, Novello S, Fusco A, Solmi M, Monaco F, Veronese N, De Berardis D, de Bartolomeis A. Incidence, prevalence and clinical correlates of antidepressant-emergent mania in bipolar depression: a systematic review and meta-analysis. Bipolar Disord. 2018;20:195–227. https://doi.org/10.1111/bdi.12612.
35. Fornaro M, Maritan E, Ferranti R, et al. Lithium exposure during pregnancy and the postpartum period: a systematic review and meta-analysis of safety and efficacy outcomes. Am J Psychiatry. 2020;177:76–92.
36. Fountoulakis KN, Grunze H, Vieta E, et al. The International College of Neuro-Psychopharmacology (CINP) treatment guidelines for bipolar disorder in adults (CINP-BD-2017), part 3: the clinical guidelines. Int J Neuropsychopharmacol. 2017;20:180–95.
37. Freeman MP, Smith KW, Freeman SA, McElroy SL, Kmetz GE, Wright R, Keck PE Jr. The impact of reproductive events on the course of bipolar disorder in women. J Clin Psychiatry. 2002;63:284–7. https://doi.org/10.4088/jcp.v63n0403.
38. Freeman EW, Stout AL, Endicott J, Spiers P. Treatment of premenstrual syndrome with a carbohydrate-rich beverage. Int J Gynaecol Obstet Off Organ Int Fed Gynaecol Obstet. 2002a;77:253–4. https://doi.org/10.1016/s0020-7292(02)00033-4.
39. Frey BN, Minuzzi L. Comorbid bipolar disorder and premenstrual dysphoric disorder: real patients, unanswered questions. Arch Womens Ment Health. 2013;16:79–81. https://doi.org/10.1007/s00737-012-0313-z.
40. Frey BN, Simpson W, Wright L, Steiner M. Sensitivity and specificity of the Mood Disorder Questionnaire as a screening tool for bipolar disorder during pregnancy and the postpartum period. J Clin Psychiatry. 2012;73:1456–61.
41. Frey BN, Allega OR, Eltayebani M, Syan SK, Mendes-Ribeiro J, Minuzzi L. A DSM-5-based tool to monitor concurrent mood and premenstrual symptoms: the McMaster Premenstrual and Mood Symptom Scale (MAC-PMSS). BMC Womens Health. 2022a;22:96. https://doi.org/10.1186/s12905-022-01678-1.
42. Frey BN, Martinez-Aguayo JC, Blier P, Soares CN. Provisional diagnosis of premenstrual dysphoric disorder among women with mood disorders. J Clin Psychiatry. 2022b;83(4)
43. Ghaemi SN, Rosenquist KJ, Ko JY, et al. Antidepressant treatment in bipolar versus unipolar depression. Am J Psychiatry. 2004;161:163–5.
44. Gilden J, Poels EM, Lambrichts S, Vreeker A, Boks MP, Ophoff RA, Kahn RS, Kamperman AM, Bergink V. Bipolar episodes after reproductive events in women with bipolar I disorder: a study of 919 pregnancies. J Affect Disord. 2021;295:72–9.
45. Gitlin MJ. Antidepressants in bipolar depression: an enduring controversy. Int J Bipolar Disord. 2018;6:25. https://doi.org/10.1186/s40345-018-0133-9.
46. Glover V, Liddle P, Taylor A, Adams D, Sandler M. Mild hypomania (the highs) can be a feature of the first postpartum week: association with later depression. Br J Psychiatry. 1994;164:517–21.
47. Goldberg JF, DelBello MP, Swartz HA. Expanded treatment options and addressing unmet needs in the diagnosis and treatment of bipolar disorder. J Clin Psychiatry. 2022;83(6):MS21058AH5. https://doi.org/10.4088/JCP.MS21058AH5.

48. Goodwin GM, Haddad PM, Ferrier IN, et al. Evidence-based guidelines for treating bipolar disorder: revised third edition recommendations from the British Association for Psychopharmacology. J Psychopharmacol. 2016;30:495–553.
49. Gordon-Smith K, Perry A, Di Florio A, Forty L, Fraser C, Casanova Dias M, et al. Symptom profile of postpartum and non-postpartum manic episodes in bipolar I disorder: a within-subjects study. Psychiatry Res. 2020;284:112748. https://doi.org/10.1016/j.psychres.2020.112748.
50. Health Canada. Health Product InfoWatch. Government of Canada. 2017. https://www.canada.ca/en/health-canada/services/drugs-health-products/medeffect-canada/health-product-infowatch/health-product-infowatch-april-2017-page-2.html. Accessed 31 Aug 2024.
51. Hirschfeld RM, Williams JB, Spitzer RL, et al. Development and validation of a screening instrument for bipolar spectrum disorder: the Mood Disorder Questionnaire. Am J Psychiatry. 2000;157(11):1873–5.
52. Hofmeister S, Bodden S. Premenstrual syndrome and premenstrual dysphoric disorder. Am Fam Physician. 2016;94:236–40.
53. Hu LY, Shen CC, Hu YW, et al. The risk of developing bipolar disorder following symptomatic menopausal transition: a nationwide population-based study. J Affect Disord. 2016;206:268–73.
54. Huhta JC, Linask K. When should we prescribe high-dose folic acid to prevent congenital heart defects? Curr Opin Cardiol. 2015;30(1):125–31. https://doi.org/10.1097/HCO.0000000000000138.
55. Huybrechts KF, Hernández-Díaz S, Patorno E, Desai RJ, Mogun H, Dejene SZ, Cohen JM, Panchaud A, Cohen L, Bateman BT. Antipsychotic use in pregnancy and the risk for congenital malformations. JAMA Psychiatry. 2016;73(9):938–46. https://doi.org/10.1001/jamapsychiatry.2016.1520.
56. Imaz ML, Soy D, Torra M, et al. Case report: clinical and pharmacokinetic profile of lithium monotherapy in exclusive breastfeeding. a follow-up case series. Front Pharmacol. 2021;12:647414. https://doi.org/10.3389/fphar.2021.647414.
57. Inglis A, Hippman C, Carrion P, Honer W, Austin J. Mania and depression in the perinatal period among women with a history of major depressive disorders. Arch Womens Ment Health. 2014;17:137–43.
58. Jaeschke RR, Dudek D, Topór-Mądry R, Drozdowicz K, Datka W, Siwek M, Rybakowski J. Postpartum depression: bipolar or unipolar? Analysis of 434 Polish postpartum women. Braz J Psychiatry. 2016;39:154–9. https://doi.org/10.1590/1516-4446-2016-1921.
59. Jairaj C, Seneviratne G, Bergink V, Sommer IE, Dazzan P. Postpartum psychosis: a proposed treatment algorithm. J Psychopharmacol (Oxford, England). 2023;37(10):960–70. https://doi.org/10.1177/02698811231181573.
60. Joffe H, Soares CN, Cohen LS. Assessment and treatment of hot flushes and menopausal mood disturbance. Psychiatr Clin North Am. 2003;26(3):563–80. https://doi.org/10.1016/s0193-953x(03)00045-5.
61. Joffe H, Crawford SL, Freeman MP, et al. Independent contributions of nocturnal hot flashes and sleep disturbance to depression in estrogen-deprived women. J Clin Endocrinol Metab. 2016;101:3847–55.
62. Kancheva Landolt N, Ivanov K. Short report: cognitive behavioral therapy - a primary mode for premenstrual syndrome management: systematic literature review. Psychol Health Med. 2021;26:1282–93. https://doi.org/10.1080/13548506.2020.1810718.
63. Kashanian M, Mazinani R, Jalalmanesh S, Babayanzad Ahari S. Pyridoxine (vitamin B6) therapy for premenstrual syndrome. Int J Gynaecol Obstet Off Organ Int Fed Gynaecol Obstet. 2007;96:43–4. https://doi.org/10.1016/j.ijgo.2006.09.014.
64. Kawa I, Carter JD, Joyce PR, Doughty CJ, Frampton CM, Wells JE, Walsh AE, Olds RJ. Gender differences in bipolar disorder: age of onset, course, comorbidity, and symptom presentation. Bipolar Disord. 2005;7:119–25. https://doi.org/10.1111/j.1399-5618.2004.00180.x.
65. Kim JW, Kim HJ, Kim JE, et al. Menopause and the incidence of bipolar disorder: a nationwide cohort study. J Psychiatr Res. 2022;146:26–33.

66. Kleinstäuber M, Witthöft M, Hiller W. Cognitive-behavioral and pharmacological interventions for premenstrual syndrome or premenstrual dysphoric disorder: a meta-analysis. J Clin Psychol Med Settings. 2012;19:308–19. https://doi.org/10.1007/s10880-012-9299-y.
67. Kuehner C, Nayman S. Premenstrual exacerbations of mood disorders: findings and knowledge gaps. Curr Psychiatry Rep. 2021;23:78. https://doi.org/10.1007/s11920-021-01286-0.
68. Lam RW, Kennedy SH, Adams C, Bahji A, Beaulieu S, Bhat V, Blier P, Blumberger DM, Brietzke E, Chakrabarty T, Do A, Frey BN, Giacobbe P, Gratzer D, Grigoriadis S, Habert J, Husain MI, Ismail Z, McGirr A, McIntyre RS, Michalak EE, Müller DJ, Parikh SV, Quilty LS, Ravindran AV, Ravindran N, Renaud J, Rosenblat JD, Samaan Z, Saraf G, Schade K, Schaffer A, Sinyor M, Soares CN, Swainson J, Taylor VH, Tourjman SV, Uher R, van Ameringen M, Vazquez G, Vigod S, Voineskos D, Yatham LN, Milev RV. Canadian network for mood and anxiety treatments (CANMAT) 2023 update on clinical guidelines for management of major depressive disorder in adults: Réseau canadien pour les traitements de l'humeur et de l'anxiété (CANMAT) 2023 : Mise à jour des lignes directrices cliniques pour la prise en charge du trouble dépressif majeur chez les adultes. Can J Psychiatry Rev Can Psychiatr [Epub ahead of print]. 2024. https://doi.org/10.1177/07067437241245384.
69. Lewis KJS, Di Florio A, Forty L, Gordon-Smith K, Perry A, Craddock N, et al. Mania triggered by sleep loss and risk of postpartum psychosis in women with bipolar disorder. J Affect Disord. 2018;225:624–9. https://doi.org/10.1016/j.jad.2017.08.054.
70. Li L, Wu J, Gong T. Bipolar disorder in women with premenstrual dysphoric disorder: a meta-analysis. J Psychiatr Res. 2022;148:110–8.
71. Li D-J, Tsai S-J, Bai Y-M, Su T-P, Chen T-J, Liang C-S, Chen M-H. Risks of major affective disorders following a diagnosis of premenstrual dysphoric disorder: a nationwide longitudinal study. Asian J Psychiatry. 2023;79:103355. https://doi.org/10.1016/j.ajp.2022.103355.
72. Liang S, Xie P, Liu J, et al. Prevalence and clinical correlates of premenstrual dysphoric disorder among Han Chinese women with bipolar disorder. J Affect Disord. 2024;307:219–26.
73. Liu B, Zhang Y, Fang H, Liu J, Liu T, Li L. Efficacy and safety of long-term antidepressant treatment for bipolar disorders - a meta-analysis of randomized controlled trials. J Affect Disord. 2017a;223:41–8. https://doi.org/10.1016/j.jad.2017.07.023.
74. Liu X, Agerbo E, Li J, Meltzer-Brody S, Bergink V, Munk-Olsen T. Depression and anxiety in the postpartum period and risk of bipolar disorder: a Danish nationwide register-based cohort study. J Clin Psychiatry. 2017b;78(5):e476. https://doi.org/10.4088/JCP.16m10970.
75. Lopez LM, Kaptein AA, Helmerhorst FM. Oral contraceptives containing drospirenone for premenstrual syndrome. Cochrane Database Syst Rev. 2012:CD006586. https://doi.org/10.1002/14651858.CD006586.pub4.
76. Ma S, Song SJ. Oral contraceptives containing drospirenone for premenstrual syndrome. Cochrane Database Syst Rev. 2023;6 https://doi.org/10.1002/14651858.CD006586.pub5.
77. Malhi GS, Bassett D, Boyce P, et al. Royal Australian and New Zealand College of Psychiatrists clinical practice guidelines for mood disorders. Aust N Z J Psychiatry. 2015;49(12):1087–206.
78. Management of Premenstrual Syndrome: Green-top Guideline No. 48 (2017) BJOG Int J Obstet Gynaecol 124–e105. https://doi.org/10.1111/1471-0528.14260.
79. Marsh WK, Templeton A, Ketter TA, Rasgon NL. Increased frequency of depressive episodes during the menopausal transition in women with bipolar disorder: preliminary report. J Psychiatr Res. 2008;42:247–51. https://doi.org/10.1016/j.jpsychires.2006.12.006.
80. Marsh WK, Ketter TA, Crawford SL, Johnson JV, Kroll-Desrosiers AR, Rothschild AJ. Progression of female reproductive stages associated with bipolar illness exacerbation. Bipolar Disord. 2012;14:515–26. https://doi.org/10.1111/j.1399-5618.2012.01026.x.
81. Marsh WK, Gershenson B, Rothschild AJ. Symptom severity of bipolar disorder during the menopausal transition. Int J Bipolar Disord. 2015;3:35. https://doi.org/10.1186/s40345-015-0035-z.
82. Masters GA, Brenckle L, Sankaran P, Person SD, Allison J, Moore Simas TA, Ko JY, Robbins CL, Marsh W, Byatt N. Positive screening rates for bipolar disorder in pregnant and

postpartum women and associated risk factors. Gen Hosp Psychiatry. 2019;61:53–9. https://doi.org/10.1016/j.genhosppsych.2019.09.002.
83. Masters GA, Hugunin J, Xu L, Ulbricht CM, Moore Simas TA, Ko JY, Byatt N. Prevalence of bipolar disorder in perinatal women: a systematic review and meta-analysis. J Clin Psychiatry. 2022;83(5):21r14045. https://doi.org/10.4088/JCP.21r14045.
84. Mendes-Ribeiro J, Juruena M, Caropreso L, Eltayebani MM, Streiner DL. Psychometric instruments and women's mental health. In: Rennó Jr J, Valadares G, Cantilino A, Mendes-Ribeiro J, Rocha R, Geraldo da Silva A, editors. Women's mental health. Cham: Springer; 2020. p. 35–45. https://doi.org/10.1007/978-3-030-29081-8_4.
85. Merikangas KR, Jin R, He JP, et al. Prevalence and correlates of bipolar spectrum disorder in the world mental health survey initiative. Arch Gen Psychiatry. 2011;68(3):241–51.
86. Merrill L, Mittal L, Nicoloro J, et al. Screening for bipolar disorder during pregnancy. Arch Womens Ment Health. 2015;18:579–83. https://doi.org/10.1007/s00737-015-0527-y.
87. Morgan ML, Cook IA, Rapkin AJ, Leuchter AF. Estrogen augmentation of antidepressants in perimenopausal depression: a pilot study. J Clin Psychiatry. 2005;66:774–80.
88. Morrison MF, Kallan MJ, Ten Have T, Katz I, Tweedy K, Battistini M. Lack of efficacy of estradiol for depression in postmenopausal women: a randomized, controlled trial. Biol Psychiatry. 2004;55:406–12.
89. Munk-Olsen T, Laursen TM, Pedersen CB, Mors O, Mortensen PB. New parents and mental disorders. JAMA. 2006;296:2582–9. https://doi.org/10.1001/jama.296.21.2582.
90. Munk-Olsen T, Laursen TM, Meltzer-Brody S, Mortensen PB, Jones I. Psychiatric disorders with postpartum onset: possible early manifestations of bipolar affective disorders. Arch Gen Psychiatry. 2012;69(4):428–34. https://doi.org/10.1001/archgenpsychiatry.2011.157.
91. Musial N, Ali Z, Grbevski J, Veerakumar A, Sharma P. Perimenopause and first-onset mood disorders: a closer look. Focus (American Psychiatric Publishing). 2021;19(3):330–7. https://doi.org/10.1176/appi.focus.20200041.
92. Nappi RE. The 2022 hormone therapy position statement of the North American Menopause Society: no news is good news. Lancet Diabetes Endocrinol. 2022;10:832–4.
93. Nelson HD. Menopause. Lancet. 2008;371:760–70. https://doi.org/10.1016/S0140-6736(08)60346-3.
94. No authors listed. Screening and diagnosis of mental health conditions during pregnancy and postpartum: ACOG clinical practice guideline no. 4. Obstet Gynecol. 2023;141(6):1232–61. https://doi.org/10.1097/AOG.0000000000005200.
95. Pacchiarotti I, León-Caballero J, Murru A, et al. Mood stabilizers and antipsychotics during breastfeeding: focus on bipolar disorder. Eur Neuropsychopharmacol. 2016;26:1562–78.
96. Panay N. Treatment of premenstrual syndrome: a decision-making algorithm. Menopause Int. 2012;18:90–2. https://doi.org/10.1258/mi.2012.012019.
97. Patorno E, Huybrechts KF, Bateman BT, Cohen JM, Desai RJ, Mogun H, Cohen LS, Hernandez-Diaz S. Lithium use in pregnancy and the risk of cardiac malformations. N Engl J Med. 2017;376(23):2245–54. https://doi.org/10.1056/NEJMoa1612222.
98. Pawlby S, Fernyhough C, Meins E, et al. Mind-mindedness and maternal responsiveness in infant-mother interactions in mothers with severe mental illness. Psychol Med. 2010;40(11):1861–9.
99. Payne JL, Roy-Byrne PP, Stetler CA. Mood disorders during the reproductive life cycle. J Clin Psychiatry. 2009;70(12):e38.
100. Perich T, Ussher J. Stress predicts depression symptoms for women living with bipolar disorder during the menopause transition. Menopause. 2021;29:231–5. https://doi.org/10.1097/GME.0000000000001894.
101. Perich TA, Mitchell PB, Meade T, et al. The impact of reproductive events on the course of bipolar disorder in women. J Affect Disord. 2017a;223:84–92.
102. Perich TA, Roberts G, Frankland A, Sinbandhit C, Meade T, Austin MP, Mitchell PB. Clinical characteristics of women with reproductive cycle-associated bipolar disorder symptoms. Aust N Z J Psychiatry. 2017b;51:161–7. https://doi.org/10.1177/0004867416670015.
103. Perich T, Ussher J, Fraser I, Perz J. Quality of life and psychological symptoms for women with bipolar disorder - a comparison between reproductive, menopause transition and post-menopause phases. Maturitas. 2021;143:72–7. https://doi.org/10.1016/j.maturitas.2020.09.002.

104. Perry A, Gordon-Smith K, Di Florio A, Craddock N, Jones L, Jones I. Mood episodes in pregnancy and risk of postpartum recurrence in bipolar disorder: the Bipolar Disorder Research Network Pregnancy Study. J Affect Disord. 2021;294:714–22. https://doi.org/10.1016/j.jad.2021.07.067.
105. Reid RL, Soares CN. Premenstrual dysphoric disorder: contemporary diagnosis and management. J Obstet Gynaecol Can. 2018;40:215–23. https://doi.org/10.1016/j.jogc.2017.05.018.
106. Reilly T, Bishop JR, Lin PY, Soares CN. Prevalence of premenstrual dysphoric disorder: a meta-analysis. Arch Womens Ment Health. 2024;27(1):25–37.
107. Roddy Mitchell A, Gordon H, Lindquist A, Walker SP, Homer CSE, Middleton A, Cluver CA, Tong S, Hastie R. Prevalence of perinatal depression in low- and middle-income countries: a systematic review and meta-analysis. JAMA Psychiatry. 2023;80(5):425–31. https://doi.org/10.1001/jamapsychiatry.2023.0069.
108. Rollins NC, Bhandari N, Hajeebhoy N, Horton S, Lutter CK, Martines JC, Piwoz EG, Richter LM, Victora CG, Lancet Breastfeeding Series Group. Why invest, and what it will take to improve breastfeeding practices? Lancet. 2016;387(10017):491–504. https://doi.org/10.1016/S0140-6736(15)01044-2.
109. Schier de Fraga F, Wan-Dall BSL, Garcia GHO, Pandolfo H, Sequinel AMTDS, Alvin P, Serman EJ, do Amaral VF. Antenatal screening of depressive and manic symptoms in south Brazilian childbearing women: a transversal study in advance of the pandemic scenario. PLoS One. 2021;16(12). https://doi.org/10.1371/journal.pone.0261874.
110. Schmidt PJ, Nieman L, Danaceau MA, Tobin MB, Roca CA, Murphy JH, Rubinow DR. Estrogen replacement in perimenopause-related depression: a preliminary report. Am J Obstet Gynecol. 2000;183:414–20. https://doi.org/10.1067/mob.2000.106004.
111. Sepede G. Mood disorders and hormonal fluctuations: insights into premenstrual dysphoric disorder. J Affect Disord. 2020;264:112–8.
112. Sepede G, Sarchione F, Matarazzo I, Di Giannantonio M, Salerno RM. Premenstrual dysphoric disorder without comorbid psychiatric conditions: a systematic review of therapeutic options. Clin Neuropharmacol. 2016;39:241–61. https://doi.org/10.1097/WNF.0000000000000173.
113. Sharma V, Xie B. Screening for postpartum bipolar disorder: validation of the mood disorder questionnaire. J Affect Disord. 2011;131(1–3):408–11. https://doi.org/10.1016/j.jad.2010.11.026.
114. Sharma V, Khan M, Smith A. A closer look at treatment resistant depression: is it due to a bipolar diathesis? J Affect Disord. 2005;84:251–7. https://doi.org/10.1016/j.jad.2005.02.018.
115. Sharma V, Khan M, Corpse C, Sharma P. Missed bipolarity and psychiatric comorbidity in women with postpartum depression. Bipolar Disord. 2008;10:742–7.
116. Sharma V, Xie B, Campbell MK, Penava D, Hampson E, Mazmanian D, Pope CJ. A prospective study of diagnostic conversion of major depressive disorder to bipolar disorder in pregnancy and postpartum. Bipolar Disord. 2014;16(1):16–21. https://doi.org/10.1111/bdi.12128.
117. Sharma V, Doobay M, Baczynski C. Bipolar postpartum depression: an update and recommendations. J Affect Disord. 2017;219:105–11. https://doi.org/10.1016/j.jad.2017.05.014.
118. Sharma V, Sharma P, Sharma S. Managing bipolar disorder during pregnancy and the postpartum period: a critical review of current practice. Expert Rev Neurother. 2020a;20(4):373–83. https://doi.org/10.1080/14737175.2020.1743684.
119. Sharma V, Singh P, Baczynski C, Khan M. A closer look at the nosological status of the highs (hypomanic symptoms) in the postpartum period. Arch Womens Ment Health. 2020b;24(1):55–62. Available from: http://resolver.scholarsportal.info.libaccess.lib.mcmaster.ca/resolve/14341816/v24i0001/55_aclatnhsitpp.xml.
120. Sharma V, Singh P, Baczynski C, Khan M. A closer look at the nosological status of the highs (hypomanic symptoms) in the postpartum period. Arch Womens Ment Health. 2021;24(1):55–62. https://doi.org/10.1007/s00737-020-01023-1.
121. Sharma V, Mazmanian D, Eccles H. Relationship of premenstrual dysphoric disorder with bipolar disorder: a systematic review. J Clin Psychiatry. 2022;83:22r14416. https://doi.org/10.4088/JCP.22r14416.

122. Slyepchenko A, Frey BN, Lafer B, Nierenberg AA, Sachs GS, Dias RS. Increased illness burden in women with comorbid bipolar and premenstrual dysphoric disorder: data from 1,099 women from STEP-BD study. Acta Psychiatr Scand. 2017a;136:473–82. https://doi.org/10.1111/acps.12797.
123. Slyepchenko A, Minuzzi L, Frey BN, et al. Premenstrual dysphoric disorder and bipolar disorder: a review of comorbidity and treatment implications. J Psychiatr Res. 2017b;90:63–70.
124. Slyepchenko A, Minuzzi L, Frey BN. Comorbid premenstrual dysphoric disorder and bipolar disorder: a review. Front Psych. 2021a;12:719241. https://doi.org/10.3389/fpsyt.2021.719241.
125. Slyepchenko A, Minuzzi L, Frey BN, et al. The clinical correlates of comorbid premenstrual dysphoric disorder and bipolar disorder. J Affect Disord. 2021b;282:69–76.
126. Smith M, Frey BN. Treating comorbid premenstrual dysphoric disorder in women with bipolar disorder. J Psychiatry Neurosci. 2016;41(2):E22–3. https://doi.org/10.1503/jpn.150073.
127. Soares CN, Cohen LS. The perimenopause and mood disturbances: an update. CNS Spectr. 2001;6:167–74.
128. Soares CN, Taylor V. Effects and management of the menopausal transition in women with depression and bipolar disorder. J Clin Psychiatry. 2007;68(Suppl 9):16–21.
129. Soares CN, Almeida OP, Joffe H, Cohen LS. Efficacy of estradiol for the treatment of depressive disorders in perimenopausal women: a double-blind, randomized, placebo-controlled trial. Arch Gen Psychiatry. 2001;58:529–34. https://doi.org/10.1001/archpsyc.58.6.529.
130. Soules MR, Sherman S, Parrott E, Rebar R, Santoro N, Utian W, Woods N. Executive summary: Stages of Reproductive Aging Workshop (STRAW). Climacteric. 2001;4:267–72.
131. Straub L, Hernández-Díaz S, Bateman BT, Wisner KL, Gray KJ, Pennell PB, Lester B, McDougle CJ, Suarez EA, Zhu Y, Zakoul H, Mogun H, Huybrechts KF. Association of antipsychotic drug exposure in pregnancy with risk of neurodevelopmental disorders: a national birth cohort study. JAMA Intern Med. 2022;182(5):522–33. https://doi.org/10.1001/jamainternmed.2022.0375.
132. Syan SK, Minuzzi L, Costescu D, et al. Neurobiological features of premenstrual dysphoric disorder and bipolar disorder: a pilot study. J Psychiatr Res. 2018;105:124–31.
133. Teatero ML, Mazmanian D, Sharma V. Effects of the menstrual cycle on bipolar disorder. Bipolar Disord. 2014a;16:22–36. https://doi.org/10.1111/bdi.12138.
134. Teatero ML, Mazmanian D, Sharma V. The prevalence and determinants of premenstrual dysphoric disorder in bipolar disorder. J Affect Disord. 2014b;166:14–20.
135. Tebeka S, Godin O, Mazer N, Bellivier F, Courtet P, Etain B, Gard S, Leboyer M, Llorca PM, Loftus J, Olié E, Passerieux C, Polosan M, Schwan R, Belzeaux R, Dubertret C, FondaMental Advanced Centers of Expertise in Bipolar Disorders (FACE-BD) Collaborators. Clinical characteristics of bipolar disorders with postpartum depressive onset. Prog Neuro-Psychopharmacol Biol Psychiatry. 2021;107:110225. https://doi.org/10.1016/j.pnpbp.2020.110225.
136. The 2022 hormone therapy position statement of the North American Menopause Society. Menopause (New York, N.Y.). 2022;29(7):767-794. https://doi.org/10.1097/GME.0000000000002028
137. Thomson M, Sharma V. Between a rock-a-bye and a hard place: mood disorders during the perinatal period. CNS Spectr. 2000;22:49–64.
138. Thys-Jacobs S, Starkey P, Bernstein D, Tian J. Calcium carbonate and the premenstrual syndrome: effects on premenstrual and menstrual symptoms. Am J Obstet Gynecol. 1998;179:444–52. https://doi.org/10.1016/s0002-9378(98)70377-1.
139. Tomson T, Battino D, Bromley R, Kochen S, Meador KJ, Pennell PB, Thomas SV. Breastfeeding while on treatment with antiseizure medications: a systematic review from the ILAE Women Task Force. Epileptic Disord. 2022;24(6):1020–32. https://doi.org/10.1684/epd.2022.1492.
140. Truong D, Marsh W. Bipolar disorder in the menopausal transition. Curr Psychiatry Rep. 2019;21:1–7.

141. Uguz F. Second-generation antipsychotics during the lactation period: a comparative systematic review on infant safety. J Clin Psychopharmacol. 2016;36:244–52.
142. VanderKruik R, Barreix M, Chou D, Allen T, Say L, Cohen LS, Barbour K, Cecatti JG, Cottler S, Fawole O, Firoz T, Gadama L, Ghérissi A, Gyte G, Hindin M, Jayathilaka A, Kalamar A, Kone Y, Lange I, Magee LA, Mathur A, Binns AMC, Morgan M, Munjanja S, Gichuhi GN, Petzold M, Sullivan E, Taulo F, Tunçalp Ö, von Dadelszen P. The global prevalence of postpartum psychosis: a systematic review. BMC Psychiatry. 2017;17:1–9. https://doi.org/10.1186/s12888-017-1427-7.
143. Vigod SN, Frey BN, Soares CN, Steiner M. Approach to premenstrual dysphoria for the mental health practitioner. Psychiatr Clin North Am. 2010;33:257–72. https://doi.org/10.1016/j.psc.2010.01.008.
144. Viguera AC, Nonacs R, Cohen LS, Tondo L, Murray A, Baldessarini RJ. Risk of recurrence of bipolar disorder in pregnant and nonpregnant women after discontinuing lithium maintenance. Am J Psychiatry. 2000;157:179–84.
145. Viguera AC, Whitfield T, Baldessarini RJ, Newport DJ, Stowe Z, Reminick A, Zurick A, Cohen LS. Risk of recurrence in women with bipolar disorder during pregnancy: prospective study of mood stabilizer discontinuation. Am J Psychiatry. 2007;164(12):1817–24.
146. Wesseloo R, Kamperman AM, Munk-Olsen T, Pop VJ, Kushner SA, Bergink V. Risk of postpartum relapse in bipolar disorder and postpartum psychosis: a systematic review and meta-analysis. Am J Psychiatry. 2016;173:117–27. https://doi.org/10.1176/appi.ajp.2015.15010124.
147. Wesseloo R, Liu X, Clark CT, et al. Risk of postpartum episodes in women with bipolar disorder after lamotrigine or lithium use during pregnancy: a population-based cohort study. J Affect Disord. 2017a;218:394–7.
148. Wesseloo R, Wierdsma AI, Van Kamp IL, et al. Lithium dosing strategies during pregnancy and the postpartum period. Br J Psychiatry. 2017b;211:31–6.
149. Whedon JM, Kizhakke Veettil A, Rugo NA, et al. Bioidentical estrogen for menopausal depressive symptoms: a systematic review and meta-analysis. J Womens Health (Larchmt). 2017;26:18–28.
150. Wisner KL, Sit DK, McShea MC, Rizzo DM, Zoretich RA, Hughes CL, et al. Onset timing, thoughts of self-harm, and diagnoses in postpartum women with screen-positive depression findings. JAMA Psychiatry. 2013;70:490–8. https://doi.org/10.1001/jamapsychiatry.2013.300.
151. Wittchen H-U. Bipolar disorder in women with premenstrual dysphoric disorder. J Clin Psychiatry. 2022;83(3)
152. Wyatt KM, Dimmock PW, Jones PW, O'Brien PMS. Efficacy of vitamin B-6 in the treatment of premenstrual syndrome: systematic review. BMJ. 1999;318:1375–81. https://doi.org/10.1136/bmj.318.7195.1375.
153. Yatham LN, Kennedy SH, Parikh SV, Schaffer A, Bond DJ, Frey BN, Sharma V, Goldstein BI, Rej S, Beaulieu S, Alda M, MacQueen G, Milev RV, Ravindran A, O'Donovan C, McIntosh D, Lam RW, Vazquez G, Kapczinski F, McIntyre RS, Kozicky J, Kanba S, Lafer B, Suppes T, Calabrese JR, Vieta E, Malhi G, Post RM, Berk M. Canadian Network for Mood and Anxiety Treatments (CANMAT) and International Society for Bipolar Disorders (ISBD) 2018 guidelines for the management of patients with bipolar disorder. Bipolar Disord. 2018;20(2):97–170. https://doi.org/10.1111/bdi.12609.
154. Yonkers KA, Simoni MK. Premenstrual disorders. Am J Obstet Gynecol. 2018;218:68–74. https://doi.org/10.1016/j.ajog.2017.05.045.
155. Yonkers KA, O'Brien PMS, Eriksson E. Premenstrual syndrome. Lancet. 2008;371:1200–10. https://doi.org/10.1016/S0140-6736(08)60527-9.
156. Zimmerman M, Galione JN, Ruggero CJ, Chelminski I, Dalrymple K, Young D. Are screening scales for bipolar disorder good enough to be used in clinical practice? Compr Psychiatry. 2011;52(6):600–6.

Chapter 9
Senior's Mental Health and Latent Stage in Bipolar Disorder

Dante Duarte, Anne-Marie Di Passa, Shelby Prokop-Millar, and Horodjei Yaya

Clinical Tips

- Clinicians should be aware of the risk factors for latent-stage bipolar disorder in older patients. For example, older adults with a late-onset depression diagnosis warrant careful attention.
- Bipolar disorder in the elderly is associated with medical comorbidities, functional impairments, and neurodegenerative factors, all of which require thoughtful consideration when developing treatment regimens.

Authors Anne-Marie Di Passa, Shelby Prokop-Millar and Horodjei Yaya have equally contributed to this chapter.

D. Duarte (✉)
Department of Psychiatry and Behavioural Neurosciences, McMaster University, Hamilton, ON, Canada

Seniors Mental Health Program, Department of Psychiatry and Neurosciences, McMaster University, Hamilton, ON, Canada
e-mail: dduarte@stjosham.on.ca

A.-M. Di Passa · S. Prokop-Millar
Department of Psychiatry and Behavioural Neurosciences, McMaster University, Hamilton, ON, Canada

Peter Boris Centre for Addictions Research, St Joseph's Healthcare Hamilton, Hamilton, ON, Canada

H. Yaya
Peter Boris Centre for Addictions Research, St Joseph's Healthcare Hamilton, Hamilton, ON, Canada

T. de Azevedo Cardoso et al. (eds.), *Latent Bipolar Disorder*,
https://doi.org/10.1007/978-3-032-01297-5_9

- If a potential case of latent-stage bipolar disorder is determined, it is also important to screen for neurocognitive disorders, such as behavioral frontotemporal dementia.

9.1 Bipolar Disorder in the Elderly

As discussed in earlier chapters, bipolar disorder (BD) can often be misdiagnosed as major depressive disorder (MDD) in its early stages. Elderly populations also face such misdiagnoses, likely due to BD presenting with an early age of onset, with most individuals experiencing an onset of illness before the age of 30 [7]. In the late 1980s, late-onset BD was defined as an onset of BD after age 50, which was estimated to affect approximately 10% of those who acquired the disorder [72]. Almost two decades later, a study of 87 senior BD inpatients presented results indicating that only 2% of individuals exhibited an onset after 60 [20]. Thus, late-onset BD appeared to be a less common phenomenon in the elderly, with most patients with BD showing signs and symptoms well before the age of 50.

In a 2014 review of 18 studies [22], Dols and colleagues reported an astounding 44.2% of older adults with BD experienced late-onset mania—that is, experienced manic symptoms only after age of 50. Is it possible that such individuals were in the latent stage of BD and had yet to develop mania? The conceptualization of latent-stage BD provides a critical framework for understanding the progression of BD from its infancy to full-blown stages. The latent-stage bipolar framework can be applied to the traditional conceptualizations of "early-" versus "late-" onset BD (Fig. 9.1).

The length of the latent stage versus the active stage is an important factor to examine. Consider patient A—an 82-year-old patient with BD who developed early-onset BD at the age of 30. That is, his active stage is longer than his latent stage. Now consider patient B—an 82-year-old patient with BD who developed BD at 60. His latent stage was longer than his current active stage. If the length of the latent stage is prolonged into late adulthood (>50 years old) and thus is late-onset BD, would patient B have a poorer prognosis? The short answer is we do not know, as literature on BD in the elderly remains sparse. Some data suggests that cognitive functioning is significantly more impaired in older adults with BD who experienced late-onset versus early-onset BD [58]. Moreover, late-onset BD in elderly patients has also been associated with neurovascular complications [16] and severe cognitive impairments [37].

Fig. 9.1 (continued) After consulting a mental health clinic, Samira and her husband were informed that she was experiencing a manic episode. Following psychiatric evaluation, Samira was given a diagnosis of late-onset BD. Her diagnosis would be classified as late-onset, as she began experiencing manic symptoms and/or a BD diagnosis after the age of 50. According to the latent-stage BD framework, Samira's latent stage began around age 20 and continued until her 60th birthday, when she transitioned to the active stage. In cases of late-onset BD, the latent stage may persist for years before progressing to the active stage

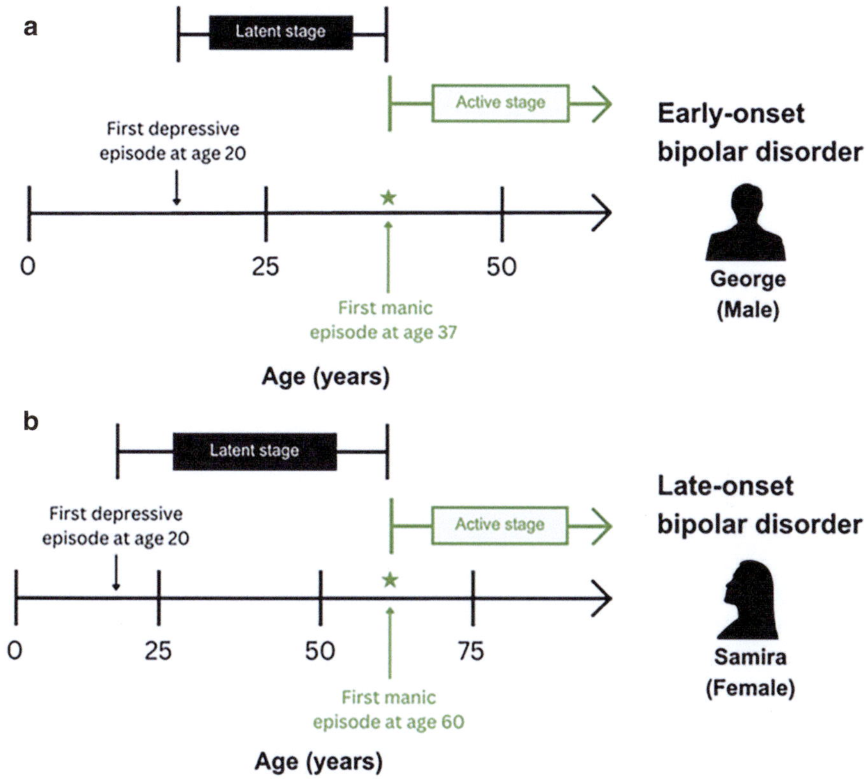

Fig. 9.1 Applying the latent bipolar framework to early-onset and late-onset bipolar disorder (**a**) A fictitious case of early-onset bipolar disorder. George was a university student who first experienced a major depressive episode at the age of 20. After consulting his family doctor, he was diagnosed with major depressive disorder (MDD) and began therapy to treat his condition. Although George felt he somewhat benefited from therapy, he continued to express feelings of a low mood and experienced recurring depressive symptoms over the years. At 37, George's family grew increasingly concerned about his unusual behavior. His mother reported to his family doctor that he had stopped sleeping at night, claiming he "didn't need it," and that he was much more talkative than usual. After being referred to a psychiatrist, George was diagnosed with bipolar disorder (BD) and began taking lithium to treat his manic symptoms. George's case exemplifies early-onset BD, as his manic symptoms and diagnosis occurred before the age of 50. Applying the latent BD framework, the "latent stage" refers to the period when George exhibited symptoms (e.g., a major depressive episode) without yet receiving a BD diagnosis, primarily due to the absence of manic symptoms. The onset of his manic symptoms at age 37 marked the transition to the "active stage," during which his symptom presentation warranted a BD diagnosis. (**b**) A fictitious case of late-onset bipolar disorder. Samira, a nursing student, experienced her first major depressive episode at the age of 20. She found herself struggling to fall asleep, feeling "numb," and began to withdraw from her friends by ignoring their messages. Unsure of how to cope, Samira contacted her family doctor for help and was prescribed escitalopram to manage her depressive symptoms. Over the years, she attended counselling sessions, during which she received an MDD diagnosis. Throughout her life, Samira turned to therapy as a trusted coping mechanism during flare-ups, feeling that escitalopram was only somewhat effective. Shortly after her 60th birthday, Samira's husband observed a notable change in her behavior: she was increasingly agitated, spoke very quickly, and would spend hundreds of dollars on clothes and furniture.

Table 9.1 Health complications in older adults with bipolar disorder

Medical complications	Functional impairments	Neurodegenerative factors
Higher rates of endocrine, metabolic, and respiratory illness compared to patients with MDD [28] Higher cardiovascular mortality rates compared to HC [68] Higher mortality rates [2] Greater risk of dementia [2] Cognitive impairment [42, 59, 65] and reduced cognitive functioning [17]	Difficulty with interpersonal relationships [17] Diminished psychosocial functioning [17] Poor social functioning [46] Lack of autonomy [17] Financial issues [17] Deficits in occupational functioning [17] Impaired executive functioning [14]	Reduced caudate volume compared to younger BD patients [12] Decreased FA in the ventral corpus callosum relative to HC [30] Decreased grey matter in the right anterior insula, caudate nucleus, nucleus accumbens, ventral putamen, and frontal orbital cortex (vs. HC; [30]) Smaller hippocampal and amygdala volumes (vs. HC) [69] Reduced grey matter in the interior frontal lobe (vs. HC) [11]

Abbreviations: *BD* bipolar disorder, *FA* fractional anisotropy, *HC* healthy controls, *MDD* major depressive disorder

BD is a challenging psychiatric disorder with a high rate of burden [56]. In older adults, this burden is amplified. With the added complication of age, BD can give rise to numerous health complications in older adults. Older adults with BD experience higher mortality rates, reduced cognitive functioning, and increased neurodegeneration relative to their healthy—or even unipolar depressed—counterparts. A detailed summary of medical complications, functional impairments, and neurodegenerative factors in older adults with BD is presented in Table 9.1.

Considering the high prevalence of medical comorbidities, functional impairments, and increased risk of mortality in older adults with active bipolar disorder, identifying the risk factors of the conversion from latent to active stage BD (i.e., MDD to BD) is a critical and time-sensitive preventative measure. We will discuss risk factors for conversion from MDD to BD in the elderly in Sect. 9.3.

9.2 Rates of Conversion from Depression to Bipolar Disorder in the Elderly

9.2.1 Conversion from MDD to BD: A Case of Misdiagnosis or Latent-Stage Bipolar Disorder?

Several individuals who experience recurrent depressive episodes are later re-diagnosed with bipolar disorder. What may prompt this change? First, let us consider the following two scenarios:

- *Scenario A*: The rarer or more unusual symptoms of bipolar disorder were missed by clinicians, leading to a misdiagnosis of MDD, which was later corrected to BD. This would suggest a general underdiagnosis of BD.
- *Scenario B*: It is a case of latent bipolar disorder, in which the individual initially presented with symptoms warranting a diagnosis of depression (i.e., during their latent phase), with no signs or symptoms of bipolar disorder. Then, with the assistance of some environmental or genetic trigger, the patient fully transitioned to active-stage bipolar, whereby clinicians were able to confidently confirm a diagnosis of BD.

In light of scenario A, consider the study by Lee and colleagues. In 2014, a Korean study [34] investigated a group of 65 elderly patients with recurrent MDD. After administering a questionnaire to detect symptoms of bipolarity, 11 (16.9%) were considered to have bipolar spectrum disorder (BSD)—a classification system recognizing two dimensions of bipolarity: (1) normal to psychotic and (2) depression to mania. The authors emphasize the importance of considering these dimensions to help reduce the current rate of underdiagnosis in BD [3] by highlighting differential aspects of bipolarity. Therefore, it is possible the conversion from MDD to BD is the result of differential symptoms of BD being misdiagnosed, leading to an underdiagnosis of BD in psychiatry.

To consider scenario B, let us explore the following case study: A case study of MDD to BD conversion in an elderly male by Lu et al. [35]. The case study is visually depicted in Fig. 9.2.

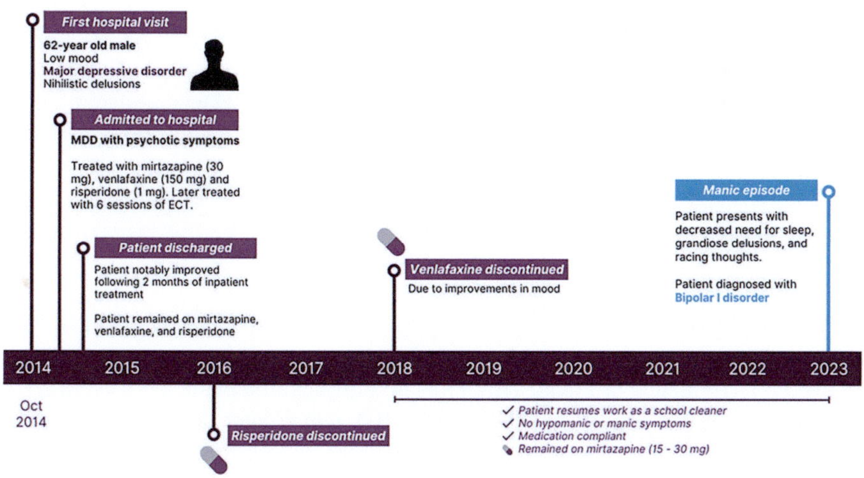

Fig. 9.2 A case study of MDD to BD conversion in an elderly male. (The data presented in this figure is derived from Lu et al. [35])

A Case Study of MDD to BD Conversion in an Elderly Male

In October 2014, a 62-year-old Chinese male visited the hospital with complaints of a deteriorating mood. He had recently been diagnosed with major depressive disorder by a private psychiatrist and had no known physical health issues. The hospital staff noticed the patient's strong nihilistic delusions, and he was later admitted to the hospital for major depressive disorder with psychotic symptoms. He was treated with a combination of mirtazapine (30 mg), venlafaxine (150 mg), and risperidone (1 mg), and later six sessions of electroconvulsive therapy (ECT). Two months later, the patient had notably improved and was discharged. The patient remained on the dose of mirtazapine, venlafaxine, and risperidone for 2 years following discharge. In 2016, the patient stopped taking risperidone (reason not provided). In 2018, he discontinued venlafaxine due to improvements in his mood. He continued to take mirtazapine (30 mg) every night. Over the next 5 years, the patient remained on mirtazapine, sometimes altering between 15 and 30 mg depending on his stress levels, and was monitored routinely at his 6-month follow-ups. During this period, the patient started working again as a school cleaner, did not display any hypomanic or manic symptoms, and was compliant with his medication. In May 2023, at 71 years old, the patient's family brought him to the hospital following a sudden change in his behavior over the previous 2 weeks. The patient was presenting with symptoms of mania—a decreased need for sleep, grandiose delusions, and racing thoughts. The patient had no known family history of mania and did not take any new medications or drugs that would have resulted in a significant behavioral change. After a medical evaluation of blood tests and MRI scans, the results were negative for organic causes that could explain these behavioral changes, so the organic cause was ruled out. The patient was taken off mirtazapine and started a combination of olanzapine (20 mg) and valproic acid (500 mg) to treat the manic episode. The patient was then diagnosed with bipolar I disorder. This case is reported by Lu et al. [35].

The case study presented by Lu et al. [35] provides support for scenario B, considering the patient had recurrent 6-month follow-ups over the course of 9 years and showed no hypomanic or manic symptoms up until his first manic episode in 2023 [35]. It is likely this patient had latent-stage BD, which later manifested its active form. It is important for psychiatrists and clinicians to be informed of the approximate conversion rates from MDD to BD in their elderly patients. However, considering that only 6–8% of new BD cases are in individuals over the age of 60 [29], researchers may be less inclined to explore MDD to BD conversion rates in this population. In fact, there are few studies to date that have examined conversion rates from MDD to BD in older adults. Although few in number, these studies are broken down in Table 9.2.

Table 9.2 Rates of conversion from MDD to BD in the older adults

	Sample characteristics		Rates of conversion				
First author (year)	Sample source	Sample size (N) by age	Follow-up period (yrs)	Key findings	Risk of conversion (IR, HR, etc.)	95% CI	*p*
Elefante et al. [25]	Inpatients and outpatients with LOD (age of onset >60) vs. TOD (age of onset <60)	*Age ≥ 65* (*N* = 57)	1.5	LOD patients had a faster rate of conversion (3×) compared to those with TOD	HR: 3.05	1.07–8.67	0.037
Patel et al. [48]	Community members who accessed mental health care for unipolar depression	*Age 56–65* (*N* = 1869)	Mean: 4.3	Older adults (56–65 yrs) had the lowest IR of developing BD compared to younger age groups	IR: 8.3 (per 1000 person-years) HR: 0.65[a]	0.50–0.85[a]	0.002[a]
Rhee et al. [53]	Individuals registered with MD on a national population-based registry	*Age 50–59* (*N* = 97,825) *Age 60–69* (*N* = 81,340) *Age > 70* (*N* = 26,643)	5	Older adults with MDD had a lower risk of developing BD compared to younger age groups	HR: 0.67 (50–59 yrs) HR: 0.31 (60–69 yrs) HR: 0.12 (> 70 yrs) *Ref. group (40–49 yrs)*	0.57–0.80 0.24–0.40 0.02–0.89	NR NR NR
Kim et al. [33]	Individuals registered with MD from nationwide database	*Age 50–59* (*N* = 198,772) *Age 60–69* (*N* = 151,851) *Age 70–79* (*N* = 119,870) *Age ≥ 80* (*N* = 32,476)	1	Older adults with MDD had lower incidence rates of converting to BD relative to younger age groups	IR: 46.74 (50–59 yrs) IR: 36.73 (60–69 yrs) IR: 41.61 (70–79 yrs) IR: 50.47 (≥ 80 yrs)	44.87–48.69 34.98–38.57 39.60–43.74 46.24–55.09	NR NR NR NR

Abbreviations: *BD* bipolar disorder, *HR* hazard ratio, *IOC* incidence of conversion, *IR* incidence rate, *LOD* late-onset depression, *MD* major depression, *MDD* major depressive disorder, *NR* not reported, *TOD* traditional-onset depression, *yrs* years

[a]Results were adjusted

Overall, the risk of conversion appears to be lower in older adults compared to younger age groups [33, 48, 53]. However, the findings by Elefante et al. [25] reported that individuals with late-onset depression (i.e., age of onset after 60) exhibited a conversion rate from MDD to BD three times higher compared to those with traditional onset depression (i.e., age of onset before 60; [25]). Therefore, though the risk of conversion from MDD to BD appears to be generally lower in older adults compared to younger age groups, clinicians should still take precautions when dealing with older patients who exhibit recurrent or new-onset depressive episodes, as this may be an indicative marker of a higher risk of conversion.

9.3 Risk Factors of Major Depressive Disorder Conversion to Bipolar Disorder in the Elderly

Returning to the issue of misdiagnosing BD as MDD in older adults, it is important to consider that some individuals may experience early-onset depression that is only correctly diagnosed later in life. Several factors contribute to this phenomenon, including the under-recognition of depressive symptoms, societal stigma surrounding mental health, and the development of coping mechanisms.

Now, you might wonder how clinicians can avoid a delayed diagnosis of MDD. Well, some people develop coping mechanisms or adaptive strategies to manage their depressive symptoms, especially if they have experienced depression earlier in life. These coping strategies could involve self-reliance, seeking social support, or engaging in activities that distract from or alleviate depressive feelings [5]. While these coping mechanisms may work effectively in the short term, they could also mask underlying depressive symptoms and delay recognition and diagnosis until later in life, when the individual's coping resources become depleted or less effective [5].

In addition to the delayed diagnosis of depression in older adults, there is also the possibility that individuals in this age group may have had latent bipolar disorder that only becomes diagnosed later in life. Some older adults who were previously diagnosed with MDD may actually have had underlying BD that was not recognized earlier. This delayed diagnosis of bipolar disorder in older adults may be attributed to several factors. In this section, we will discuss risk factors that lead to the conversion from MDD to BD in older adults.

9.3.1 Family History of Bipolar Disorder

One of the primary risk factors for the conversion from MDD to BD in the elderly population is a family history of BD. Numerous studies have emphasized how robust genetic factors play a role in the onset of BD in seniors [57]. In a retrospective study conducted by Moorhead and Young [43], they used a UK psychiatric case registry to assess the age of onset among patients diagnosed with bipolar I disorder [43]. Researchers discovered that within the subset of patients displaying mania or bipolar disorder alongside neurological lesions, another contributing risk factor to the disorder, genetic predisposition, remains significant in geriatric bipolar disorders [43]. Research has found that within the subset of older bipolar disorder patients with neurological comorbidities, there remains a high prevalence of positive family history among first-degree relatives [43, 57]. These findings highlight the importance of conducting comprehensive family assessments when evaluating elderly individuals with MDD, as a positive family history may warrant closer monitoring and potential consideration of BD as a diagnosis.

9.3.2 The Discontinuation of Lithium

Antidepressants are frequently prescribed to geriatric patients to treat MDD. However, for those patients who do not respond well to them, a combination of antidepressants and lithium is often considered as an alternative. Lithium, a mood stabilizer, has been used to enhance the effectiveness of antidepressant medication and has seen a significant rise since its initial description in an open-label trial [18]. Studies have revealed that lithium can enhance the effects of various antidepressants, such as selective serotonin reuptake inhibitors (SSRIs) [10]. Furthermore, there have been no reports of serious side effects associated with the combination of lithium and antidepressants [44, 55], and as a result, this approach has been advocated as a primary strategy for individuals with treatment-resistant depression [9]. However, various studies, such as the study conducted by Bauer et al. [9], have shown the adverse effects of discontinuing lithium, which can lead to the risk of mood disorder recurrence, especially in MDD and BD.

Dr. Bauer and his team initiated a double-blind, placebo-controlled trial to explore the efficacy of adding lithium to antidepressant medication in the ongoing treatment of unipolar major depression [9]. Within this study, a total of 75 subjects who had not responded to antidepressants were enrolled. The average duration of antidepressant treatment before incorporating lithium was 46.1 days. Throughout the subsequent 6-week acute treatment phase with lithium augmentation, participants remained on the same antidepressant regimen. Of those diagnosed with MDD, with no evidence of bipolar disorder or suicidality, and exhibiting inadequate response to antidepressants over 1 month, 41 out of 75 individuals (54.7%) displayed signs of improvement following open-label lithium treatment for a duration of 8–10 weeks.

Following this initial phase, 30 patients underwent further assessment, with one participant opting to withdraw from the study. Of the remaining 29 subjects, 14 were randomly assigned to continue lithium therapy, and 15 were randomly assigned to transition to a placebo while maintaining antidepressant treatment for an additional 4 months. Upon lithium discontinuation, seven out of the 15 patients in the placebo group (46.7%) experienced a relapse, with five of these individuals (71.4%) experiencing depressive symptoms and two (28.6%) displaying manic features. Tragically, one participant (6.7%) from the placebo group died by suicide. Consequently, two out of the initial 30 individuals diagnosed with unipolar depression (6.7%), both of whom were from the placebo group (13.3%), received a subsequent diagnosis of bipolar disorder. These developments occurred within a span of 4 months, with an average duration of 4 weeks following the discontinuation of lithium treatment.

Many studies have found a high risk of conversion from MDD to BD after lithium discontinuation; however, in Dr. Bauer and colleagues' study, the conversion rate of switching from MDD to BD was substantially higher—70 times greater, to be exact. These patients may have exhibited latent bipolar disorder, initially presenting with symptoms resembling unipolar depression and undergoing antidepressant treatment without lithium protection. Generally, individuals with depression who fail to respond to antidepressant therapy may harbor an elevated risk of BD.

9.3.3 Cerebrovascular Disease

Cerebrovascular disease is another risk factor for converting from MDD to BD in older adults. It encompasses a range of conditions impacting blood vessels and blood flow to the brain, including blood clots and stroke [15]. Specifically, cerebrovascular diseases include stroke, transient ischemic attack (TIA), aneurysm, and vascular malformation. In the elderly, BD, particularly secondary mania resulting from medical comorbidities or neurological causes [24], has been documented in 17–43% of manic cases [26]. This form of bipolar disorder has been associated with a higher prevalence of cerebral organic disorders, such as cerebrovascular disease, dementia, space-occupying lesions, infections, and head injury [26]. In a study conducted by Fujikawa et al. [26], they discovered a higher prevalence of silent cerebral infarctions in patients diagnosed with BD after age 50 and in those with MDD, compared to individuals with early-onset MDD. As such, these findings must be interpreted in the context of higher cerebrovascular risk factors in late-onset BD individuals, which may predict a poorer prognosis compared to those with early-onset bipolar disorder [62].

A Case Study of Cerebrovascular Risk Factor in Late-Onset BD in an Elderly Woman

E., a 72-year-old woman, began experiencing severe major depressive episodes at 58, leading to three inpatient admissions over 3 years (two at 58, one at 61). During the third admission, she exhibited psychotic symptoms, mainly suspiciousness and persecutory delusions. Despite treatment with imipramine and fluoxetine, her depressive symptoms did not improve, but she responded well to electroconvulsive therapy (ECT). Her family history includes two sisters with a history of major depressive disorder. At 61, after discharge, she developed talkativeness, restlessness, and an elevated mood typical of a hypomanic episode. She was started on lithium, but frequent depressive episodes persisted. At 62, she underwent 15 sessions of bilateral ECT due to severe depression. Over 6 years, E. remained on regular maintenance pharmacological antidepressant treatment. At 68, she experienced a full-blown manic phase while using nortriptyline and lithium. During this manic episode, she needed constant supervision and was unable to carry out her usual activities. Symptoms lasted nearly a month and remitted after reducing the nortriptyline dose and adjusting the lithium dosage. Over the last 3 years, she has often experienced rapid mood shifts from depression to hypomania, with one manic and two hypomanic episodes. There were also major depressive episodes, one requiring hospital admission in 2005. During that admission, she was prescribed olanzapine and lamotrigine, but depressive symptoms remitted only after unilateral ECT administrations. Since then, E. has been under regular maintenance ECT treatment. She has a history of hypertension, hypercholesterolemia, subclinical hypothyroidism, and psoriasis. However, neurological symptoms such as falls and facial paresis began at 66. At 70, a brain MRI revealed hypersignal lesions in T2 and FLAIR in subcortical and periventricular white matter hyperintensities (WHM). The full case is reported elsewhere [73].

The case study by Zanetti et al. [73] provides support that cerebrovascular disease, like brain lesions, may contribute to the conversion of MDD to BD in older adults. In E's case, T2 weighted MRI images revealed WMH, which are bright lesions resulting from localized alterations in cerebral tissue composition [8, 73]. Several studies have shown that these lesions are often ischemic among elderly individuals with depression [64]. Vascular abnormalities affecting areas in the brain critical for mood regulation may contribute to depressive syndrome [1]. Therefore, it is plausible that ischemic white matter lesions could play a role in developing late-onset BD following MDD. In numerous studies, it has been demonstrated that the majority of patients experiencing late-onset BD go through a significant period of latency, often spanning years, from the emergence of the first depressive symptom to the onset of the first manic episode [60, 61, 73]. Hence, these findings suggest that brain lesions may contribute to the transition from MDD to bipolar illness.

Going back to E's case, it is possible that the development of WMH over time played a crucial role in the conversation between MDD and BD. This is because E did not have any family history of BD, and the use of tricyclic antidepressants (i.e., imipramine and fluoxetine) during the early stages of her MDD did not trigger any manic episodes. Hence, these details suggest that during E's depressive episodes, it is possible that she had latent bipolar disorder, and her manic episodes only became apparent during the progression of WHM associated with cerebrovascular disease.

Discoveries like these could be instrumental in raising awareness about the potential connection between cerebrovascular disease and the development of manic episodes in older adults, which presents additional complexities and challenges in management. In the next section, we will explore how to differentiate between latent bipolar disorder and dementia in older adults, considering the close association between cerebrovascular disease and dementia.

9.4 How to Differentiate Latent-Stage Bipolar and Dementia as a Diagnosis

To properly identify latent-stage bipolar versus dementia as a diagnosis, it is important to reflect on the current literature pertaining to BD and dementia as a whole.

The global prevalence of dementia was estimated to be 57.4 million as of 2019 and is predicted to rise to 152.8 million by 2050 [27]. With the cost of dementia worldwide believed to be $1313.4 billion USD as of 2019, when accounting for 55.2 million individuals inflicted by the condition [70].

There are a multitude of disorders that fall under the classification of "dementia." Such disorders include Alzheimer's disease, vascular dementia, dementia with Lewy bodies, and frontotemporal dementia, among others. Symptoms of dementia comprise a decrease in one's capacity to function on a daily basis (e.g., the inability to care for oneself) and two or more impairments to one's cognition (e.g., executive function and memory), as well as a noticeable deterioration in one's functional abilities as compared to their state before the onset of their current condition [4].

A diagnosis of BD increases one's risk of developing dementia by almost three times [66]. The more episodes one has, the more at risk they are for developing dementia [66].

Individuals with behavioral variant frontotemporal dementia (bvFTD) can be mistaken for having BD and vice versa, as both disorders can present with similar symptom profiles [36]. Such symptoms include anhedonia, irritability, lack of interest, and impulsivity, to name a few [36]. BvFTD was misdiagnosed as a psychiatric condition 52.7% of the time, as compared to Alzheimer's disease and two other presentations of FTD, non-fluent primary progressive aphasia and semantic variant primary progressive aphasia [71]. Such disorders as bvFTD were originally misdiagnosed as schizophrenia and BD [71].

Interestingly, it has been speculated that BD may eventually progress into FTD in some patients [54]. Papazacharias et al. [47] touched on the idea of BD potentially being a "prodromal state" in the lead-up to the development of FTD. Mendez et al. [38] suggested that late-onset BD may also be a prodromal manifestation of bvFTD in a subset of patients as well.

As stated above, frontotemporal dementia (FTD) is one of the many disorders that fall under the classification of dementia. The prevalence of FTD varies based on the age of the population investigated [31]. For those younger than 65 years of age, the prevalence of FTD is 10.2%. Whereas for those 65 years of age and older, the prevalence of FTD is 2.7%. There are several different presentations of FTD that can occur such as bvFTD, non-fluent primary progressive aphasia, semantic variant primary progressive aphasia, etc. But, for the purpose of this chapter, bvFTD will be the primary focus of our discussion [45, 51].

The average age of onset for bvFTD is approximately 58 years old [50]. Furthermore, three of the six diagnostic features listed must be present for an individual to receive a diagnosis: apathy, compulsions, disinhibition, hyperorality, executive dysfunction, and lack of empathy [45].

To better identify latent-stage BD versus dementia, the remaining part of this chapter will compare the clinical presentations of bvFTD to latent-stage BD, with an emphasis on the current literature pertaining to BD. For a brief breakdown of the findings, please refer to Table 9.3.

Table 9.3 Differences between behavioral variant frontotemporal dementia and bipolar disorder

	Behavior	Cognitive	Neurophysiology
Bipolar disorder	NA	Performed better on VF (in mood episode) Greater executive dysfunction, VM, WM, and attention (when in a mood episode) Appear to stay stagnant over time	Greater GM reduction in the VLPFC
Behavioral variant frontotemporal dementia	Hyperorality + dietary changes Ritualistic + compulsive behaviors	Greater executive dysfunction, specifically in AC, VF, WCSTc (in comparison to euthymic BD) Greater ToM impairment (in comparison to euthymic BD) Appear to progress over time particularly in nonverbal and verbal memory in the RAD—NAB and MMSE	Greater and/or unique GM reductions in CC, FG, SMA, DLPFC, IG, FMA, PSL, and ITL

Abbreviations: AC abstraction capacity, *BD* bipolar disorder, *CC* cingulate cortex, *DLPFC* dorsolateral prefrontal cortex, *FG* fusiform gyrus, *FMA* frontal medial area, *GM* grey matter, *IG* inferior gyrus, *ITL* inferior temporal lobe, *MMSE* Mini Mental State Examination, *NA* not applicable, *PSL* parietal superior lobe, *RAD–NAB* Registry for Alzheimer's Disease–Neuropsychological Assessment Battery, *SMA* supplementary motor area, *ToM* Theory of Mind, *TPN* temporo-parietal network, *VF* verbal fluency, *VIC* verbal inhibitory control, *VLPFC* ventrolateral prefrontal cortex, *VM* verbal memory, *WCSTc* Wisconsin Card Sorting Task categories, *WM* working memory

9.4.1 Behavioral Differences

There are two distinct behaviors found within bvFTD that are not present within BD or are incredibly unlikely to be that could help a clinician identify latent-stage BD over bvFTD. Such behaviors include marked dietary changes and/or hyperorality and ritualistic and/or compulsive behaviors that are typically related to bvFTD [23, 36, 45].

Hyperorality and dietary changes are symptoms found within bvFTD [52]. Fifty-nine percent of those with bvFTD will experience hyperorality. Though a less common presentation of bvFTD when compared to apathy (84%), it can allow for a clearer differentiation, when present, from BD. An individual with bvFTD may begin placing inedible objects within their mouth and even attempt to consume the object. Food preferences may change, such as a preference towards carbohydrates, and the patient may begin to engage in binge eating behavior, with the patient continuously eating past the point of satiety [39, 49, 52].

Ritualistic and compulsive behaviors are commonly found within bvFTD. Approximately 60–64% of those with bvFTD will experience repetitive behaviors throughout the course of their illness, including ritualistic and/or obsessive-compulsive-like behaviors [40, 41]. With 47% of those with bvFTD experiencing such behaviors during the initial presentation of the disorder. Such behaviors include stereotyped speech, hoarding, compulsive cleaning, repeated movements, and checking.

9.4.2 Cognition

Though bvFTD and BD have a multitude of similarities behaviorally speaking, there are potential differences found within cognition that can assist clinicians in distinguishing latent-stage BD and bvFTD more clearly.

When examining differences between bvFTD and BD within euthymia, it appears that those with bvFTD have severe impairments within theory of mind and executive functioning as compared to BD [6, 54]. Specifically, within abstraction capacity, verbal inhibitory control, verbal fluency, and the Wisconsin Card Sorting Task categories.

In respect to BD in an active mood episode (whether depressive or manic), individuals with BD seem to perform better than bvFTD within verbal fluency as well, especially within animal naming [54, 67]. However, this is not true for verbal memory, attention, executive function, and working memory, where individuals with bvFTD performed better than those with BD in an active mood episode.

Cognitive symptoms within individuals with late-onset BD seem to be maintained over time and to not progress further over an average 33-month period, according to a meta-analysis by Szmulewicz et al. [63]. For bvFTD, a significant reduction in scores on both the Consortium to Establish a Registry for Alzheimer's

Disease—Neuropsychological Assessment Battery (particularly within nonverbal and verbal memory, as well as naming; there was no significant reduction found in visuoconstruction, category fluency, and recognition) and the Mini-Mental-State-Examination was found after an average 13-month follow-up in a study by Diehl-Schmid et al. [21]. Though the reduction in scores was significant, the results within certain cognitive tasks were quite heterogeneous, resulting in high standard deviations.

9.4.3 Neurophysiology

Unfortunately, there are only two articles that address the matter of utilizing imaging to distinguish between bvFTD and BD. Based on their findings via the use of either magnetic resonance imaging (MRI) or combined MRI and positron emission tomography (PET), reductions in grey matter seem to be significantly worse in individuals with bvFTD as opposed to older adults with BD.

Alterations within temporal grey matter were found to be greater within individuals with bvFTD. Particularly, larger volume reductions within grey matter, specifically in the inferior lobe, and metabolic dysfunction were evident within the temporal region [6, 19]. Frontal grey matter reductions were also greater in bvFTD, but only in specific regions such as the dorsolateral prefrontal cortex, inferior gyrus, and frontal medial area. However, grey matter reductions within the ventrolateral prefrontal cortex were more significant in older adults with BD. Interestingly, Delvecchio et al. [19] found that the areas within the temporo-parietal network had volume loss that was distinctive in individuals with bvFTD. Baez et al. [6] also found that individuals with bvFTD had remarkable volume loss compared to individuals with BD in the superior parietal lobe, fusiform gyrus, supplementary motor area, and cingulate cortex.

9.4.4 Case Study Review: Frontotemporal Dementia Mistaken for Latent-Stage Bipolar?

As broken down in the case study conducted by Kerstein et al. [32], the patient evaluated appeared to be potentially displaying symptoms mimicking latent-stage BD within an older adult, though it was determined to be FTD in the end. This case study highlights the importance of being able to clinically distinguish between the two disorders/concepts.

The patient appeared to have a profile similar to that of latent-stage BD in an older adult, as covered in this chapter. The patient exhibited risk factors of latent-stage BD within an older adult, such as a family history of BD and a potential case of late-onset depression (though it is unclear when what was thought to be hypomanic symptoms began), eventually "converting" to BD II.

As explained, two out of the four risk factors of latent-stage BD in an older adult were present in the patient. However, as seen in this case, it is still important to also assess the patient for FTD if suspected latent-stage BD is present, as they carry common symptom profiles. To allow for a more clear-cut diagnosis, a clinician should consider requesting diagnostic imaging and a neuropsychological evaluation to be conducted on the patient. Table 9.3 highlights what a clinician should specifically look for when differentiating between the two conditions.

Case Study: Frontotemporal Dementia Mistaken for Latent-Stage Bipolar?

A Caucasian male, 65 years of age, presented to a psychiatric clinic. Upon evaluation, medical professionals concluded that the patient was likely experiencing bipolar II disorder. The patient's mother was diagnosed with bipolar disorder and was treated with lithium. Three years prior to his evaluation, the patient had been struggling at work, feeling consistently fatigued and depressed, as well as overwhelmed and anhedonic. In the 2 months after his retirement, the patient seemed to improve, helping out at his church, engaging in childcare, doing work around his yard, and helping a friend with construction at their home. The patient began to find it difficult adapting to his new life after retirement, specifically being around his wife more often than before. As a result, the patient lost 25 pounds and would typically only sleep for 2–3 hours per night. At evaluation the patient was labile but had no psychotic features; he also seemed to be absorbed with his current circumstance. Though unhappy about it, the patient described himself as being incredibly active as well as more talkative and energetic. The patient was originally brought into the clinic for his attraction to a teenager; the patient also mentioned having an increased libido. In the past, the patient did mention experiencing times in which he would irresponsibly spend, have sleepless nights, work more, and eat less. The patient was prescribed 600 mg of lithium carbonate, 1 mg of risperidone, and 1–2 mg of lorazepam. Two months into taking lithium, it was discontinued as the patient was not adherent. Eventually, the patient's risperidone was switched to 15 mg of aripiprazole (and was moved down to 2 mg months later). Throughout treatment, the patient lacked motivation and was anhedonic. At this point in time, the patient was finally assessed for dementia. The Mini-Mental State Examination was utilized, in which the patient scores a 20/30, representative of dementia. A neuropsychological assessment was administered in which the following cognitive deficits were found within working memory, executive functioning (incredibly impaired), processing speed, and visuospatial functioning. A diagnostic interview was employed, where it became clear that the patient was both impulsive and apathetic, likely related to his remarkable impairments within executive functioning. Magnetic resonance imaging did not show anything of note. The patient was diagnosed with frontotemporal dementia.

The data in this case study is derived from Kerstein et al. [32].

9.5 Conclusions

Following a comprehensive review of current evidence, older adults appear to be at a lower risk of experiencing latent-stage BD relative to their younger counterparts. Nonetheless, it is still important to determine the potential risks and differential diagnoses of latent-stage BD in older populations. Most evidence suggests that a diagnosis of late-onset depression, a family history of BD, the discontinuation of lithium, and cerebrovascular diseases are the greatest risk factors for the development of latent-stage BD. Clinicians may encounter challenges in their diagnostic practices due to the considerable overlap between symptoms of latent-stage BD and neurocognitive conditions (i.e., bvFTD). Fortunately, several independent behavioral, cognitive, and neurophysiological indicators have begun to emerge, thereby assisting in this needed distinction.

9.6 Clinical Considerations

9.6.1 How to Identify a Potential Case of Latent-Stage Bipolar Disorder in Older Adults?

- A late-onset depression (i.e., age of onset after 60) diagnosis.
- Family history of bipolar disorder.
- Discontinuation of lithium leading to a diagnosis of bipolar disorder.
- Cerebral vascular disease and a diagnosis of bipolar disorder.

9.6.2 How to Identify a Potential Case of Latent-Stage Bipolar Disorder Versus Behavioral Frontotemporal Dementia (bvFTD)?

- Hyperorality, such as placing inedible objects in the mouth (seen in bvFTD).
- Dietary changes, such as consuming high amounts of carbohydrates (seen in bvFTD).
- Engage in ritualistic and compulsive behaviors, such as hoarding (seen in bvFTD).
- Patients with bvFTD experience greater executive dysfunction than euthymic patients with bipolar disorder. However, this switches when a bipolar patient is in a mood episode (manic or depressive).
- Patients with bipolar disorder in a mood episode (manic or depressive) appear to perform better in verbal fluency than patients with bvFTD.
- Patients with bipolar disorder appear to have greater grey matter reductions to the ventrolateral prefrontal cortex.

- Patients with bvFTD appear to have greater and/or unique grey matter reductions overall, specifically within the dorsolateral prefrontal cortex, inferior gyrus, frontal medial area, parietal superior lobe, and inferior temporal lobe.

9.7 Future Perspectives

In considering the future of bipolar disorder research, it is crucial to integrate genetic sequencing and neuroimaging to discover new biomarkers and improve diagnostic accuracy and treatment methods. Additionally, advances in imaging techniques like fMRI and PET scans could provide critical insights into brain changes and identify new intervention targets. Furthermore, expanding longitudinal studies will help understand how the progression of the disorder and how genetic and environmental factors contribute to the development of BD symptoms. Overall, a multidisciplinary approach combining psychiatry, neuroscience, and technology is essential for developing effective treatments and gaining a comprehensive understanding of bipolar disorder in the elderly.

References

1. Alexopoulos GS, Meyers BS, Young RC, Campbell S, Silbersweig D, Charlson M. "Vascular depression" hypothesis. Arch Gen Psychiatry. 1997;54(10):915–22. https://doi.org/10.1001/archpsyc.1997.01830220033006.
2. Almeida OP, McCaul K, Hankey GJ, Yeap BB, Golledge J, Flicker L. Risk of dementia and death in community-dwelling older men with bipolar disorder. Br J Psychiatry J Ment Sci. 2016;209(2):121–6. https://doi.org/10.1192/bjp.bp.115.180059.
3. Angst J. The bipolar spectrum. Br J Psychiatry J Ment Sci. 2007;190:189–91. https://doi.org/10.1192/bjp.bp.106.030957.
4. Arvanitakis Z, Shah RC, Bennett DA. Diagnosis and management of dementia: review. JAMA. 2019;322(16):1589–99. https://doi.org/10.1001/jama.2019.4782.
5. Aziz R, Steffens DC. What are the causes of late-life depression? Psychiatr Clin North Am. 2013;36(4):497–516. https://doi.org/10.1016/j.psc.2013.08.001.
6. Baez S, Pinasco C, Roca M, Ferrari J, Couto B, García-Cordero I, Ibañez A, Cruz F, Reyes P, Matallana D, Manes F, Cetcovich M, Torralva T. Brain structural correlates of executive and social cognition profiles in behavioral variant frontotemporal dementia and elderly bipolar disorder. Neuropsychologia. 2019;126:159–69. https://doi.org/10.1016/j.neuropsychologia.2017.02.012.
7. Baldessarini RJ, Bolzani L, Cruz N, Jones PB, Lai M, Lepri B, Perez J, Salvatore P, Tohen M, Tondo L, Vieta E. Onset-age of bipolar disorders at six international sites. J Affect Disord. 2010;121(1–2):143–6. https://doi.org/10.1016/j.jad.2009.05.030.
8. Barkhof F, Scheltens P. Imaging of white matter lesions. Cerebrovasc Dis. 2002;13 Suppl 2:21–30. https://doi.org/10.1159/000049146.
9. Bauer M, Bschor T, Kunz D, Berghöfer A, Ströhle A, Müller-Oerlinghausen B. Double-blind, placebo-controlled trial of the use of lithium to augment antidepressant medication in continuation treatment of unipolar major depression. Am J Psychiatry. 2000;157(9):1429–35. https://doi.org/10.1176/appi.ajp.157.9.1429.

10. Baumann P, Nil R, Souche A, Montaldi S, Baettig D, Lambert S, Uehlinger C, Kasas A, Amey M, Jonzier-Perey M. A double-blind, placebo-controlled study of citalopram with and without lithium in the treatment of therapy-resistant depressive patients: a clinical, pharmacokinetic, and pharmacogenetic investigation. J Clin Psychopharmacol. 1996;16(4):307–14. https://doi.org/10.1097/00004714-199608000-00006.
11. Beyer JL, Kuchibhatla M, Payne ME, Macfall J, Cassidy F, Krishnan KRR. Gray and white matter brain volumes in older adults with bipolar disorder. Int J Geriatr Psychiatry. 2009;24(12):1445–52. https://doi.org/10.1002/gps.2285.
12. Beyer JL, Kuchibhatla M, Payne M, Moo-Young M, Cassidy F, MacFall J, Krishnan KRR. Caudate volume measurement in older adults with bipolar disorder. Int J Geriatr Psychiatry. 2004;19(2):109–14. https://doi.org/10.1002/gps.1030.
13. Bschor T, Bauer M. Efficacy and mechanisms of action of lithium augmentation in refractory major depression. Curr Pharm Des. 2006;12(23):2985-92. https://doi.org/10.2174/138161206777947650. PMID: 16918427.
14. Caixeta L, Soares VLD, Vieira RT, Soares CD, Caixeta V, Ferreira SB, Aversi-Ferreira TA. Executive function is selectively impaired in old age bipolar depression. Front Psychol. 2017;8:194. https://doi.org/10.3389/fpsyg.2017.00194.
15. Caplan LR, Simon RP, Hassani S. Cerebrovascular disease—stroke∗. In: Zigmond MJ, Wiley CA, Chesselet M-F, editors. Neurobiology of brain disorders. Second ed. Academic; 2023. p. 457–76. https://doi.org/10.1016/B978-0-323-85654-6.00044-7.
16. Cassidy F, Carroll BJ. Vascular risk factors in late onset mania. Psychol Med. 2002;32(2):359–62. https://doi.org/10.1017/s0033291701004718.
17. Comes M, Rosa A, Reinares M, Torrent C, Vieta E. Functional impairment in older adults with bipolar disorder. J Nerv Ment Dis. 2017;205(6):443–7. https://doi.org/10.1097/NMD.0000000000000683.
18. Dé Montigny C, Grunberg F, Mayer A, Deschenes JP. Lithium induces rapid relief of depression in tricyclic antidepressant drug non-responders. Br J Psychiatry J Ment Sci. 1981;138:252–6. https://doi.org/10.1192/bjp.138.3.252.
19. Delvecchio G, Mandolini GM, Arighi A, Prunas C, Mauri CM, Pietroboni AM, Marotta G, Cinnante CM, Triulzi FM, Galimberti D, Scarpini E, Altamura AC, Brambilla P. Structural and metabolic cerebral alterations between elderly bipolar disorder and behavioural variant frontotemporal dementia: a combined MRI-PET study. Aust N Z J Psychiatry. 2019;53(5):413–23. https://doi.org/10.1177/0004867418815976.
20. Depp CA, Jin H, Mohamed S, Kaskow J, Moore DJ, Jeste DV. Bipolar disorder in middle-aged and elderly adults: is age of onset important? J Nerv Ment Dis. 2004;192(11):796–9. https://doi.org/10.1097/01.nmd.0000145055.45944.d6.
21. Diehl-Schmid J, Bornschein S, Pohl C, Förstl H, Kurz A, Jahn T. Cognitive decline in the behavioral variant of frontotemporal dementia. Int Psychogeriatr. 2011;23(2):230–7. https://doi.org/10.1017/S104161021000164X.
22. Dols A, Kupka RW, van Lammeren A, Beekman AT, Sajatovic M, Stek ML. The prevalence of late-life mania: a review. Bipolar Disord. 2014;16(2):113–8. https://doi.org/10.1111/bdi.12104.
23. Ducharme S, Price BH, Larvie M, Dougherty DD, Dickerson BC. Clinical approach to the differential diagnosis between behavioral variant frontotemporal dementia and primary psychiatric disorders. Am J Psychiatry. 2015;172(9):827–37. https://doi.org/10.1176/appi.ajp.2015.14101248.
24. El Moussaoui N. Secondary mania in older adults: a case report and review of literature. Eur Psychiatry. 2023;66(Suppl 1):S707. https://doi.org/10.1192/j.eurpsy.2023.1479.
25. Elefante C, Brancati GE, Petrucci A, Gemmellaro T, Toni C, Lattanzi L, Perugi G. Risk of conversion to bipolar disorder in patients with late-onset major depression. Int Clin Psychopharmacol. 2022;37(6):234–41. https://doi.org/10.1097/YIC.0000000000000421.
26. Fujikawa T, Yamawaki S, Touhouda Y. Silent cerebral infarctions in patients with late-onset mania. Stroke. 1995;26(6):946–9. https://doi.org/10.1161/01.str.26.6.946.

27. GBD 2019 Dementia Forecasting Collaborators. Estimation of the global prevalence of dementia in 2019 and forecasted prevalence in 2050: an analysis for the Global Burden of Disease Study 2019. Lancet Public Health. 2022;7(2):e105–25. https://doi.org/10.1016/S2468-2667(21)00249-8.
28. Gildengers AG, Whyte EM, Drayer RA, Soreca I, Fagiolini A, Kilbourne AM, Houck PR, Reynolds CF, Frank E, Kupfer DJ, Mulsant BH. Medical burden in late-life bipolar and major depressive disorders. Am J Geriatr Psychiatry. 2008;16(3):194–200. https://doi.org/10.1097/JGP.0b013e318157c5b1.
29. Gomes J, Sousa A, Afonso H, Lima G. Late onset bipolar disorder: clinical characterization. Eur Psychiatry. 2017;41(S1):S116–6. https://doi.org/10.1016/j.eurpsy.2017.01.1900.
30. Haller S, Xekardaki A, Delaloye C, Canuto A, Lövblad KO, Gold G, Giannakopoulos P. Combined analysis of grey matter voxel-based morphometry and white matter tract-based spatial statistics in late-life bipolar disorder. J Psychiatry Neurosci. 2011;36(6):391–401. https://doi.org/10.1503/jpn.100140.
31. Hogan DB, Jetté N, Fiest KM, Roberts JI, Pearson D, Smith EE, Roach P, Kirk A, Pringsheim T, Maxwell CJ. The prevalence and incidence of frontotemporal dementia: a systematic review. Canadian J Neurol Sci. 2016; 43: 96–109. https://doi.org/10.1017/cjn.2016.25.
32. Kerstein AH, Schroeder RW, Baade LE, Lincoln J, Khan AY. Frontotemporal dementia mimicking bipolar disorder. J Psychiatr Pract. 2013;19(6):498–500. https://doi.org/10.1097/01.pra.0000438190.04786.16.
33. Kim EY, Kim NW, Kim MJ, Yang BR, Rhee SJ, Park CHK, Lee HJ, Kim SH, Ahn YM. Rate of diagnostic conversion to bipolar disorder in adults with unipolar depression and psychopharmacological treatment in the Republic of Korea: a nationwide register-based study. J Affect Disord. 2020;273:240–6. https://doi.org/10.1016/j.jad.2020.03.159.
34. Lee C-I, Jung Y-E, Kim M-D, Hong S-C, Bahk W-M, Yoon B-H. The prevalence of bipolar spectrum disorder in elderly patients with recurrent depression. Neuropsychiatr Dis Treat. 2014;10:791–5. https://doi.org/10.2147/NDT.S63073.
35. Lu VJM, Zhang MW, Tan GM-Y, Ying J. From unipolar to bipolar: the diagnostic evolution in an elderly man. Case Rep Psychiatry. 2023;2023:6609793. https://doi.org/10.1155/2023/6609793.
36. Maia da Silva MN, Porto FH d G, Lopes PMG, Sodré de Castro Prado C, Frota NAF, Alves CHL, Alves GS. Frontotemporal dementia and late-onset bipolar disorder: the many directions of a busy road. Front Psych. 2021;12:768722. https://doi.org/10.3389/fpsyt.2021.768722.
37. Martino DJ, Strejilevich SA, Manes F. Neurocognitive functioning in early-onset and late-onset older patients with euthymic bipolar disorder. Int J Geriatr Psychiatry. 2013;28(2):142–8. https://doi.org/10.1002/gps.3801.
38. Mendez MF, Parand L, Akhlaghipour G. Bipolar disorder among patients diagnosed with frontotemporal dementia. J Neuropsychiatry Clin Neurosci. 2020;32(4):376–84. https://doi.org/10.1176/appi.neuropsych.20010003.
39. Miller BL, Darby AL, Swartz JR, Yener GG, Mena I. Dietary changes, compulsions and sexual behavior in frontotemporal degeneration. Dementia. 1995;6(4):195–9. https://doi.org/10.1159/000106946.
40. Mitchell E, Tavares TP, Palaniyappan L, Finger EC. Hoarding and obsessive-compulsive behaviours in frontotemporal dementia: clinical and neuroanatomic associations. Cortex. 2019;121:443–53. https://doi.org/10.1016/j.cortex.2019.09.012.
41. Moheb N, Charuworn K, Ashla MM, Desarzant R, Chavez D, Mendez MF. Repetitive behaviors in frontotemporal dementia: compulsions or impulsions? J Neuropsychiatry Clin Neurosci. 2019;31(2):132–6. https://doi.org/10.1176/appi.neuropsych.18060148.
42. Montejo L, Torrent C, Jiménez E, Martínez-Arán A, Blumberg HP, Burdick KE, Chen P, Dols A, Eyler LT, Forester BP, Gatchel JR, Gildengers A, Kessing LV, Miskowiak KW, Olagunju AT, Patrick RE, Schouws S, Radua J, Bonnín CDM, et al. Cognition in older adults with bipolar disorder: an ISBD task force systematic review and meta-analysis based on a com-

prehensive neuropsychological assessment. Bipolar Disord. 2022;24(2):115–36. https://doi.org/10.1111/bdi.13175.
43. Moorhead SRJ, Young AH. Evidence for a late onset bipolar-I disorder sub-group from 50 years. J Affect Disord. 2003;73(3):271–7. https://doi.org/10.1016/s0165-0327(01)00476-1.
44. Nelson JC. Combined drug treatment strategies for major depression. Psychiatr Ann. 1998;28(4):197–203. https://doi.org/10.3928/0048-5713-19980401-05.
45. Olney NT, Spina S, Miller BL. Frontotemporal dementia. Neurol Clin. 2017;35(2):339–74. https://doi.org/10.1016/j.ncl.2017.01.008.
46. Orhan M, Korten N, Stek M, Comijs H, Schouws S, Dols A. The relationship between cognitive and social functioning in older patients with bipolar disorder. J Affect Disord. 2018;240:177–82. https://doi.org/10.1016/j.jad.2018.07.055.
47. Papazacharias A, Lozupone M, Barulli MR, Capozzo R, Imbimbo BP, Veneziani F, De Blasi R, Nardini M, Seripa D, Panza F, Logroscino G. Bipolar disorder and frontotemporal dementia: an intriguing association. J Alzheimers Dis. 2017;55(3):973–9. https://doi.org/10.3233/JAD-160860.
48. Patel R, Reiss P, Shetty H, Broadbent M, Stewart R, McGuire P, Taylor M. Do antidepressants increase the risk of mania and bipolar disorder in people with depression? A retrospective electronic case register cohort study. BMJ Open. 2015;5(12):e008341. https://doi.org/10.1136/bmjopen-2015-008341.
49. Peet BT, Castro-Suarez S, Miller BL. The neuropsychiatric features of behavioral variant frontotemporal dementia. Adv Exp Med Biol. 2021;1281:17–31. https://doi.org/10.1007/978-3-030-51140-1_2.
50. Pressman PS, Miller BL. Diagnosis and management of behavioral variant frontotemporal dementia. Biol Psychiatry. 2014;75(7):574–81. https://doi.org/10.1016/j.biopsych.2013.11.006.
51. Puppala GK, Gorthi SP, Chandran V, Gundabolu G. Frontotemporal dementia—current concepts. Neurol India. 2021;69(5):1144–52. https://doi.org/10.4103/0028-3886.329593.
52. Rascovsky K, Hodges JR, Knopman D, Mendez MF, Kramer JH, Neuhaus J, van Swieten JC, Seelaar H, Dopper EGP, Onyike CU, Hillis AE, Josephs KA, Boeve BF, Kertesz A, Seeley WW, Rankin KP, Johnson JK, Gorno-Tempini M-L, Rosen H, et al. Sensitivity of revised diagnostic criteria for the behavioural variant of frontotemporal dementia. Brain J Neurol. 2011;134(Pt 9):2456–77. https://doi.org/10.1093/brain/awr179.
53. Rhee SJ, Ohlsson H, Sundquist J, Sundquist K, Kendler KS. Predictors of diagnostic conversion from major depression to bipolar disorder: a Swedish national longitudinal study. Psychol Med. 2023;53(16):7805–16. https://doi.org/10.1017/S0033291723001848.
54. Roman Meller M, Patel S, Duarte D, Kapczinski F, de Azevedo Cardoso T. Bipolar disorder and frontotemporal dementia: a systematic review. Acta Psychiatr Scand. 2021;144(5):433–47. https://doi.org/10.1111/acps.13362.
55. Rouillon F, Gorwood P. The use of lithium to augment antidepressant medication. J Clin Psychiatry. 1998;59 Suppl 5:32–9; discussion 40-41.
56. Sajatovic M. Bipolar disorder: disease burden. Am J Manag Care. 2005;11(3 Suppl):S80–4.
57. Sajatovic M, Chen P. Geriatric bipolar disorder. Psychiatr Clin North Am. 2011;34(2):319–33., vii. https://doi.org/10.1016/j.psc.2011.02.007.
58. Sajatovic M, Strejilevich SA, Gildengers AG, Dols A, Al Jurdi RK, Forester BP, Kessing LV, Beyer J, Manes F, Rej S, Rosa AR, Schouws SN, Tsai S-Y, Young RC, Shulman KI. A report on older-age bipolar disorder from the International Society for Bipolar Disorders Task Force. Bipolar Disord. 2015;17(7):689–704. https://doi.org/10.1111/bdi.12331.
59. Schouws SNTM, Comijs HC, Dols A, Beekman ATF, Stek ML. Five-year follow-up of cognitive impairment in older adults with bipolar disorder. Bipolar Disord. 2016;18(2):148–54. https://doi.org/10.1111/bdi.12374.
60. Shulman K, Post F. Bipolar affective disorder in old age. Br J Psychiatry J Ment Sci. 1980;136:26–32. https://doi.org/10.1192/bjp.136.1.26.

61. Stone K. Mania in the elderly. Br J Psychiatry J Ment Sci. 1989;155:220–4. https://doi.org/10.1192/bjp.155.2.220.
62. Subramaniam H, Dennis MS, Byrne EJ. The role of vascular risk factors in late onset bipolar disorder. Int J Geriatr Psychiatry. 2007;22(8):733–7. https://doi.org/10.1002/gps.1730.
63. Szmulewicz A, Valerio MP, Martino DJ. Longitudinal analysis of cognitive performances in recent-onset and late-life bipolar disorder: a systematic review and meta-analysis. Bipolar Disord. 2020;22(1):28–37. https://doi.org/10.1111/bdi.12841.
64. Thomas AJ, O'Brien JT, Davis S, Ballard C, Barber R, Kalaria RN, Perry RH. Ischemic basis for deep white matter hyperintensities in major depression: a neuropathological study. Arch Gen Psychiatry. 2002;59(9):785–92. https://doi.org/10.1001/archpsyc.59.9.785.
65. Tsai S-Y, Lee H-C, Chen C-C, Huang Y-L. Cognitive impairment in later life in patients with early-onset bipolar disorder. Bipolar Disord. 2007;9(8):868–75. https://doi.org/10.1111/j.1399-5618.2007.00498.x.
66. Velosa J, Delgado A, Finger E, Berk M, Kapczinski F, de Azevedo Cardoso T. Risk of dementia in bipolar disorder and the interplay of lithium: a systematic review and meta-analyses. Acta Psychiatr Scand. 2020;141(6):510–21. https://doi.org/10.1111/acps.13153.
67. Vijverberg EGB, Schouws S, Meesters PD, Verwijk E, Comijs H, Koene T, Schreuder C, Beekman A, Scheltens P, Stek M, Pijnenburg Y, Dols A. Cognitive deficits in patients with neuropsychiatric symptoms: a comparative study between behavioral variant frontotemporal dementia and primary psychiatric disorders. J Clin Psychiatry. 2017;78(8):e940–6. https://doi.org/10.4088/JCP.16m11019.
68. Westman J, Hällgren J, Wahlbeck K, Erlinge D, Alfredsson L, Osby U. Cardiovascular mortality in bipolar disorder: a population-based cohort study in Sweden. BMJ Open. 2013;3(4):e002373. https://doi.org/10.1136/bmjopen-2012-002373.
69. Wijeratne C, Sachdev S, Wen W, Piguet O, Lipnicki DM, Malhi GS, Mitchell PB, Sachdev PS. Hippocampal and amygdala volumes in an older bipolar disorder sample. Int Psychogeriatr. 2013;25(1):54–60. https://doi.org/10.1017/S1041610212001469.
70. Wimo A, Seeher K, Cataldi R, Cyhlarova E, Dielemann JL, Frisell O, Guerchet M, Jönsson L, Malaha AK, Nichols E, Pedroza P, Prince M, Knapp M, Dua T. The worldwide costs of dementia in 2019. Alzheimers Dement. 2023;19(7):2865–73. https://doi.org/10.1002/alz.12901.
71. Woolley JD, Khan BK, Murthy NK, Miller BL, Rankin KP. The diagnostic challenge of psychiatric symptoms in neurodegenerative disease: rates of and risk factors for prior psychiatric diagnosis in patients with early neurodegenerative disease. J Clin Psychiatry. 2011;72(2):126–33. https://doi.org/10.4088/JCP.10m06382oli.
72. Yassa R, Nair NP, Iskandar H. Late-onset bipolar disorder. Psychiatr Clin North Am. 1988;11(1):117–31.
73. Zanetti MV, Cordeiro Q, Busatto GF. Late onset bipolar disorder associated with white matter hyperintensities: a pathophysiological hypothesis. Prog Neuro-Psychopharmacol Biol Psychiatry. 2007;31(2):551–6. https://doi.org/10.1016/j.pnpbp.2006.10.004.

Chapter 10
Impulsivity and Latent Bipolar Disorder

Igor Wischneski, Sarah Aline Roza, José Bento da Silva Neto, and Thiago Henrique Roza

10.1 Introduction

A variety of definitions for impulsivity have been proposed over the years, most pertaining to a tendency to act prematurely, with insufficient forethought, frequently in a risky or inappropriate fashion, and often resulting in undesired outcomes [1]. Many psychometric techniques have been developed to measure impulsivity and its different domains, with the self-report Barratt Impulsiveness Scale (BIS-11) being the most used instrument in the studies discussed in this chapter [2]. The 11th revision of this scale divides impulsivity in three major domains: motor impulsivity, the tendency to act on the spur of the moment; attentional impulsivity, an intolerability to complex cognitive actions; and non-planning impulsivity, a lack of consideration for the consequences of one's actions [2]. An alternative to the three domain structure of the BIS-11 has been proposed by Khan et al. in 2019—cognitive impulsivity measures the presence or lack of awareness of factors present before the action and its consequences; behavioral impulsivity, on the other hand, measures factors present during the time an impulsive action occurs [3].

I. Wischneski
Laboratory of Digital Psychiatry, Universidade Federal do Paraná, Curitiba, PR, Brazil

Department of Psychiatry, School of Public Health, São José dos Pinhais, PR, Brazil

S. A. Roza
Laboratory of Digital Psychiatry, Universidade Federal do Paraná, Curitiba, PR, Brazil

Department of Psychology, Universidade Tuiuti do Paraná, Curitiba, PR, Brazil

J. B. da Silva Neto
Laboratory of Digital Psychiatry, Universidade Federal do Paraná, Curitiba, PR, Brazil

T. H. Roza (✉)
Laboratory of Digital Psychiatry, Universidade Federal do Paraná, Curitiba, PR, Brazil

Department of Psychiatry, Universidade Federal do Paraná, Curitiba, PR, Brazil

T. de Azevedo Cardoso et al. (eds.), *Latent Bipolar Disorder*,
https://doi.org/10.1007/978-3-032-01297-5_10

Other psychometric techniques often used to measure, directly and indirectly, aspects of impulsivity and related traits include: the Balloon Analogue Risk Task , which measures risk-taking behavior [4]; the Behavioral Inhibition/Behavioral Activation scales , especially pertaining to low behavioral inhibition [5]; the Immediate and Delayed Memory Task software, a comparatively more objective way to measure impulsivity when comparing with self-report scales like the BIS-11 [6]; the Iowa Gambling Task , focused on measuring decision-making deficits [7]; the Cambridge Gambling Task (CGT), used to access impulsivity as a whole [8]; Go/No-go tasks, measuring motor impulsivity [9]; the Single Key Impulsivity Paradigm , a measure of reward delay and response inhibition [10]; the Stop Signal Task (SSK), which measures inhibitory control [11]; and the Urgency, Premeditation, Perseverance, Sensation Seeking, Positive Urgency Impulsive Behavior Scale, which divides impulsivity in five different domains and also measures it as a whole [12].

10.2 Impulsivity in Bipolar Disorder

Bipolar disorder (BD) has been linked to impulsivity in multiple studies, using a variety of methodologies and psychometric techniques, proving that patients with BD tend to be more impulsive than healthy controls [13–16]. Impulsivity in BD can be divided into state- and trait-based impulsivity; state-based impulsivity refers to the impulsivity present during a mood episode, whether manic, depressed, or mixed, while trait-based impulsivity refers to the impulsivity present during euthymia, mood episodes, and during periods with subthreshold symptoms [17, 18]. State-based impulsivity is more pronounced during episodes of mania than depression, affecting predominantly the motor impulsivity score [19], with even modest manic symptoms during depressive episodes predicting higher impulsivity [20]. Trait-based impulsivity seems to affect all dimensions of impulsivity when patients with BD are compared to controls, and it is presumably present even in a latent stage of the disease [13, 15]. High trait-based impulsivity is more prevalent in males and positively correlates with increased state-based impulsivity during mood episodes and more frequent mood swings [21]. State-based impulsivity might be best evaluated with objective tests, rather than subjective, self-report scales like the BIS-11, as indicated by the tendency for BIS-11 scores to be stable regardless of mood episode, while objective tests of response inhibition, continuous performance tasks, and delayed reward tasks are significantly more impaired during mania when compared to any other mood state [22, 23].

A recent meta-analysis reviewed studies about impulsivity that used a wide range of different neurocognitive tests, and found that, overall, patients with BD have worse response inhibition scores, are less capable of delaying gratification, and make optimal choices less often than controls; this same study, however, did not find differences between patients with BD and controls when it comes to risk-taking behavior [24]. A study that followed 120 patients with BD during euthymia through

54 weeks indicated that the BIS-11 dimension most correlated with a worsened prognosis is the attentional impulsivity dimension [25].

Impulsive patients with BD have a worse prognosis [15], a higher number of hospitalizations [26], more functional impairment, lower cognitive functioning [27], lower quality of life [28, 29], less resilience to adversity [30], an earlier onset of disease, more suicide attempts [15], more substance abuse [15, 31], poorer response to treatment, and a shorter time between mood episodes [15, 32], are less adherent to treatment [33], and have worse financial control in their personal lives [34]. Impulsive patients with BD are also at a higher risk for high blood pressure and obesity when compared to non-impulsive patients with BD [35].

Patients with BD that have a comorbid anxiety disorder present significantly increased impulsivity, with higher anxiety scores being directly related to higher impulsivity scores [13, 36, 37]. Childhood trauma predicts higher impulsivity scores and a greater risk for suicide attempts [38]. In youths with BD, a smaller sleep duration and greater changes in sleep duration between school days and weekends predict higher impulsivity [39].

10.2.1 Latent BD and Impulsivity

Patients with BD often present with subsyndromal symptoms before the diagnosis of a first mood episode. A meta-analysis encompassing 1078 patients showed that sleep, energy, and cognitive disturbances, as well as milder versions of mood episodes, are the most common prodromal symptoms [40], presenting months before the diagnosis, often in a periodic nature [41]. Even though this meta-analysis showed a relatively low prevalence of impulsivity as a prodromal manifestation in patients with BD, it is a well-established fact that comorbidities traditionally related with high impulsivity increase the risk for a BD diagnosis, such as conduct disorder [42, 43], Attention-deficit/hyperactivity disorder (ADHD), especially when combined with conduct disorders) [44, 45], and a past history of criminal behavior [46].

As expected, some studies point toward an increased risk of developing BD in patients with high impulsivity scores [47–49], especially if impulsivity, increased aggression, and behavioral disinhibition are already present during early childhood, before the age of 3 years [50, 51]. Unaffected relatives of patients with BD score significantly higher than healthy controls in the BIS-11, SSK, and CGT, even when controlling for other conditions traditionally related to high impulsivity, such as individuals with high scores in the Hypomanic Personality Scale, indicating an average increase in impulsivity in this high-risk group [52]. Furthermore, unaffected relatives of patients with BD display more aggressive behaviors compared to healthy controls, especially when executive dysfunction is present, but to a lesser degree when compared to patients with BD [53]. Another proposed high-risk group with increased impulsivity comprises highly reward-sensitive individuals, more prone to reward and risk-seeking behaviors [54].

Many studies tried to classify individuals at-risk of BD into subgroups [55–58]; the subgroup most related to impulsivity seems to be the subset of patients with cyclothymic-hypersensitive temperament, characterized by rapid mood shifts, a higher prevalence of conduct disorders, irritability, aggressiveness, and suicidality, symptoms included in the spectrum of impulsiveness [59]. These patients have a worse prognosis compared to other BD subgroups, with more mood episodes, a lower likelihood of employment, lower levels of education, and more comorbidities [60]. Cyclothymic patients also tend to have higher mean scores on anger and hostility measures [61].

10.2.2 Neurophysiological Basis for Impulsivity in BD

The glycogen synthetase kinase-3, a widely studied enzyme in the context of neurodegeneration, BD, and lithium usage, has been related to impulsivity in patients with BD. A study showed that certain polymorphisms of this enzyme are related to increased impulsivity scores [62]. Higher BIS-11 scores were inversely related to the volume of the anterior medial frontal region of the brain in a small study with 20 patients with BD and 27 controls [63]. Early life stress is related to lower dopamine signaling in the accumbens nucleus, which, in turn, is related to higher impulsivity [64]. Furthermore, a study with 24 euthymic patients with BD and 24 controls revealed a lower integrity of the right cingulum in patients with BD who had higher impulsivity [65].

The response to safe rewards in the dorsolateral prefrontal cortex is inversely related to trait impulsiveness in patients with BD, while they have a more pronounced activation of the lateral prefrontal cortex when presented with a prospect of a risky reward, the opposite pattern of healthy controls, explaining the preference for high-risk and high-reward scenarios in this population, a tendency of behavior strongly correlated with impulsiveness. Both of these regions are hyperactivated during the processing of rewards in patients with BD when compared to controls, indicating that rewards have a greater hedonic impact in this population, predisposing patients with BD to reward-seeking behaviors and, thus, impulsivity [66]. Furthermore, patients with BD have an impaired responsivity of the ventral striatum to reward stimuli [67], indicating a need for more intense rewards, possibly contributing to risk-seeking behavior.

A recent study with 46 patients with BD and 60 healthy controls studied multiple brain regions and networks with a whole-brain multivariate method called source-based morphometry, focusing on how impulsivity affects different brain regions; this study indicated a reduction in gray matter in a parietal-occipital-cerebellar network related to attentional and cognitive processes specifically in impulsive patients with BD [68].

10.2.3 Aggressiveness, Criminality, and Impulsivity in BD

Conviction history in BD is related to impairments in response inhibition, but not in the ability to delay rewards; criminal history is most associated with predominantly manic episodes and the presence of a previous suicide attempt [69]. Childhood maltreatment, negligence, and emotional neglect, as well as comorbidity with substance abuse, post-traumatic stress disorder, antisocial and borderline personality disorders, and current affective episode, were shown to increase trait aggression in patients with BD as measured by the Brown-Goodwin Aggression Scale [70, 71]. Impulsivity as a trait seems to expose patients with BD to more anger-inducing events, predisposing an aggressive response and increasing overall levels of stress [72]. In inpatient settings, BD increases by 2.81 times the risk for aggression, usually directed to staff, especially in younger and psychotic patients [73]. Furthermore, patients with major depressive disorder (MDD) and cluster B personality traits, traits traditionally related to higher aggressiveness, have a higher chance of converting their diagnosis from MDD to BD when compared to patients with MDD and no cluster B personality traits [74, 75].

A study with 58 patients with BD indicated that substance abuse and personality traits are better predictors than current affective symptoms when it comes to predicting future aggression [76]. The inverse is also true—aggressive behavior in childhood predicts substance use disorder (SUD) in later stages of life [77].

A recent study with 799 patients with BD showed that about a quarter of them had a high risk of developing or had already been aggressive to others; the use of atypical antipsychotics, serotonin and norepinephrine reuptake inhibitors treatment, substance abuse, rapid cycling, irritability, lack of insight, impulsivity, and psychotic symptoms predicted aggressiveness [78].

10.2.4 Suicidality, Self-Harm, and Impulsivity in BD

Patients with BD that had prior suicide attempts have higher impulsivity scores [33], especially motor impulsivity, when compared to patients with BD without prior suicide attempts; these patients also have a higher chance of showing aggressive behaviors, have a higher chance of having white matter abnormalities in the internal capsule, and generally have smaller corpus callosum volumes [63, 79]. Impulsivity is also related to an increase in previous history of self-harm, which, in turn, is related to lower levels of global functioning, more severe depressive symptoms, and higher self-reported emotional dysregulation [80].

Impulsivity alone, however, is not able to reliably predict a tendency for suicidal behaviors and should always be evaluated alongside aggressive traits and hostility to predict higher chances of a future suicide attempt [81, 82]. Emotional dysregulation is also linked to suicidal ideation—the worse the score in emotional regulation scales, the higher the risk for a suicide attempt [83]. Higher number of hospital admissions, lower level of education, higher number of mood episodes, and a reported poorer controllability of suicidal thoughts are also associated with a higher risk for suicide attempts in patients with BD [84]. Insomnia not only increases impulsivity but also independently increases risk for suicidality [85]. Comorbid SUDs also predict higher rates of suicide attempts [86]. Prior suicide attempts and a history of self-harm should always be included in the evaluation of suicide risk in patients with BD, as they substantially increase the risk for suicide [87]. Furthermore, a study with 3021 adolescents showed that increased suicidality is a risk factor for diagnosis conversion from MDD to BD, with an odds ratio of 2.31 [88].

10.2.5 Substance Abuse and Impulsivity in BD

Substance abuse, just like BD, predicts higher impulsivity regardless of other diagnoses [89]. Patients with BD have a comorbid SUD score higher in the BIS-11 scale when compared to isolated BD, particularly in the non-planning and motor impulsivity dimensions, regardless of current mood episode [89–91]. In a study with 98 patients with BD who did not met diagnostic criteria for SUDs at the time of the study, history of prior substance abuse was not related to an increase in BIS-11 scores [92], indicating that state-based impulsivity might be more relevant than trait based impulsivity when it comes to predicting substance abuse. Indeed, impulsivity in euthymic patients with BD and SUDs is comparable to impulsivity in patients with BD without SUDs during a manic episode when using objective measures of performance impulsivity [89, 93]. SUDs are also a risk factor for diagnosis conversion from other psychiatric illnesses to BD [94, 95].

Specifically in the BD + alcohol use disorder comorbidity, a preliminary study with 78 individuals showed uniquely reduced levels of GABA and glutamate in the prefrontal cortex, and those levels were related to increased impulsivity and cravings [96]. SUD comorbidity predicts a higher suicide attempt rate and increased hostility and aggression scores [97] and is more prevalent in male subjects and patients with an earlier onset of disease [77].

10.2.6 Gambling Disorder and Impulsivity in BD

Patients with gambling disorder (GD) without BD have very similar impulsivity scores when compared to patients with BD, differing only in positive urgency, a domain in which patients with BD have higher scores [98]. Patients with BD have three to six times the prevalence of GD when compared to the general population [99, 100], with GD being substantially more prevalent in males and in patients with comorbid SUDs [101]. GD is more associated with type 2 disorder, rapid cycling, and history of suicidal ideation and attempts [102]. Problem gambling is also related to lower education, being unmarried, and being sedentary [100].

Gambling is often used by patients with mood disorders as a tool to regulate mood, with gambling urges being more prevalent both during hypomanic/manic states and during depressive states [103–105]; the role of gambling as a regulator of negative affect explains the similar prevalences of GD in major depression and BD found by some studies [101, 106].

10.2.7 Hypersexuality, Risky Sexual Behavior, and Impulsivity in BD

Risky sexual behavior can be defined as sexual behavior with a high risk of having undesired outcomes, such as pregnancy and sexually transmitted diseases. Unsurprisingly, risky sexual behavior is more prevalent during manic and hypomanic mood episodes, as well as in patients with more grandiose and expansive temperaments during euthymia [107, 108]. BD is the psychiatric disorder with the most risk of contracting HIV and other sexually transmitted diseases [109–112], as well as being the psychiatric disorder that most predicts a continuous exposition of sexual partners even after the knowledge of one's diagnosis of being HIV-positive [113], all of these risks being significantly increased during mania and hypomania and in patients with a comorbid SUD [114, 115]. Furthermore, during hypomanic, manic, or mixed episodes, male patients with BD report more sex with multiple partners and prostitutes, while female patients with BD report trading sex for goods and services [115]. In a 15-month follow-up study, more total weeks in mania and cocaine use were significantly related to risky sexual behavior [116].

Female patients with BD have a higher risk of sexual assault when compared to female patients with other psychiatric conditions [117]. Sexual addiction in patients with BD is related not only to higher impulsivity but also to comorbidity with personality disorders [118]. Patients with BD type I have a higher desired frequency of intercourse and a higher occurrence of repeated sexual intercourse when compared to patients with BD type II [119]. Patients with BD report lower sexual satisfaction, avoid more sexual contact, have more difficulty communicating sexual needs, and suffer more from vaginismus and premature ejaculation during mood episodes [120].

Of note, pubertal children might present with hypersexuality as one of the first symptoms of mania [121]; these children are more often females, do not live with both parents, have a lower socioeconomic status, have comorbid conduct and substance abuse disorders, and have a history of prior sexual abuse [122]. Offspring of patients with BD, a well-established risk group for BD, engage more in risky sexual behavior, report more abortions, have more unprotected sex, and have an early initiation in sexual activity when compared to offspring of healthy controls [123]. Risky sexual behavior, a positive history of sexually transmitted diseases, and initiating sexual activity before the age of 16 years are risk factors for the development of mania [124].

10.2.8 Compulsive Shopping and Impulsivity in BD

Compulsive shopping disorder is an emerging phenomenon, recently recognized as an addictive behavior, characterized by problematic shopping activities (with significant loss of time in the activity) and excessive spending on consumer items that are not necessary or not used for their intended purposes [125, 126]. This disorder may manifest through offline purchasing behaviors (in stores, for example) or online behaviors (shopping websites) [125, 126]. The diagnostic characteristics of the disorder also include difficulty in self-control over shopping behaviors (in terms of frequency, intensity, duration, and context), as well as increased priority given to the act of shopping, so that consumption activities interfere with other interests, leisure activities, professional duties, or daily responsibilities [125]. Compulsive shopping disorder is also associated with significant impairment and/or suffering that can affect different areas of the individual's life (personal, family, social, educational, and occupational, among others). Oftentimes, there is an accumulation of purchased items, which, in some cases, may suggest a comorbid diagnosis of hoarding disorder [125]. These problematic behaviors, which may be chronic or episodic, commonly arise during adolescence or emerging adulthood, which may be associated with the first stages in life when the individual is independent to decide on his/her own on how to spend money [126].

As discussed in other sections of this chapter, BD is often associated with substantial impulsive and disinhibited behaviors linked to high-risk consequences [127, 128]. Even though there is a scarcity of data concerning problematic shopping behaviors as predictors of a future diagnosis of BD, these impulsive behaviors may manifest earlier in comparison to other traditional symptoms of BD or may occur during a depressive episode (in a patient that, in the future, may present clear clinical manifestations of BD) [129].

Patients with BD usually present higher scores in compulsive buying and shopping measures compared to healthy controls [130]. Uncontrolled spending (which may take the form of spending large amounts of money in short periods of time, or compulsive buying practices) is one of the most common risk-taking behaviors in patients with BD experiencing a manic/hypomanic episode [114]. During manic episodes, the patient may embark on extravagant and impractical schemes, spending money uncontrollably and facing adverse consequences as a result [131]. Moreover, during hypomania, these individuals are also prone to new endeavors, risky ideas, and possibilities, with little to no planning in several cases, which often result in overspending [131]. Nevertheless, it is important to highlight that impulsive behaviors, such as problematic shopping, may be present during asymptomatic phases of BD [34].

In addition to the objective financial difficulties associated with compulsive buying, caregivers often report that impulsive spending practices are an important source of stress and anxiety in patients with BD [132]. Financial difficulties are also an important issue in BD for other reasons. For instance, severe mental health problems lead to difficulties in productivity and the capacity to earn money on a regular basis [131].

Importantly, patients with BD are often reluctant to accept advice and supervision when facing a manic/hypomanic episode, which may be associated with an inflated sense of self, also expressed in the seeking for fame and financial success [114]. Because of these characteristics, these individuals are more likely to develop strong beliefs about goal attainment (e.g., if I try hard enough, I should be able to excel in anything I attempt, including financial investments) and life achievements, which may be poorly rooted in reality [114].

Considering this context, in addition to the adequate pharmacological treatment of BD, it is important to consider the clinical management of problematic shopping practices in these patients [127]. In this sense, it is essential to consider the role of psychological treatments, especially cognitive behavioral therapy and mindfulness interventions, which may help patients through psychoeducation practices, as well as regulation of emotions, beliefs, thoughts, and behaviors related to the problematic and impulsive behaviors [133].

10.3 Clinical Relevance of These Findings

Impulsivity is increased both as a trait and as a state in patients with BD, being more prominent during mania [17, 18]. During latent stages of BD, impulsivity is not as prevalent as subsyndromal mood symptoms or mood lability [40], but it predicts a significantly worsened prognosis when present, with more comorbidities, more functional impairment, more substance abuse, more suicide attempts, more risky sexual behavior, more behavioral addictions, and more aggressive behaviors [15, 31, 33, 71, 118]. The presence of impulsivity in high-risk groups for BD, such as offspring of patients with BD, demands a closer and more intense monitoring of the patient. As seen by the many structural and genetic differences between impulsive and nonimpulsive patients with BD [62, 63, 65, 66, 68], as well as the plethora of psychometric techniques available for accessing impulsivity, screening protocols might emerge in the future as more studies focus on this uncommon, albeit severely impaired, subgroup.

10.4 Future Perspectives

Latent BD is a field that seldom benefits from cross-sectional studies, requiring a longitudinal approach to investigate possible risk factors. More studies are needed to consolidate the many risk factors involved in the development of BD; once this is done, screening protocols can be developed to precisely identify youth at risk for BD, and early interventions can start to be studied, with the goal to prevent unfavorable outcomes and delay disease onset.

References

1. Evenden JL. Varieties of impulsivity. Psychopharmacology. 1999;146(4):348–61.
2. Patton JH, Stanford MS, Barratt ES. Factor structure of the Barratt impulsiveness scale. J Clin Psychol. 1995;51(6):768–74.
3. Kahn JP, Cohen RF, Etain B, Aubin V, Bellivier F, Belzeaux R, et al. Reconsideration of the factorial structure of the Barratt Impulsiveness Scale (BIS-11): assessment of impulsivity in a large population of euthymic bipolar patients. J Affect Disord. 2019;253:203–9.
4. White TL, Lejuez CW, de Wit H. Test-retest characteristics of the Balloon Analogue Risk Task (BART). Exp Clin Psychopharmacol. 2008;16(6):565–70.
5. Carver CS, White TL. Behavioral inhibition, behavioral activation, and affective responses to impending reward and punishment: the BIS/BAS scales. J Pers Soc Psychol. 1994;67(2):319–33.
6. Dougherty DM, Marsh DM, Mathias CW. Immediate and delayed memory tasks: a computerized behavioral measure of memory, attention, and impulsivity. Behav Res Methods Instrum Comput. 2002;34(3):391–8.
7. Bull PN, Tippett LJ, Addis DR. Decision making in healthy participants on the Iowa Gambling Task: new insights from an operant approach. Front Psychol. 2015;6:391.
8. Romeu RJ, Haines N, Ahn WY, Busemeyer JR, Vassileva J. A computational model of the Cambridge gambling task with applications to substance use disorders. Drug Alcohol Depend. 2020;206:107711.
9. Gomez P, Ratcliff R, Perea M. A model of the go/no-go task. J Exp Psychol Gen. 2007;136(3):389–413.
10. Dougherty DM, Mathias CW, Marsh DM, Jagar AA. Laboratory behavioral measures of impulsivity. Behav Res Methods. 2005;37(1):82–90.
11. Lipszyc J, Schachar R. Inhibitory control and psychopathology: a meta-analysis of studies using the stop signal task. J Int Neuropsychol Soc. 2010;16(6):1064–76.
12. Dugré JR, Giguére CÉ, Percie du Sert O, Potvin S, Dumais A, Consortium Signature. The psychometric properties of a short UPPS-P impulsive behavior scale among psychiatric patients evaluated in an emergency setting. Front Psych. 2019;10:139.
13. Çörekçioğlu S, Cesur E, Devrim Balaban Ö. Relationship between impulsivity, comorbid anxiety and neurocognitive functions in bipolar disorder. Int J Psychiatry Clin Pract. 2021;25(1):62–72.
14. Reddy LF, Lee J, Davis MC, Altshuler L, Glahn DC, Miklowitz DJ, et al. Impulsivity and risk taking in bipolar disorder and schizophrenia. Neuropsychopharmacology. 2014;39(2):456–63.
15. Swann AC, Lijffijt M, Lane SD, Steinberg JL, Moeller FG. Increased trait-like impulsivity and course of illness in bipolar disorder. Bipolar Disord. 2009;11(3):280–8.
16. Dervic K, Garcia-Amador M, Sudol K, Freed P, Brent DA, Mann JJ, et al. Bipolar I and II versus unipolar depression: clinical differences and impulsivity/aggression traits. Eur Psychiatry. 2015;30(1):106–13.
17. Santana RP, Kerr-Gaffney J, Ancane A, Young AH. Impulsivity in bipolar disorder: state or trait? Brain Sci [Internet]. 2022;12(10). Available from: https://doi.org/10.3390/brainsci12101351.
18. Halvorson MA, Pedersen SL, Feil MC, Lengua LJ, Molina BSG, King KM. Impulsive states and impulsive traits: a study of the multilevel structure and validity of a multifaceted measure of impulsive states. Assessment. 2021;28(3):796–812.
19. Swann AC, Steinberg JL, Lijffijt M, Moeller FG. Impulsivity: differential relationship to depression and mania in bipolar disorder. J Affect Disord. 2008;106(3):241–8.
20. Swann AC, Moeller FG, Steinberg JL, Schneider L, Barratt ES, Dougherty DM. Manic symptoms and impulsivity during bipolar depressive episodes. Bipolar Disord. 2007;9(3):206–12.
21. Benazzi F. Impulsivity in bipolar-II disorder: trait, state, or both? Eur Psychiatry. 2007;22(7):472–8.

22. Strakowski SM, Fleck DE, DelBello MP, Adler CM, Shear PK, McElroy SL, et al. Characterizing impulsivity in mania. Bipolar Disord. 2009;11(1):41–51.
23. Strakowski SM, Fleck DE, DelBello MP, Adler CM, Shear PK, Kotwal R, et al. Impulsivity across the course of bipolar disorder. Bipolar Disord. 2010;12(3):285–97.
24. Ramírez-Martín A, Ramos-Martín J, Mayoral-Cleries F, Moreno-Küstner B, Guzman-Parra J. Impulsivity, decision-making and risk-taking behaviour in bipolar disorder: a systematic review and meta-analysis. Psychol Med. 2020;50(13):2141–53.
25. Rote J, Dingelstadt AML, Aigner A, Bauer M, Fiebig J, König B, et al. Impulsivity predicts illness severity in long-term course of bipolar disorder: a prospective approach. Aust N Z J Psychiatry. 2018;52(9):876–86.
26. Rosa AR, Reinares M, Franco C, Comes M, Torrent C, Sánchez-Moreno J, et al. Clinical predictors of functional outcome of bipolar patients in remission. Bipolar Disord. 2009;11(4):401–9.
27. Jiménez E, Arias B, Castellví P, Goikolea JM, Rosa AR, Fañanás L, et al. Impulsivity and functional impairment in bipolar disorder. J Affect Disord. 2012;136(3):491–7.
28. Kim YS, Cha B, Lee D, Kim SM, Moon E, Park CS, et al. The relationship between impulsivity and quality of life in euthymic patients with bipolar disorder. Psychiatry Investig. 2013;10(3):246–52.
29. Victor SE, Johnson SL, Gotlib IH. Quality of life and impulsivity in bipolar disorder. Bipolar Disord. 2011;13(3):303–9.
30. Choi JW, Cha B, Jang J, Park CS, Kim BJ, Lee CS, et al. Resilience and impulsivity in euthymic patients with bipolar disorder. J Affect Disord. 2015;170:172–7.
31. Henna E, Hatch JP, Nicoletti M, Swann AC, Zunta-Soares G, Soares JC. Is impulsivity a common trait in bipolar and unipolar disorders? Bipolar Disord. 2013;15(2):223–7.
32. Dawson EL, Shear PK, Howe SR, Adler CM, DelBello MP, Fleck DE, et al. Impulsivity predicts time to reach euthymia in adults with bipolar disorder. Bipolar Disord. 2014;16(8):846–56.
33. Depp CA, Moore RC, Dev SI, Mausbach BT, Eyler LT, Granholm EL. The temporal course and clinical correlates of subjective impulsivity in bipolar disorder as revealed through ecological momentary assessment. J Affect Disord. 2016;193:145–50.
34. Cheema MK, MacQueen GM, Hassel S. Assessing personal financial management in patients with bipolar disorder and its relation to impulsivity and response inhibition. Cogn Neuropsychiatry. 2015;20(5):424–37.
35. Naiberg MR, Newton DF, Collins JE, Bowie CR, Goldstein BI. Impulsivity is associated with blood pressure and waist circumference among adolescents with bipolar disorder. J Psychiatr Res. 2016;83:230–9.
36. Bellani M, Hatch JP, Nicoletti MA, Ertola AE, Zunta-Soares G, Swann AC, et al. Does anxiety increase impulsivity in patients with bipolar disorder or major depressive disorder? J Psychiatr Res. 2012;46(5):616–21.
37. Taylor CT, Hirshfeld-Becker DR, Ostacher MJ, Chow CW, LeBeau RT, Pollack MH, et al. Anxiety is associated with impulsivity in bipolar disorder. J Anxiety Disord. 2008;22(5):868–76.
38. De Filippis R, Carbone EA, D'Angelo M, Liuzza MT, De Fazio P, Steardo L Jr. The mediation role of impulsivity between childhood trauma and dissociative symptomatology in bipolar disorder. Riv Psichiatr. 2023;58(2):84–92.
39. Gershon A, Johnson SL, Thomas L, Singh MK. Double trouble: weekend sleep changes are associated with increased impulsivity among adolescents with bipolar I disorder. Bipolar Disord. 2019;21(2):132–41.
40. Van Meter AR, Burke C, Youngstrom EA, Faedda GL, Correll CU. The bipolar prodrome: meta-analysis of symptom prevalence prior to initial or recurrent mood episodes. J Am Acad Child Adolesc Psychiatry. 2016;55(7):543–55.
41. Hunt J, Schwarz CM, Nye P, Frazier E. Is there a bipolar prodrome among children and adolescents? Curr Psychiatry Rep. 2016;18(4):35.

42. Morcillo C, Duarte CS, Sala R, Wang S, Lejuez CW, Kerridge BT, et al. Conduct disorder and adult psychiatric diagnoses: associations and gender differences in the U.S. adult population. J Psychiatr Res. 2012;46(3):323–30.
43. Shankman SA, Lewinsohn PM, Klein DN, Small JW, Seeley JR, Altman SE. Subthreshold conditions as precursors for full syndrome disorders: a 15-year longitudinal study of multiple diagnostic classes. J Child Psychol Psychiatry. 2009;50(12):1485–94.
44. Biederman J, Petty CR, Dolan C, Hughes S, Mick E, Monuteaux MC, et al. The long-term longitudinal course of oppositional defiant disorder and conduct disorder in ADHD boys: findings from a controlled 10-year prospective longitudinal follow-up study. Psychol Med. 2008;38(7):1027–36.
45. Biederman J, Faraone S, Milberger S, Guite J, Mick E, Chen L, et al. A prospective 4-year follow-up study of attention-deficit hyperactivity and related disorders. Arch Gen Psychiatry. 1996;53(5):437–46.
46. Zimmermann P, Brückl T, Nocon A, Pfister H, Lieb R, Wittchen HU, et al. Heterogeneity of DSM-IV major depressive disorder as a consequence of subthreshold bipolarity. Arch Gen Psychiatry. 2009;66(12):1341–52.
47. Alloy LB, Urošević S, Abramson LY, Jager-Hyman S, Nusslock R, Whitehouse WG, et al. Progression along the bipolar spectrum: a longitudinal study of predictors of conversion from bipolar spectrum conditions to bipolar I and II disorders. J Abnorm Psychol. 2012;121(1):16–27.
48. Hernandez M, Marangoni C, Grant MC, Estrada J, Faedda GL. Parental reports of prodromal psychopathology in pediatric bipolar disorder. Curr Neuropharmacol. 2017;15(3):380–5.
49. Alloy LB, Bender RE, Wagner CA, Whitehouse WG, Abramson LY, Hogan ME, et al. Bipolar spectrum-substance use co-occurrence: Behavioral approach system (BAS) sensitivity and impulsiveness as shared personality vulnerabilities. J Pers Soc Psychol. 2009;97(3):549–65.
50. Hirshfeld-Becker DR, Biederman J, Faraone SV, Violette H, Wrightsman J, Rosenbaum JF. Temperamental correlates of disruptive behavior disorders in young children: preliminary findings. Biol Psychiatry. 2002;51(7):563–74.
51. Fergus EL, Miller RB, Luckenbaugh DA, Leverich GS, Findling RL, Speer AM, et al. Is there progression from irritability/dyscontrol to major depressive and manic symptoms? A retrospective community survey of parents of bipolar children. J Affect Disord. 2003;77(1):71–8.
52. Wessa M, Kollmann B, Linke J, Schönfelder S, Kanske P. Increased impulsivity as a vulnerability marker for bipolar disorder: evidence from self-report and experimental measures in two high-risk populations. J Affect Disord. 2015;178:18–24.
53. Simonetti A, Kurian S, Saxena J, Verrico CD, Soares JC, Sani G, et al. Cognitive correlates of impulsive aggression in youth with pediatric bipolar disorder and bipolar offspring. J Affect Disord. 2021;287:387–96.
54. Carroll AL, Damme KSF, Alloy LB, Bart CP, Ng TH, Titone MK, et al. Risk for bipolar spectrum disorders associated with positive urgency and orbitofrontal cortical grey matter volume. Neuroimage Clin. 2022;36:103225.
55. Faedda GL, Baldessarini RJ, Marangoni C, Bechdolf A, Berk M, Birmaher B, et al. An International Society of Bipolar Disorders task force report: precursors and prodromes of bipolar disorder. Bipolar Disord. 2019;21(8):720–40.
56. Ahmed AO, Green BA, Clark CB, Stahl KC, McFarland ME. Latent structure of unipolar and bipolar mood symptoms. Bipolar Disord. 2011;13(5–6):522–36.
57. Arathimos R, Fabbri C, Vassos E, Davis KAS, Pain O, Gillett A, et al. Latent subtypes of manic and/or irritable episode symptoms in two population-based cohorts. Br J Psychiatry. 2022;221(6):722–31.
58. Pignon B, Peyre H, Noblins E, Rolland B, Thomas P, Vaiva G, et al. A latent class analysis of manic and psychotic symptoms. J Nerv Ment Dis. 2020;208(9):721–8.
59. Kochman FJ, Hantouche EG, Ferrari P, Lancrenon S, Bayart D, Akiskal HS. Cyclothymic temperament as a prospective predictor of bipolarity and suicidality in children and adolescents with major depressive disorder. J Affect Disord. 2005;85(1–2):181–9.

60. Syrstad VEG, Oedegaard KJ, Fasmer OB, Halmoy A, Haavik J, Dilsaver S, et al. Cyclothymic temperament: associations with ADHD, other psychopathology, and medical morbidity in the general population. J Affect Disord. 2020;260:440–7.
61. Dolenc B, Dernovšek MZ, Sprah L, Tavcar R, Perugi G, Akiskal HS. Relationship between affective temperaments and aggression in euthymic patients with bipolar mood disorder and major depressive disorder. J Affect Disord. 2015;174:13–8.
62. Jiménez E, Arias B, Mitjans M, Goikolea JM, Roda E, Ruíz V, et al. Association between GSK3β gene and increased impulsivity in bipolar disorder. Eur Neuropsychopharmacol. 2014;24(4):510–8.
63. Matsuo K, Nielsen N, Nicoletti MA, Hatch JP, Monkul ES, Watanabe Y, et al. Anterior genu corpus callosum and impulsivity in suicidal patients with bipolar disorder. Neurosci Lett. 2010;469(1):75–80.
64. Sanchez EO, Bangasser DA. The effects of early life stress on impulsivity. Neurosci Biobehav Rev. 2022;137:104638.
65. Scholz V, Houenou J, Kollmann B, Duclap D, Poupon C, Wessa M. Dysfunctional decision-making related to white matter alterations in bipolar I disorder. J Affect Disord. 2016;194:72–9.
66. Mason L, O'Sullivan N, Montaldi D, Bentall RP, El-Deredy W. Decision-making and trait impulsivity in bipolar disorder are associated with reduced prefrontal regulation of striatal reward valuation. Brain. 2014;137(Pt 8):2346–55.
67. Trost S, Diekhof EK, Zvonik K, Lewandowski M, Usher J, Keil M, et al. Disturbed anterior prefrontal control of the mesolimbic reward system and increased impulsivity in bipolar disorder. Neuropsychopharmacology. 2014;39(8):1914–23.
68. Lapomarda G, Pappaianni E, Siugzdaite R, Sanfey AG, Rumiati RI, Grecucci A. Out of control: an altered parieto-occipital-cerebellar network for impulsivity in bipolar disorder. Behav Brain Res. 2021;406:113228.
69. Swann AC, Lijffijt M, Lane SD, Kjome KL, Steinberg JL, Moeller FG. Criminal conviction, impulsivity, and course of illness in bipolar disorder. Bipolar Disord. 2011;13(2):173–81.
70. Drachman R, Colic L, Sankar A, Spencer L, Goldman DA, Villa LM, et al. Rethinking "aggression" and impulsivity in bipolar disorder: risk, clinical and brain circuitry features. J Affect Disord. 2022;303:331–9.
71. Garno JL, Gunawardane N, Goldberg JF. Predictors of trait aggression in bipolar disorder. Bipolar Disord. 2008;10(2):285–92.
72. Molz AR, Black CL, Shapero BG, Bender RE, Alloy LB, Abramson LY. Aggression and impulsivity as predictors of stress generation in bipolar spectrum disorders. J Affect Disord. 2013;146(2):272–80.
73. Barlow K, Grenyer B, Ilkiw-Lavalle O. Prevalence and precipitants of aggression in psychiatric inpatient units. Aust N Z J Psychiatry. 2000;34(6):967–74.
74. Bartz de Ávila G, Montezano BB, Dias de Mattos Souza L, de Azevedo Cardoso T, Azevedo da Silva R, Mondin TC, et al. Personality disorders as predictors for the conversion from major depressive disorder to bipolar disorder: a prospective cohort study. Psychiatry Res Commun. 2022;2(3):100068.
75. Mesbah R, de Bles N, Rius-Ottenheim N, van der Does AJW, Penninx BWJH, van Hemert AM, et al. Anger and cluster B personality traits and the conversion from unipolar depression to bipolar disorder. Depress Anxiety. 2021;38(6):671–81.
76. Johnson SL, Carver CS. Emotion-relevant impulsivity predicts sustained anger and aggression after remission in bipolar I disorder. J Affect Disord. 2016;189:169–75.
77. Grunebaum MF, Galfalvy HC, Nichols CM, Caldeira NA, Sher L, Dervic K, et al. Aggression and substance abuse in bipolar disorder. Bipolar Disord. 2006;8(5 Pt 1):496–502.
78. Fico G, Janiri D, Pinna M, Sagué-Vilavella M, Gimenez Palomo A, Oliva V, et al. Affective temperaments mediate aggressive dimensions in bipolar disorders: a cluster analysis from a large, cross-sectional, international study. J Affect Disord. 2023;323:327–35.

79. Reich R, Gilbert A, Clari R, Burdick KE, Szeszko PR. A preliminary investigation of impulsivity, aggression and white matter in patients with bipolar disorder and a suicide attempt history. J Affect Disord. 2019;247:88–96.
80. Weintraub MJ, Van de Loo MM, Gitlin MJ, Miklowitz DJ. Self-harm, affective traits, and psychosocial functioning in adults with depressive and bipolar disorders. J Nerv Ment Dis. 2017;205(11):896–9.
81. Michaelis BH, Goldberg JF, Davis GP, Singer TM, Garno JL, Wenze SJ. Dimensions of impulsivity and aggression associated with suicide attempts among bipolar patients: a preliminary study. Suicide Life Threat Behav. 2004 Summer;34(2):172–6.
82. Perroud N, Baud P, Mouthon D, Courtet P, Malafosse A. Impulsivity, aggression and suicidal behavior in unipolar and bipolar disorders. J Affect Disord. 2011;134(1–3):112–8.
83. Kulacaoglu F, Izci F. The effect of emotional dysregulation and impulsivity on suicidality in patients with bipolar disorder. Psychiatr Danub. 2022 Winter;34(4):706–14.
84. Jiménez E, Arias B, Mitjans M, Goikolea JM, Ruíz V, Brat M, et al. Clinical features, impulsivity, temperament and functioning and their role in suicidality in patients with bipolar disorder. Acta Psychiatr Scand. 2016;133(4):266–76.
85. Palagini L, Cipollone G, Masci I, Caruso D, Paolilli F, Perugi G, et al. Insomnia symptoms predict emotional dysregulation, impulsivity and suicidality in depressive bipolar II patients with mixed features. Compr Psychiatry. 2019;89:46–51.
86. Potash JB, Kane HS, Chiu YF, Simpson SG, MacKinnon DF, McInnis MG, et al. Attempted suicide and alcoholism in bipolar disorder: clinical and familial relationships. Am J Psychiatry. 2000;157(12):2048–50.
87. Johnson SL, Carver CS, Tharp JA. Suicidality in bipolar disorder: the role of emotion-triggered impulsivity. Suicide Life Threat Behav. 2017;47(2):177–92.
88. Pfennig A, Ritter PS, Höfler M, Lieb R, Bauer M, Wittchen HU, et al. Symptom characteristics of depressive episodes prior to the onset of mania or hypomania. Acta Psychiatr Scand. 2016;133(3):196–204.
89. Swann AC, Dougherty DM, Pazzaglia PJ, Pham M, Moeller FG. Impulsivity: a link between bipolar disorder and substance abuse. Bipolar Disord. 2004;6(3):204–12.
90. Bauer IE, Meyer TD, Sanches M, Spiker D, Zunta-Soares G, Soares JC. Are self-rated and behavioural measures of impulsivity in bipolar disorder mainly related to comorbid substance use problems? Cogn Neuropsychiatry. 2017;22(4):298–314.
91. Ozten M, Erol A, Karayilan S, Kapudan H, Orsel ES, Kumsar NA. Impulsivity in bipolar and substance use disorders. Compr Psychiatry. 2015;59:28–32.
92. Powers RL, Russo M, Mahon K, Brand J, Braga RJ, Malhotra AK, et al. Impulsivity in bipolar disorder: relationships with neurocognitive dysfunction and substance use history. Bipolar Disord. 2013;15(8):876–84.
93. Kathleen Holmes M, Bearden CE, Barguil M, Fonseca M, Serap Monkul E, Nery FG, et al. Conceptualizing impulsivity and risk taking in bipolar disorder: importance of history of alcohol abuse. Bipolar Disord. 2009;11(1):33–40.
94. Ratheesh A, Cotton SM, Betts JK, Chanen A, Nelson B, Davey CG, et al. Prospective progression from high-prevalence disorders to bipolar disorder: exploring characteristics of pre-illness stages. J Affect Disord. 2015;183:45–8.
95. Bukh JD, Andersen PK, Kessing LV. Rates and predictors of remission, recurrence and conversion to bipolar disorder after the first lifetime episode of depression—a prospective 5-year follow-up study. Psychol Med. 2016;46(6):1151–61.
96. Prisciandaro JJ, Tolliver BK, Prescot AP, Brenner HM, Renshaw PF, Brown TR, et al. Unique prefrontal GABA and glutamate disturbances in co-occurring bipolar disorder and alcohol dependence. Transl Psychiatry. 2017;7(7):e1163.
97. Elizabeth Sublette M, Carballo JJ, Moreno C, Galfalvy HC, Brent DA, Birmaher B, et al. Substance use disorders and suicide attempts in bipolar subtypes. J Psychiatr Res. 2009;43(3):230–8.

98. Shakeel MK, Hodgins DC, Goghari VM. A comparison of self-reported impulsivity in gambling disorder and bipolar disorder. J Gambl Stud. 2019;35(1):339–50.
99. Cox BJ, Yu N, Afifi TO, Ladouceur R. A national survey of gambling problems in Canada. Can J Psychiatr. 2005;50(4):213–7.
100. McIntyre RS, McElroy SL, Konarski JZ, Soczynska JK, Wilkins K, Kennedy SH. Problem gambling in bipolar disorder: results from the Canadian Community Health Survey. J Affect Disord. 2007;102(1–3):27–34.
101. Kennedy SH, Welsh BR, Fulton K, Soczynska JK, McIntyre RS, O'Donovan C, et al. Frequency and correlates of gambling problems in outpatients with major depressive disorder and bipolar disorder. Can J Psychiatr. 2010;55(9):568–76.
102. Jones L, Metcalf A, Gordon-Smith K, Forty L, Perry A, Lloyd J, et al. Gambling problems in bipolar disorder in the UK: prevalence and distribution. Br J Psychiatry. 2015;207(4):328–33.
103. Shead NW, Hodgins DC. Probability discounting of gains and losses: implications for risk attitudes and impulsivity. J Exp Anal Behav. 2009;92(1):1–16.
104. Rømer Thomsen K, Callesen MB, Linnet J, Kringelbach ML, Møller A. Severity of gambling is associated with severity of depressive symptoms in pathological gamblers. Behav Pharmacol. 2009;20(5–6):527–36.
105. McElroy SL, Pope HG Jr, Keck PE Jr, Hudson JI, Phillips KA, Strakowski SM. Are impulse-control disorders related to bipolar disorder? Compr Psychiatry. 1996;37(4):229–40.
106. Quilty LC, Watson C, Robinson JJ, Toneatto T, Bagby RM. The prevalence and course of pathological gambling in the mood disorders. J Gambl Stud. 2011;27(2):191–201.
107. Kopeykina I, Kim HJ, Khatun T, Boland J, Haeri S, Cohen LJ, et al. Hypersexuality and couple relationships in bipolar disorder: a review. J Affect Disord. 2016;195:1–14.
108. Dvorak RD, Wray TB, Kuvaas NJ, Kilwein TM. Mania and sexual risk: associations with behavioral self-regulation. J Affect Disord. 2013;150(3):1076–81.
109. Chen SF, Wang LY, Chiang JH, Shen YC. Bipolar disorder is associated with an increased risk of sexually transmitted infections: a nationwide population-based cohort study. Sex Transm Dis. 2018;45(11):735–40.
110. Marengo E, Martino DJ, Igoa A, Fassi G, Scápola M, Urtueta Baamonde M, et al. Sexual risk behaviors among women with bipolar disorder. Psychiatry Res. 2015;230(3):835–8.
111. Volavka J, Convit A, Czobor P, Douyon R, O'Donnell J, Ventura F. HIV seroprevalence and risk behaviors in psychiatric inpatients. Psychiatry Res. 1991;39(2):109–14.
112. Sacks MH, Silberstein C, Weiler P, Perry S. HIV-related risk factors in acute psychiatric inpatients. Hosp Community Psychiatry. 1990;41(4):449–51.
113. Meade CS, Bevilacqua LA, Key MD. Bipolar disorder is associated with HIV transmission risk behavior among patients in treatment for HIV. AIDS Behav. 2012;16(8):2267–71.
114. Fletcher K, Parker G, Paterson A, Synnott H. High-risk behaviour in hypomanic states. J Affect Disord. 2013;150(1):50–6.
115. Meade CS, Graff FS, Griffin ML, Weiss RD. HIV risk behavior among patients with co-occurring bipolar and substance use disorders: associations with mania and drug abuse. Drug Alcohol Depend. 2008;92(1–3):296–300.
116. Meade CS, Fitzmaurice GM, Sanchez AK, Griffin ML, McDonald LJ, Weiss RD. The relationship of manic episodes and drug abuse to sexual risk behavior in patients with co-occurring bipolar and substance use disorders: a 15-month prospective analysis. AIDS Behav. 2011;15(8):1829–33.
117. Ozcan NK, Boyacıoğlu NE, Enginkaya S, Dinç H, Bilgin H. Reproductive health in women with serious mental illnesses. J Clin Nurs. 2014;23(9–10):1283–91.
118. Di Nicola M, Tedeschi D, Mazza M, Martinotti G, Harnic D, Catalano V, et al. Behavioural addictions in bipolar disorder patients: role of impulsivity and personality dimensions. J Affect Disord. 2010;125(1–3):82–8.
119. Mazza M, Harnic D, Catalano V, Di Nicola M, Bruschi A, Bria P, et al. Sexual behavior in women with bipolar disorder. J Affect Disord. 2011;131(1–3):364–7.

120. Lam D, Donaldson C, Brown Y, Malliaris Y. Burden and marital and sexual satisfaction in the partners of bipolar patients. Bipolar Disord. 2005;7(5):431–40.
121. Geller B, Zimerman B, Williams M, Bolhofner K, Craney JL, Delbello MP, et al. Diagnostic characteristics of 93 cases of a prepubertal and early adolescent bipolar disorder phenotype by gender, puberty and comorbid attention deficit hyperactivity disorder. J Child Adolesc Psychopharmacol. 2000 Autumn;10(3):157–64.
122. Krantz M, Goldstein T, Rooks B, Merranko J, Liao F, Gill MK, et al. Sexual risk behavior among youth with bipolar disorder: identifying demographic and clinical risk factors. J Am Acad Child Adolesc Psychiatry. 2018;57(2):118–24.
123. Nijjar R, Ellenbogen MA, Hodgins S. Personality, coping, risky behavior, and mental disorders in the offspring of parents with bipolar disorder: a comprehensive psychosocial assessment. J Affect Disord. 2014;166:315–23.
124. Ramrakha S, Caspi A, Dickson N, Moffitt TE, Paul C. Psychiatric disorders and risky sexual behaviour in young adulthood: cross sectional study in birth cohort. BMJ. 2000;321(7256):263–6.
125. Müller A, Laskowski NM, Thomas TA, Antons S, Tahmassebi N, Steins-Loeber S, et al. Update on treatment studies for compulsive buying-shopping disorder: a systematic review. J Behav Addict. 2023;12(3):631–51.
126. Black DW. Compulsive shopping: a review and update. Curr Opin Psychol. 2022;46:101321.
127. Yatham LN, Kennedy SH, Parikh SV, Schaffer A, Bond DJ, Frey BN, et al. Canadian Network for Mood and Anxiety Treatments (CANMAT) and International Society for Bipolar Disorders (ISBD) 2018 guidelines for the management of patients with bipolar disorder. Bipolar Disord. 2018;20(2):97–170.
128. McIntyre RS, Berk M, Brietzke E, Goldstein BI, López-Jaramillo C, Kessing LV, et al. Bipolar disorders. Lancet. 2020;396(10265):1841–56.
129. Kapczinski F, Montezano BB, de Azevedo Cardoso T. Latent bipolar disorder. Lancet. 2023;401(10394):2109.
130. Kesebir S, Işitmez S, Gündoğar D. Compulsive buying in bipolar disorder: is it a comorbidity or a complication? J Affect Disord. 2012;136(3):797–802.
131. Richardson T, Jansen M, Fitch C. Financial difficulties in bipolar disorder part 2: psychological correlates and a proposed psychological model. J Ment Health. 2021;30(1):3–11.
132. Beentjes TAA, Goossens PJJ, Poslawsky IE. Caregiver burden in bipolar hypomania and mania: a systematic review. Perspect Psychiatr Care. 2012;48(4):187–97.
133. Muhtadie L, Johnson SL, Carver CS, Gotlib IH, Ketter TA. A profile approach to impulsivity in bipolar disorder: the key role of strong emotions. Acta Psychiatr Scand. 2014;129(2):100–8.

Chapter 11
The Role of Biological Rhythms Disruption in Latent Bipolar Disorder

Melissa Alves Braga Oliveira, Danyella Richter, and Adriane R. Rosa

11.1 Neurobiology of Circadian Rhythms and Bipolar Disorder

Multiple hypotheses have been proposed over time to explain the development of major psychiatric disorders, such as bipolar disorder (BD). Their emergence is probably influenced by a complex interaction of predisposing factors and other risk factors, exacerbated by the burden of the illness and compensatory mechanisms. Disturbances in circadian rhythms and the sleep–wake cycle are among these factors, being described in individuals with mood disorders since the 1950s, and often serving as key diagnostic criteria [1]. In BD, alterations in circadian rhythms represent a core feature of the disorder, and among the most common manifestations are

M. A. B. Oliveira
Laboratory of Chronobiology and Sleep, Hospital de Clínicas de Porto Alegre, Universidade Federal do Rio Grande do Sul, Porto Alegre, RS, Brazil

D. Richter
Laboratory of Molecular Psychiatry, Hospital de Clínicas de Porto Alegre, Porto Alegre, RS, Brazil

Postgraduate Program of Psychiatry and Behavioral Sciences, Universidade Federal do Rio Grande do Sul (UFRGS), Porto Alegre, RS, Brazil

A. R. Rosa (✉)
Laboratory of Molecular Psychiatry, Hospital de Clínicas de Porto Alegre, Porto Alegre, RS, Brazil

Postgraduate Program of Psychiatry and Behavioral Sciences, Universidade Federal do Rio Grande do Sul (UFRGS), Porto Alegre, RS, Brazil

Department of Pharmacology, Institute of Basic Health Science, Universidade Federal do Rio Grande do Sul (UFRGS), Porto Alegre, RS, Brazil

T. de Azevedo Cardoso et al. (eds.), *Latent Bipolar Disorder*,
https://doi.org/10.1007/978-3-032-01297-5_11

the reduction in the amplitude of activity–rest rhythm, phase advance or delay on sleep timing, as well as sleep fragmentation [2].

While the circadian system is primarily known for regulating sleep–wake cycles, it is also intricately linked to molecular and cellular processes believed to underlie mood disorders. Consequently, disruptions in circadian rhythms, whether genetic or environmental, could lead to mood disturbances [3]. However, first, it is important to understand how the circadian timing system is organized. It consists of a robust system that is organized in a hierarchical manner to enable organisms to predict and synchronize their internal physiology and behavior with the 24-hour light–dark cycle [4]. The suprachiasmatic nucleus (SCN) is the small structure in the hypothalamus that functions as the central clock of our temporal system and is heavily affected by how much light we are exposed to and uses this temporal cue as the main *zeitgeber*—from German zeit "time" and geber "giver"—to daily reset to 24 hours our body time. As a conductor in an orchestra, after receiving this light information from the environment, the SCN conveys it to the clocks in our peripheral systems via humoral and neural signaling to align the timing of physiological and behavioral processes as a coordinated symphony [5]. Consequently, the body is striving for optimal health in any given circumstance (Fig. 11.1).

With regard to light exposure, mounting evidence supports the photic signal as the strongest cue to modulate circadian rhythms with effects in sleep, mood, alertness, and cognition [6]. It is noteworthy that light therapy has become an established treatment for some psychiatric disorders, such as seasonal affective disorder, but is still entering guidelines for depression in BD [7]. The photic information is signaled to retinal ganglion cells (RCGs), which are the only output neurons that link the retina to the brain. A small portion of the RCGs are intrinsically photosensitive and they project via retinohypothalamic tract to distinct brain regions, including the SCN and other nuclei involved in sleep regulation, affect, and BD like medial amygdala, lateral habenula, and subparaventricular zone. Besides, there are other important structures that are innervated by the SCN and that could represent an indirect path by which light could impact behavior such as ventrolateral preoptic area, lateral hypothalamus, ventral tegmental area, and raphe [6].

In the circadian timing system, the temporal organization also occurs at a molecular level. Inside each cell, we also have a molecular machinery that sustains circadian rhythmicity by means of cell-autonomous autoregulatory transcriptional–translational feedback loops (TTFLs) between clock genes. In the positive feedback loop, we have Brain and muscle Arnt-like protein-1 (BMAL1) that heterodimerizes with Circadian Locomotor output cycles Kaput (CLOCK) to bind to E-box enhancer elements and activate the transcription of CRYPTOCHROME (CRY) and PERIOD (PER) proteins. In the negative feedback loop, the PER/CRY complex is formed in the cytosol and is then translocated to the nucleus to repress the BMAL1/CLOCK heterodimer. The transcription of BMAL1 is also regulated by a secondary TTFL composed of REV-ERB, an orphan nuclear receptor that inhibits transcription of BMAL1 and the transactivator Rora [8].

Besides being associated with dysfunction across the neuronal system that leads to behavioral abnormalities, BD is also related to hormonal imbalances and changes

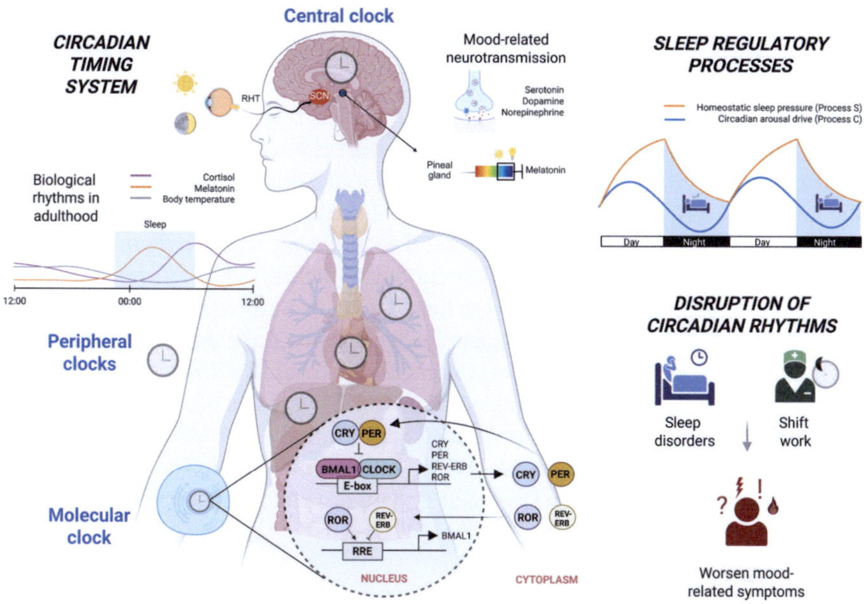

Fig. 11.1 Sleep–circadian regulation in humans. The circadian timing system is organized hierarchically from its central regulation in the suprachiasmatic nucleus (SCN), through peripheral clocks up to the cellular level by means of the molecular machinery that encompass clock genes that generate circadian rhythmicity in our body. Light is the main temporal cue capable of synchronizing our inner rhythms to the environment and biological rhythms such as sleep–wake cycles and body temperature are examples of outputs that follow a circadian pattern. Sleep regulation, in addition to having a circadian component that influences its manifestation pattern (known as process C), is also governed by a homeostatic process (process S). In this process, the greater the sleep deprivation, the higher the sleep pressure. When these processes are disrupted by irregular routines, sleep disorders, shift work, and other disturbances, mood-related symptoms may arise or worsen. SCN suprachiasmatic nucleus, RHT retinohypothalamic tract, CRY cryptochrome gene, PER period gene, BMAL1 brain and muscle ARNT-like 1, CLOCK circadian locomotor output cycles kaput, E-BOX enhancer box, ROR retinoic acid receptor, REV-ERB nuclear receptors involved in the cell-autonomous circadian transcriptional/translational feedback loops as transcriptional repressors, RRE ROR response element

in peripheral physiology. Disrupted circadian rhythms might affect a variety of cellular and physiological processes, possibly explaining the wide range of effects of BD on various dimensions of health. Many studies that made use of genetic manipulations in inbred animals have shown the relevance of altered expression of clock genes and BD phenotypes [9]. For instance, ClockΔ19-mutant mice, which present alteration in CLOCK protein, show reduced amplitude, long period, delayed phase of activity–rest rhythm [10], and display mania-like phenotype with traits that are partly reversible by lithium [11].

Some rhythmic outputs of our temporal regulation are sleep–wake cycles, cortisol and melatonin levels, body temperature, and mood symptoms, all physiological and behavioral manifestations that present daily rhythmicity [12]. The way our temporal organization reflects in our behavior can present inter-individual variation that we can address by means of chronotypes. Varying from morning to evening, the chronotype is associated with distinct physiological, genetic, and behavioral characteristics. As a consequence, individuals may present, for example, individual tendencies to allocate their activity/rest periods, which is related to dim light melatonin onset (DMLO), considered a measure of circadian phase. The earlier the individual allocates their sleep phase, the earlier the peak of melatonin production will be, and the morning/early chronotype the person should exhibit. The opposite occurs with the evening chronotype [13, 14]. Current data suggest that hyperthymic temperament is associated with a morning chronotype, whereas other affective temperaments and high-risk groups for BD are linked to an evening chronotype [9].

A bidirectional relationship exists between mood disorders and circadian rhythms. While mood disorders are frequently associated with circadian rhythms disruption, behaviors known to induce disturbances in rhythms, such as weak *zeitgebers*, shift-work, sleep disorders, travel across time zones, and irregular social schedules can worsen these disorders or trigger episodes [15]. The following section is the current evidence on sleep and rhythm disturbances among individuals at high risk of developing BD.

11.2 Sleep and Rhythm Disturbances in Individuals at High Risk of Developing BD: Evidence and Implications

Sleep and rhythm disturbances represent a well-established clinical symptom in individuals with BD. It persists during euthymic periods, as well as precedes and predicts the onset of both manic and hypomanic episodes [16–21]. According to Geoffroy and colleagues [21], patients with BD are more likely to experience longer sleep latency, longer sleep duration, poorer sleep efficiency, higher fragmentation index, and poorer interdaily stability, as determined by mean actigraphy scores. When assessed by the Pittsburgh Sleep Quality Index (PSQI) [22], they reported poorer sleep quality, more frequent sleep disturbances, and more daytime dysfunction compared with healthy controls. As stated by Giglio et al. [23], patients with BD who experience sleep disturbances have worse global functioning and quality of life in physical, psychological, social, and environmental domains when compared with patients with BD without sleep problems. Similarly, Lunsford-Avery et al. [24] found that adolescents with BD and sleep disturbance had greater psychosocial impairment, in particular, in the academic domain. Even though the scientific community increasingly focuses on prevention and enhancing prognosis to reduce the global burden of mental disorders [25], there remains a lack of understanding regarding the relationship between sleep disturbances and psychopathology in individuals at high risk of BD [26].

A selective review on studies conducted by Duffy and colleagues [27] pointed out that the experience of non-specific childhood anxiety and sleep disturbances are more prevalent among high-risk offspring compared to the general population.

These factors may serve as markers indicating an increased risk of developing mood disorders like depression and BD during adolescence and early adulthood [20, 28, 29]. The authors also state circadian and sleep disturbance as important vulnerability markers for mood disorders in high-risk youth, suggesting their monitoring for early risk syndromes [27]. On that account, Duffy and colleagues [27] advocate that an approach focused on developmental stages is crucial for correctly identifying young individuals who may be heading toward severe psychiatric disorders at an earlier stage. This developmental phase is pivotal for neurobiological and psychosocial development [27, 30]. Such an approach also allows the identification of opportunities for early and effective treatment, which is fundamental for neuroprotection and improvement of prognosis and quality of life for these individuals [27, 30, 31].

A systematic review and meta-analysis conducted by Scott et al. [26] shed light on circadian rhythms in adolescents and young adults at high risk for developing BD. The study revealed that sleep and circadian rhythm disturbances are common among individuals who exhibit early manifestations of the disorder and among offspring of patients with BD, as these specific populations display poorer sleep quality compared to the general population. Notably, pooled analyses indicated that individuals with sub-threshold manifestations of BD exhibit lower social rhythmicity and a preference for eveningness, suggesting these factors as crucial mechanisms in the neurobiological vulnerability to BD. Moreover, actigraphy data revealed dysregulated sleep rhythms in these individuals, characterized by shorter sleep duration, lower stability, greater variability, and reduced amplitude in circadian rhythms.

Nonetheless, when evaluating sleep patterns in adolescents and young adults, it is important to discern whether the symptoms primarily reflect a typical adolescent sleep pattern rather than being solely attributable to BD. Recognizing this distinction, the authors underscored that while analogous characteristics often manifest in adolescents and young adults, those with early-onset BD tend to exhibit more accentuated sleep pattern manifestations associated with the disorder compared to their counterparts [26].

According to Scott and colleagues [26], individuals with sleep and circadian rhythm disturbances are at a 40% higher risk of developing BD in the future. Hence, regulating sleep may serve as a viable intervention for individuals at risk of or recently diagnosed with BD. However, the study did not clearly identify a unique pattern of sleep disturbance linked to latent BD, nor did it investigate specific disturbances like hypersomnia and sleep variability due to limited data.

Another systematic review and meta-analysis by Ng and colleagues [32] explored sleep–wake disturbances in inter-episode BD (n = 17) and high-risk individuals (n = 5). They found weakened and less stable rest–activity cycles in individuals at high risk of developing BD. This was evidenced by lower relative amplitude and higher variability in sleep efficiency compared to the general population, underscoring the importance of treating sleep disturbances to prevent the disorder. However, aside from the small sample size, this study failed to investigate other sleep–wake parameters, thereby limiting the interpretation of the results.

A systematic review undertaken by Melo and colleagues [33] reaffirmed the prevalence of sleep disturbances among individuals with a family history of BD. Most of these included studies used subjective ($n = 17$), objective ($n = 10$), or both measures ($n = 3$) to assess sleep disturbances. Indeed, one of these studies [34] suggested that nighttime awakenings could serve as a prognostic indicator for future BD development. Additionally, a population-based study encompassing 3021 individuals indicated that alterations in sleep quality escalated the risk for developing BD [35].

Despite the apparent relationship between rhythm disturbances and BD or high risk for BD, as reported by independent systematic reviews, some methodological limitations in these studies warrant discussion. First, the number of included studies varied from 5 [32] to 76 [26]. Second, the definition of latent BD was quite heterogeneous among the studies. Third, there was variability for the assessment of biological rhythms as discussed in the next section. Finally, many of the studies were not specifically designed to study sleep disturbance in high-risk individuals or early onset of BD, being the evidence mainly derived from secondary analysis, which may have compromised the quality of data available. These methodological issues could explain, partially, some conflicting results regarding the relationship between sleep disturbances and latent BD.

11.3 Measures Used for Sleep and Rhythm Evaluation

The inconsistency found in sleep and rhythmic patterns in BD could be due to the heterogeneity in study designs and the lack of well-established protocols to assess sleep–wake cycles and other circadian rhythms. In the context of mental health, we could divide the available methods into objective and subjective tools, such as actigraphy and validated questionnaires, respectively. The correct understanding of what is being evaluated by each distinct approach is essential to guide the choice of the better method to answer the research question, leading to meaningful and reproducible results. The table below summarizes the main characteristics of the most frequently used assessment tools.

Even though polysomnography is considered the gold standard to assist in the diagnosis of sleep disturbances, the actigraphy, also known as actimetry, has been extensively used in the research scenario due to its most outstanding advantage of enabling continuous recordings, besides being a noninvasive and convenient method that does not interfere with the individuals' normal routine. These devices are commonly worn on the wrist, particularly for estimating sleep timing and duration. Based on wrist movements, it is possible to infer sleepiness/wakefulness, as well as to calculate rhythmic parameters that have been implicated in mood disorders such as mesor, acrophase, relative amplitude (RA), the individual's least active 5 consecutive hours (L5), the individual's most active 10 consecutive hours (M10), interdaily stability (IS), and intradaily variability (IV) [36, 37].

From the DLMO, phase advances and delays of the melatonin rhythm can be characterized, also allowing the diagnosis of individuals synchronized to the 24-hour light–dark rhythm or in free-running conditions. In this way, the DLMO constitutes a useful test for evaluating sleep disturbances, for measuring phase change in the psychiatric evaluation of mood disorders, in addition to being able to provide guidance on the ideal time for light therapy or administration of exogenous melatonin [38].

The Mood Rhythm Instrument (MRhI) is a self-reported questionnaire designed to assess the rhythmicity of mood symptoms. It covers somatic domains (sleep, appetite, and sexual arousal), cognitive domains (problem-solving, concentration, memory, and energy), and affective domains (sadness, irritability, anxiety, and pessimism). Notably, perceiving rhythmicity in mood-related symptoms, particularly in those from the affective domain, has been positively associated with an increased risk of psychiatric disorders [39, 40]. While the MRhI was designed to assess mood rhythmicity in clinical and epidemiological studies, the Biological Rhythms Interview of Assessment in Neuropsychiatry (BRIAN) focuses on evaluating biological rhythms in mental health clinical settings, in these domains: sleep/social, activity, and eating pattern. Higher scores in the BRIAN were found among individuals with BD in comparison with healthy individuals, reinforcing that biological rhythm impairment is a trait marker in patients with BD [41, 42].

The Morningness-Eveningness Questionnaire (MEQ) and the Munich Chronotype Questionnaire (MCTQ) are both well-established instruments that evaluate, from distinct approaches, the individual circadian typology, or also, the chronotype. The MCTQ also enables the calculation of social jetlag, which represents the misalignment of the internal biological timing and the social time, and is usually related to sleep deprivation during work days that we try to "recover" over the work-free days [43].

Finally, the PSQI is the most adopted tool for self-evaluating sleep quality. The higher the global score, the worse the sleep quality.

Characteristics of the most frequently used assessment tools

Name	References	Definition and outputs
Objective tools		
Wrist actigraphy	Ancoli-Israel et al. [44]	The actimeter is a device similar to a watch that enables long-term recording of activity–rest rhythm. Additionally, they often include sensors that measure various other parameters, such as light exposure, skin temperature, and heart rate.
DLMO	Lewy and Sack [45]	Procedure to assess circadian phase based on the peak of melatonin concentration that can be measured in plasma or saliva samples.
Subjective tools		
MRhI	Oliveira et al. [40]	Detects rhythmicity of mood-related symptoms among cognitive, affective, and somatic domains. Each item is composed of a yes/no question about the perception of rhythmicity and a time scale to point out when it peaks (in the case of an affirmative answer).

Name	References	Definition and outputs
BRIAN	Giglio et al. [46]	Assesses biological rhythms in mental health clinical settings, being composed of sleep/social rhythm, activity, and eating pattern factors.
Sleep, Circadian Rhythms and Mood questionnaire	Byrne et al. [47]	Assesses sleep quality, circadian phase, and depressed mood.
MEQ	Horne and Ostberg [48]	Classifies subjects in morning, intermediate, or evening chronotypes based on preferences in sleep and waking times, and subjective "peak" times at which individuals feel their best to perform different types of activities.
MCTQ	Roenneberg et al. [13]	Assesses, separately for workdays and work-free days, sleep schedules and calculates parameters that are used to estimate chronotype and social jetlag such as: midpoint of sleep on workdays (MSW) and on work-free days (MSF); social jetlag (calculated by the difference between MSF and MSW); and the sleep deficit (difference between sleep duration on workdays and sleep duration on work-free days).
PSQI	Buysse et al. [22]	Assesses sleep quality and sleep disturbances.

11.4 Therapeutic Strategies for Sleep Disturbances in BD

As exposed, several studies have established a robust connection between disruptions in sleep and circadian rhythms and mood episodes in BD. Consequently, there is significant interest in comprehending circadian rhythms in BD and devising diagnostic markers and treatments based on chronobiological principles. Stabilizing circadian rhythms and enhancing sleep quality can effectively manage and prevent mood episodes, offering a holistic approach to BD treatment. The variability in circadian rhythms among individuals with BD underscores the potential effectiveness of personalized treatment strategies targeting specific circadian disruptions, aligning with the broader trend in psychiatry toward personalized and precision medicine. Interventions aimed at correcting these disruptions have shown efficacy in reducing the frequency and severity of mood episodes, supporting their role in the comprehensive management of BD. This section explores therapeutic strategies targeting sleep and circadian rhythm disturbances in individuals with BD, including pharmacological treatments, behavioral interventions, and light therapy, among others [49, 50]. Here is a brief overview of these interventions and their mechanisms:

11.4.1 Pharmacological Treatments

(a) Mood stabilizers: Lithium and valproate, first-line treatment for BD, appear to exert their effects partly through chronobiological mechanisms. A systematic review of 95 studies indicated lithium's potential to delay sleep–wake phase rhythms, stabilize social rhythms, and improve sleep efficiency and duration [51]. Another study comparing chronotypes and sleep patterns in euthymic patients with BD, currently receiving (n = 149) or not receiving (n = 376) lithium, showed better sleep efficiency and increased sleep duration in those receiving lithium [52]. These findings suggest that lithium could offer benefits for circadian rhythm dysregulation in BD, potentially through its effects on related circadian genes (e.g., NR1D1, PER2, and ARNTL) and promoting the release of melatonin [49].

(b) Melatonin and Melatonin Receptor Agonists: Exogenous melatonin can exert distinct effects according to the timing of its administration. For instance, taking melatonin in the afternoon induces a phase advance, with the most significant effect occurring 4–5 hours before the onset of endogenous melatonin secretion. This phase advance is useful for correcting delayed sleep phase disorder. Conversely, administering melatonin in the morning can be beneficial for adjusting an advanced sleep phase. These effects are observed even at low doses, ranging from 0.125 to 1 mg. Both effects are referred to as the "chronobiotic" effect of melatonin, signifying its capacity to alter the characteristics of biological rhythms, including the period, amplitude, or phase of circadian rhythms. Furthermore, sleep-promoting, known as the "soporific" effect, can be achieved with melatonin's administration close to bedtime (15–30 minutes before) with initial doses at 2 mg. The soporific effect refers to melatonin's ability to promote sleep by inducing drowsiness and facilitating sleep onset [53].

Exogenous melatonin is available in various forms, including tablets, capsules, orodispersible forms, oral solutions, and sprays, with options for immediate or prolonged release. Doses typically range from 3 to 10 mg. It is generally well-tolerated, with mild adverse effects such as headache, dizziness, nausea, and drowsiness.

As a result of melatonin's effects, it has been recommended to treat three main conditions, such as delayed sleep phase syndrome and chronic insomnia disorder, and to improve sleep quality. Melatonin has been used in the treatment of patients with mood disorders in various situations, including sleep disturbances or low sleep quality, delayed sleep phase, and mood stabilization during both acute and remitted phases [53]. However, these benefits have been particularly observed in studies on unipolar depression in combination with antidepressants, although with small sample sizes.

With regard to the melatonin agonist ramelteon, their effects on sleep disturbance in patients with BD were inconclusive [49, 50]. Similarly, the limited studies assessing the effects of agomelatine for the treatment of sleep disturbance in BD have controversial results. Furthermore, there have been reports of patients experiencing a switch to mania when receiving agomelatine for the treatment of bipolar depression [49, 50]. Further randomized and placebo-controlled clinical trials, with larger samples, are necessary to define the potential benefits of melatonin and its agonists for the treatment of biological rhythms in BD.

11.4.2 Light Therapy

Light therapy is highly recommended as a primary treatment for both seasonal and non-seasonal depression (including unipolar and BD), offering significant benefits such as improved sleep, alertness, and regulation of circadian rhythms, all of which can be disrupted in depressive states.

Traditionally, light therapy is administered through direct exposure to a light box equipped with fluorescent tubes, although LED technology has largely replaced these. Other devices, such as glasses or visors, also exist but have been explored in fewer studies. In BD, studies utilizing “blue-light blocking glasses” have demonstrated a reduction in manic symptoms, with noticeable improvements observed in the initial days of treatment [54]. Conversely, for individuals with bipolar depression, exposure to bright light revealed significant reductions in depressive symptoms and higher rates of remission compared to placebo [55]. Despite these encouraging results, further prospective studies with more rigorous design and consistent follow-up, and larger samples are required to replicate the potential benefits of light therapy in BD.

Despite variations in delivery methods, light therapy appears to be well-tolerated overall, with adverse effects typically mild and transient. These effects may include headache, glare, sleep disturbances, eyestrain, nausea, agitation, and, in the case of patients with BD, manic switches. Although the risk of manic switch in BD is low, the International Society of Bipolar Disorders (ISBD) task force has recommended pre-treating patients with BD with a mood stabilizer and closely monitoring for hypomanic switches [56]. For more detailed information on usage protocols and parameters of light therapy in depressive episodes, referring to recent studies like Geoffroy and Palagini [53] is advisable.

11.4.3 Sleep Deprivation

Evidence suggests that response rates to sleep deprivation among individuals with mood disorders range from 45% to 60%. This intervention is recognized as safe and rapid, often yielding a response within 7 days [53]. Consequently, the ISBD task force has recommended considering sleep deprivation when more established treatment options fail, are not tolerated, or when a swift antidepressant response is necessary [56]. However, it is important to note that sleep deprivation is contraindicated in the acute treatment of manic episodes [56].

11.4.4 Behavioral Interventions

(a) Cognitive Behavioral Therapy for Insomnia stands as the foremost recommended treatment for chronic insomnia or insomnia disorder. Within the realm of research exploring the interplay between insomnia and psychiatric conditions, Harvey et al. [57] proposed a modified version of CBT-I tailored specifically for BD, termed CBTI-BP [57]. The protocol includes behavioral elements such as helping patients develop "winding down" activities that can take place in low-lighting settings and encourage sleep, identifying ways that patients can ensure regular sleep–wake, exercise, and mealtimes, and educating patients on the relevance of circadian rhythms in sleep.

    Overall, other authors have supported the use of CBT-I in the management of sleep disorders in patients with BD. For instance, Costa [58] and Scott [59] both reported that CBT, when used in conjunction with psychoeducation and pharmacological treatment, can reduce the frequency and duration of mood episodes, improve quality of life, and increase compliance. Furthermore, the ISBD task force has endorsed the use of the CBTI-BP protocol for treating insomnia in patients with BD during euthymic phases [56].

(b) The Interpersonal and Social Rhythm Therapy (IPSRT) is a manualized treatment, developed by Ellen Frank [60], that addresses interpersonal problems and disrupted social rhythms with the intent of stabilizing underlying biologic processes [61]. It focuses on stabilizing daily routines and sleep–wake cycles, involving monitoring and regulating social rhythms, such as mealtimes, exercise, and social interactions, to maintain a consistent daily schedule. At least three randomized clinical trials have clearly demonstrated the efficacy of the IPSRT on mood stabilizing, improving functioning, and life satisfaction in adults with BD. Based on evidence, IPSRT is also recommended for the acute treatment of bipolar depression and for the prevention of bipolar mood episodes. Furthermore, this intervention was investigated in adolescents who are at risk of developing BD. While there are potential advantages to this intervention for regulating circadian rhythms in young patients, the limited attendance of young individuals at the sessions may hinder the interpretation of the results [62].

(c) Other interventions incorporating elements targeting social rhythm disruption in BD include the Facilitated Integrated Mood Management (FIMM) program. This five-session intervention integrates traditional practices of BD-targeted psychotherapies (e.g., psychoeducation and identification of mood relapse warning signs) in the context of a single treatment program. One element focuses on stabilizing sleep/wake and daily activity times, thus holding application for improving social rhythm dysfunction in BD. Despite being promising, the effects of FIMM were modest in clinical trials [50].

In conclusion, as demonstrated throughout this section, most studies have been conducted in adults with BD. Indeed, therapeutic interventions based on circadian principles are included in contemporary professional treatment guidelines for BD. However, the ambiguous and incomplete chronobiology of BD literature, in particular, in latent BD limits utilization of these treatments, the development of standard protocols, and the means to identify optimally responsive patients with BD.

11.5 Future Perspectives

This chapter underscores the critical importance of recognizing and addressing sleep and circadian rhythm disturbances in individuals with or at risk for BD. By elucidating the complex interplay between these disturbances and the onset and progression of BD, this chapter calls for enhanced early detection methods and targeted interventions. Future research efforts should focus on refining assessment tools, advancing understanding of the underlying pathophysiological mechanisms, and developing personalized treatment strategies. Ultimately, integrating these insights into clinical practice promises to significantly improve outcomes and quality of life for individuals affected by BD.

References

1. Wirz-Justice A. Biological rhythm disturbances in mood disorders. Int Clin Psychopharmacol. 2006;21(Supplement 1):S11–5.
2. American Psychiatric Association. Diagnostic and statistical manual of mental disorders [Internet]. 5th. ed. American Psychiatric Association; 2013. [cited 2024 Jul 1]. Available from: https://psychiatryonline.org/doi/book/10.1176/appi.books.9780890425596
3. McClung CA. How might circadian rhythms control mood? Let me count the ways. Biol Psychiatry. 2013;74(4):242–9.
4. Bell-Pedersen D, Cassone VM, Earnest DJ, Golden SS, Hardin PE, Thomas TL, et al. Circadian rhythms from multiple oscillators: lessons from diverse organisms. Nat Rev Genet. 2005;6(7):544–56.
5. Patton AP, Hastings MH. The suprachiasmatic nucleus. Curr Biol. 2018;28(15):R816–22.
6. LeGates TA, Fernandez DC, Hattar S. Light as a central modulator of circadian rhythms, sleep and affect. Nat Rev Neurosci. 2014;15(7):443–54.
7. Wirz-Justice A, Terman M. CME: light therapy: why, what, for whom, how, and when (and a postscript about darkness). Praxis. 2022;111(2):56–62.
8. Chaix A, Zarrinpar A, Panda S. The circadian coordination of cell biology. J Cell Biol. 2016;215(1):15–25.
9. McCarthy MJ, Gottlieb JF, Gonzalez R, McClung CA, Alloy LB, Cain S, et al. Neurobiological and behavioral mechanisms of circadian rhythm disruption in bipolar disorder: a critical multidisciplinary literature review and agenda for future research from the ISBD task force on chronobiology. Bipolar Disord. 2022;24(3):232–63.
10. Vitaterna MH, King DP, Chang AM, Kornhauser JM, Lowrey PL, McDonald JD, et al. Mutagenesis and mapping of a mouse gene, *Clock*, essential for circadian behavior. Science. 1994;264(5159):719–25.
11. Dzirasa K, Coque L, Sidor MM, Kumar S, Dancy EA, Takahashi JS, et al. Lithium ameliorates nucleus accumbens phase-signaling dysfunction in a genetic mouse model of mania. J Neurosci. 2010;30(48):16314–23.

12. Oliveira MAB, De Abreu ACOV, Constantino DB, Tonon AC, Díez-Noguera A, Amaral FG, et al. Taking biological rhythms into account: from study design to results reporting. Physiol Behav. 2024;273:114387.
13. Roenneberg T, Wirz-Justice A, Merrow M. Life between clocks: daily temporal patterns of human chronotypes. J Biol Rhythm. 2003;18(1):80–90.
14. Adan A, Archer SN, Hidalgo MP, Di Milia L, Natale V, Randler C. Circadian typology: a comprehensive review. Chronobiol Int. 2012;29(9):1153–75.
15. Walker WH, Walton JC, DeVries AC, Nelson RJ. Circadian rhythm disruption and mental health. Transl Psychiatry. 2020;10(1):28.
16. Millar A, Espie CA, Scott J. The sleep of remitted bipolar outpatients: a controlled naturalistic study using actigraphy. J Affect Disord. 2004;80(2–3):145–53.
17. Jackson A, Cavanagh J, Scott J. A systematic review of manic and depressive prodromes. J Affect Disord. 2003;74(3):209–17.
18. Harvey AG, Schmidt DA, Scarnà A, Semler CN, Goodwin GM. Sleep-related functioning in euthymic patients with bipolar disorder, patients with insomnia, and subjects without sleep problems. Am J Psychiatry. 2005;162(1):50–7.
19. Bauer M, Grof P, Rasgon N, Bschor T, Glenn T, Whybrow PC. Temporal relation between sleep and mood in patients with bipolar disorder. Bipolar Disord. 2006;8(2):160–7.
20. Ritter PS, Marx C, Lewtschenko N, Pfeiffer S, Leopold K, Bauer M, et al. The characteristics of sleep in patients with manifest bipolar disorder, subjects at high risk of developing the disease and healthy controls. J Neural Transm. 2012;119(10):1173–84.
21. Geoffroy PA, Boudebesse C, Bellivier F, Lajnef M, Henry C, Leboyer M, et al. Sleep in remitted bipolar disorder: a naturalistic case-control study using actigraphy. J Affect Disord. 2014;158:1–7.
22. Buysse DJ, Reynolds CF, Monk TH, Berman SR, Kupfer DJ. The Pittsburgh sleep quality index: a new instrument for psychiatric practice and research. Psychiatry Res. 1989;28(2):193–213.
23. Giglio LMF, Andreazza AC, Andersen M, Cereser KM, Walz JC, Sterz L, et al. Sleep in bipolar patients. Sleep Breath. 2009;13(2):169–73.
24. Lunsford-Avery JR, Judd CM, Axelson DA, Miklowitz DJ. Sleep impairment, mood symptoms, and psychosocial functioning in adolescent bipolar disorder. Psychiatry Res. 2012;200(2–3):265–71.
25. Patel V, Saxena S, Lund C, Thornicroft G, Baingana F, Bolton P, et al. The lancet commission on global mental health and sustainable development. Lancet. 2018;392(10157):1553–98.
26. Scott J, Etain B, Miklowitz D, Crouse JJ, Carpenter J, Marwaha S, et al. A systematic review and meta-analysis of sleep and circadian rhythms disturbances in individuals at high-risk of developing or with early onset of bipolar disorders. Neurosci Biobehav Rev. 2022;135:104585.
27. Duffy A, Jones S, Goodday S, Bentall R. Candidate risks indicators for bipolar disorder: early intervention opportunities in high-risk youth. Int J Neuropsychopharmacol. 2016;19(1):pyv071.
28. Grof P, Duffy A, Alda M, Hajek T. Lithium response across generations. Acta Psychiatr Scand. 2009;120(5):378–85.
29. Duffy A, Alda M, Hajek T, Sherry SB, Grof P. Early stages in the development of bipolar disorder. J Affect Disord. 2010;121(1–2):127–35.
30. Duffy A, Carlson GA. How does a developmental perspective inform us about the early natural history of bipolar disorder? J Can Acad Child Adolesc Psychiatry. 2013;22(1):6–12.
31. McGorry PD, Nelson B, Goldstone S, Yung AR. Clinical staging: a heuristic and practical strategy for new research and better health and social outcomes for psychotic and related mood disorders. Can J Psychiatr. 2010;55(8):486–97.
32. Ng TH, Chung KF, Ho FYY, Yeung WF, Yung KP, Lam TH. Sleep–wake disturbance in interepisode bipolar disorder and high-risk individuals: a systematic review and meta-analysis. Sleep Med Rev. 2015;20:46–58.
33. Melo MCA, Garcia RF, Linhares Neto VB, Sá MB, De Mesquita LMF, De Araújo CFC, et al. Sleep and circadian alterations in people at risk for bipolar disorder: a systematic review. J Psychiatr Res. 2016;83:211–9.

34. Levenson JC, Axelson DA, Merranko J, Angulo M, Goldstein TR, Mullin BC, et al. Differences in sleep disturbances among offspring of parents with and without bipolar disorder: association with conversion to bipolar disorder. Bipolar Disord. 2015;17(8):836–48.
35. Ritter PS, Höfler M, Wittchen HU, Lieb R, Bauer M, Pfennig A, et al. Disturbed sleep as risk factor for the subsequent onset of bipolar disorder – data from a 10-year prospective-longitudinal study among adolescents and young adults. J Psychiatr Res. 2015;68:76–82.
36. Pilz LK, De Oliveira MAB, Steibel EG, Policarpo LM, Carissimi A, Carvalho FG, et al. Development and testing of methods for detecting off-wrist in actimetry recordings. Sleep. 2022;45(8):zsac118.
37. Lyall LM, Wyse CA, Graham N, Ferguson A, Lyall DM, Cullen B, et al. Association of disrupted circadian rhythmicity with mood disorders, subjective wellbeing, and cognitive function: a cross-sectional study of 91 105 participants from the UK Biobank. Lancet Psychiatry. 2018;5(6):507–14.
38. Pandi-Perumal SR, Smits M, Spence W, Srinivasan V, Cardinali DP, Lowe AD, et al. Dim light melatonin onset (DLMO): a tool for the analysis of circadian phase in human sleep and chronobiological disorders. Prog Neuro-Psychopharmacol Biol Psychiatry. 2007;31(1):1–11.
39. Pilz LK, Carissimi A, Oliveira MAB, Francisco AP, Fabris RC, Medeiros MS, et al. Rhythmicity of mood symptoms in individuals at risk for psychiatric disorders. Sci Rep. 2018;8(1):11402.
40. Alves Braga De Oliveira M, De Mendonça Filho E, Carissimi A, Lima Dos Santos Garay L, Scop M, Ruschel Bandeira D, et al. The revised mood rhythm instrument: a large multicultural psychometric study. J Clin Med. 2021;10(3):388.
41. Moro MF, Carta MG, Pintus M, Pintus E, Melis R, Kapczinski F, et al. Validation of the Italian version of the Biological Rhythms Interview of Assessment in Neuropsychiatry (BRIAN): some considerations on its screening usefulness. Clin Pract Epidemiol Ment Health. 2014;10(1):48–52.
42. Kuppili P, Menon V, Chandrasekaran V, Navin K. Biological rhythm impairment in bipolar disorder: a state or trait marker? Indian J Psychiatry. 2018;60(4):404.
43. Wittmann M, Dinich J, Merrow M, Roenneberg T. Social jetlag: misalignment of biological and social time. Chronobiol Int. 2006;23(1–2):497–509.
44. Ancoli-Israel S, Cole R, Alessi C, Chambers M, Moorcroft W, Pollak CP. The role of actigraphy in the study of sleep and circadian rhythms. Sleep. 2003;26(3):342–92.
45. Lewy AJ, Sack RL. The dim light melatonin onset as a marker for orcadian phase position. Chronobiol Int. 1989;6(1):93–102.
46. Giglio LMF, Magalhães PVDS, Andreazza AC, Walz JC, Jakobson L, Rucci P, et al. Development and use of a biological rhythm interview. J Affect Disord. 2009;118(1–3):161–5.
47. Byrne JEM, Bullock B, Murray G. Development of a measure of sleep, circadian rhythms, and mood: the SCRAM questionnaire. Front Psychol. 2017;1(8):2105.
48. Horne JA, Ostberg O. A self-assessment questionnaire to determine morningness-eveningness in human circadian rhythms. Int J Chronobiol. 1976;4(2):97–110.
49. Bellivier F, Geoffroy PA, Etain B, Scott J. Sleep- and circadian rhythm–associated pathways as therapeutic targets in bipolar disorder. Expert Opin Ther Targets. 2015;19(6):747–63.
50. Gold AK, Kinrys G. Treating circadian rhythm disruption in bipolar disorder. Curr Psychiatry Rep. 2019;21(3):14.
51. Moreira J, Geoffroy PA. Lithium and bipolar disorder: impacts from molecular to behavioural circadian rhythms. Chronobiol Int. 2016;33(4):351–73.
52. Geoffroy PA, Samalin L, Llorca PM, Curis E, Bellivier F. Influence of lithium on sleep and chronotypes in remitted patients with bipolar disorder. J Affect Disord. 2016;204:32–9.
53. Geoffroy PA, Palagini L. Biological rhythms and chronotherapeutics in depression. Prog Neuro-Psychopharmacol Biol Psychiatry. 2021;106:110158.
54. Phelps J. Dark therapy for bipolar disorder using amber lenses for blue light blockade. Med Hypotheses. 2008;70(2):224–9.

55. Sit DK, McGowan J, Wiltrout C, Diler RS, Dills JJ, Luther J, et al. Adjunctive bright light therapy for bipolar depression: a randomized double-blind placebo-controlled trial. Am J Psychiatry. 2018;175(2):131–9.
56. Gottlieb JF, Benedetti F, Geoffroy PA, Henriksen TEG, Lam RW, Murray G, et al. The chronotherapeutic treatment of bipolar disorders: a systematic review and practice recommendations from the ISBD task force on chronotherapy and chronobiology. Bipolar Disord. 2019;21(8):741–73.
57. Harvey AG, Soehner AM, Kaplan KA, Hein K, Lee J, Kanady J, et al. Treating insomnia improves mood state, sleep, and functioning in bipolar disorder: a pilot randomized controlled trial. J Consult Clin Psychol. 2015;83(3):564–77.
58. Costa RTD, Rangé BP, Malagris LEN, Sardinha A, Carvalho MRD, Nardi AE. Cognitive–behavioral therapy for bipolar disorder. Expert Rev Neurother. 2010;10(7):1089–99.
59. Scott J, Paykel E, Morriss R, Bentall R, Kinderman P, Johnson T, et al. Cognitive–behavioural therapy for severe and recurrent bipolar disorders: randomised controlled trial. Br J Psychiatry. 2006;188(4):313–20.
60. Frank E, Swartz HA, Boland E. Interpersonal and social rhythm therapy: an intervention addressing rhythm dysregulation in bipolar disorder. Dialogues Clin Neurosci. 2007;9(3):325–32.
61. Frank E, Kupfer DJ, Thase ME, Mallinger AG, Swartz HA, Fagiolini AM, et al. Two-year outcomes for interpersonal and social rhythm therapy in individuals with bipolar I disorder. Arch Gen Psychiatry. 2005;62(9):996.
62. Goldstein TR, Fersch-Podrat R, Axelson DA, Gilbert A, Hlastala SA, Birmaher B, et al. Early intervention for adolescents at high risk for the development of bipolar disorder: pilot study of Interpersonal and Social Rhythm Therapy (IPSRT). Psychotherapy. 2014;51(1):180–9.

Chapter 12
The Impact of Substance Use in Latent Bipolar Disorder

Kyara Rodrigues de Aguiar, Camila Zimmer, Vanessa Gnielka, and Devon Watts

12.1 Common Markers Between Substance Use Disorder and Bipolar Disorder

There are some common factors to both disorders, as well as characteristics of bipolar disorder (BD) that are more associated with substance use disorder (SUD) compared to others. For instance, men are recognized to have greater lifetime susceptibility to SUD in contrast to women, which is also observed in BD [15]. Among individuals with BD, the most pronounced co-occurrences with SUD are observed with alcohol use disorder (AUD) (42%), succeeded by Cannabis (20%) and other illicit substances (17%) [15].

According to a cross-sectional study that compared patients with BD with and without SUD, factors that were mainly associated with comorbid SUD in BD were BD type I diagnosis and mixed features [28]. Moreover, a familiar history of BD was significantly more frequent among subjects with comorbid SUD[28]. This corroborates the evidence of genetic association between the conditions. It is important to highlight that SUD can also impact the progression of illness in this population,

K. R. de Aguiar (✉) · C. Zimmer
Psychiatry and Behavioral Sciences, Universidade Federal do Rio Grande do Sul (UFRGS), Porto Alegre, Brazil

V. Gnielka
Post Graduate Program in Psychiatry and Behavioral Sciences, Department of Psychiatry, School of Medicine, Universidade Federal do Rio Grande do Sul (UFRGS), Porto Alegre, RS, Brazil

Mood Disorders Clinic, McMaster University, Hamilton, ON, Canada

D. Watts
Harvard Medical School, Boston, MA, USA

T. de Azevedo Cardoso et al. (eds.), *Latent Bipolar Disorder*,
https://doi.org/10.1007/978-3-032-01297-5_12

potentially leading to the emergence of a complete major affective episode [4], an increased risk of psychotic symptoms, and heightened functional impairment [5].

In this context, a Spanish cohort study followed for 23 years aimed to identify the most meaningful variables associated with SUD, AUD, and AUD in comorbidity with any other SUD (AUD + SUD) in a large sample of patients with BD through the use of a random forest model [33]. The model with the highest accuracy was the one predicting the co-occurrence of another SUD among individuals with AUD, and compared with those without SUD, correctly classifying up to 75% of the sample. In this model, a first episode of hypomanic and heterodirected aggressivity was associated with AUD + SUD in patients with BD. Among other models, a lifetime comorbid diagnosis of cluster B personality disorder and not being in a relationship predicted the presence of SUD alone when compared to non-SUD in patients with BD. Also, a first episode of depressive was associated with AUD alone when compared to AUD + SUD.

12.2 Impact of SUD in BD

It is difficult to determine whether SUD is a predisposing factor for BD, whether it is an early marker of the onset of the disease, or even whether it is a comorbid disorder that begins from a common denominator. The fact is that the interaction between SUD and BD leads to numerous problematic outcomes. The presence of SUD accounts for a higher number of lifetime mood episodes and hospitalizations [18] and lifetime medical comorbidities [27]. It is also associated with non-remission in patients with BD [44]. A study found that SUD in patients with BD is associated with impulsive-aggressive behavior, including both dimensional traits and categorical DSM diagnoses such as conduct disorder and Cluster B personality disorder [11]. SUD was also associated with all-cause mortality in BD patients in a large populational study, especially alcohol and hard drugs [14]. The same study found an association of alcohol and hard drugs use and death from accidents. Additionally, a systematic review highlights that individuals with BD and SUD comorbidity exhibit notable cognitive impairments across several domains, particularly executive functioning and memory [8]. These cognitive deficits can further complicate treatment and exacerbate symptoms, potentially impacting long-term outcomes. This suggests that interventions addressing cognitive impairments may be beneficial in managing the comorbid conditions. Substance use may also reduce adherence and effectiveness of psychopharmacological treatments, further worsening the BD course [24]. Patients with BD with multiple SUD experience exacerbated outcomes, such as heightened risk of overdose, criminal involvement, poor adherence to treatment, and diminished overall functioning [27].

Another important aspect to be addressed in the relationship between SUD and BD concerns a severe mental health outcome: suicidality. A systematic review done by the International Society for Bipolar Disorder identified that the presence of a current or lifetime comorbid SUD was associated with a higher risk of suicide attempts in patients with BD, with an odds ratio (OR) of 1.81 when all substances were considered. Significant associations were identified among studies of AUD (OR = 1.60) and illicit drug use (OR = 1.72), but not for cannabis use (OR = 1.29) [39]. Although related to suicide attempts, the presence of SUD was not significantly associated with suicide deaths in this population. Similarly, in a meta-analysis involving 7952 individuals, individuals with BD with lifetime comorbid SUDs had a higher risk of suicidal behaviors compared with those without SUDs (OR = 1.77), with no significant heterogeneity across studies [3]. This relationship was seen with both AUD and SUD, and with both abuse and dependence, demonstrating that the type of substance and the severity of the condition are less determining than previously thought. A further retrospective cross-sectional study corroborates this association, identifying that patients with lifetime suicide attempts were found to have a more frequent history of poly-SUDs [42].

12.3 SUD as a Predictor of BD

Another possible association is that SUD plays a predictive role in the development of BD throughout life. Although there is some evidence in this direction, studies on the subject are scarce. A retrospective observational cohort study developed a prognostic model of major depressive disorder (MDD) diagnostic conversion to BD within a 1-year period. Substance misuse was found as a clinical predictor of prospective transition from MDD to BD in this sample [32].

Moreover, a prospective study involving offspring of parents with BD indicated that SUD emerges early in the progression of BD among those genetically predisposed, preceding the onset of initial major depressive or fully developed manic or hypomanic episodes [5]. The rate of lifetime SUD in this population was high (23.70%), and individuals with SUD had lower global functioning scores. The condition was also associated with mood psychopathology, psychotic features, and neurodevelopmental antecedents. Considering the temporal order of psychopathological occurrences, it became evident that minor mood disorders predicted SUD, whereas BD exhibited a bidirectional relationship with SUD. Additionally, SUD foretold the subsequent emergence of psychotic symptoms. The risk of major mood disorder, including BD, was approximately three times higher in individuals with SUD compared to those without a prior SUD. A systematic review confirmed that substance use is indeed a risk factor for the development of BD, with 66.7% of studies supporting this association. The review highlighted cannabis, nonmedical use of prescription medications, nicotine, and alcohol as notable substances contributing to the risk of developing BD [19]. The frequency of cannabis use, in particular, was identified as an important variable, with greater use associated with higher risks of transitioning to BD.

Data from two extensive studies revealed a gradual decline in the age at onset of BD type I among male and female patients within a pan-European clinical sample. Additionally, these studies found a birth cohort effect in which the age at onset of

BD type I has decreased in recent cohorts, with this trend linked to increasing rates of SUD [40]. Individuals with SUD, particularly males, consistently experience an earlier onset of BD type I in this population. This suggests that SUD may either trigger earlier episodes of BD type I or share common risk factors. The findings highlight SUD as a potentially modifiable factor that could be targeted to delay BD type I onset in at-risk individuals, although more studies are needed to corroborate these data.

Older studies already sought to investigate the effects of antecedent substance abuse on the development of first-episode psychotic mania. In a sample of patients hospitalized for a first manic or mixed episode of BD, antecedent alcohol and drug abuse were associated with a shorter delay between the onset of the affective syndrome and hospitalization [41]. However, these findings were deemed preliminary due to the study's small sample size ($n = 59$) and its *post-hoc* design.

12.4 Polygenic Architecture and Genetic Overlap Between BD and SUDs: Insights from Recent Studies

BD and SUDs are complex psychiatric conditions that often co-occur, leading to significant morbidity and mortality. Twin and family studies have demonstrated that BD is highly heritable, with estimates ranging from 60% to 85% [21, 26], whereas SUDs are moderately heritable, with estimates ranging from 40% to 70% depending on the specific substance [47]. These heritability estimates are derived from twin and family studies, which compare the concordance rates of a disorder between monozygotic and dizygotic twins or the prevalence of the disorder among first-degree relatives of affected individuals. While these studies provide valuable insights into the overall genetic heritability of BD and SUDs, they do not identify specific genetic variants associated with these disorders [45].

Recent large-scale genome-wide association studies (GWASs) have begun to unravel the complex genetic underpinnings of SUDs and BD. The largest GWAS of BD to date conducted by the Psychiatric Genomics Consortium (PGC), included 41,917 BD cases and 371,549 controls of European ancestry [29]. This study identified 64 genome-wide significant risk loci, 33 of which were novel discoveries. These loci encompassed genes involved in synaptic signaling, calcium channel activity, and neurodevelopmental processes. However, these genome-wide significant loci still only explain a small portion of the total heritability of BD. Moreover, in the largest GWAS of problematic alcohol use (PAU), including 435,563 individuals of European ancestry, 29 independent risk variants were identified explaining 9% of the variance in PAU [50]. Similarly, a GWAS of cannabis use disorder (CUD) in 20,916 cases and 363,116 controls identified two genome-wide significant loci explaining 11% of the variance in CUD [16].

Despite these advances, genome-wide significant loci identified in these studies only explain a small portion of the total heritability of BD and SUDs, with many variants of small effects contributing to overall risk, rather than a few genes of large effect, highlighting the highly polygenic nature of these disorders [12]. Polygenic risk scores (PRSs), which are calculated by summing the effects of many genetic variants associated with a disorder (weighted by their effect sizes estimated from GWAS), have been used to further investigate the genetic architecture of BD and SUDs. While PRSs have shown promise in predicting risk for psychiatric disorders, their predictive power remains limited, as they only capture a portion of the genetic risk identified through GWAS [35]. Nevertheless, PRS can be useful for investigating the shared genetic architecture between disorders and identifying individuals at higher risk for developing comorbid conditions.

Interestingly, the genetic architecture of SUDs appears to differ depending on the specific trait being studied. For instance, the genetic risk for substance dependence tends to be partially distinct from the genetic risk for level of use or frequency of use. A recent study by Kranzler et al. [17] found that PAU, as measured by the Alcohol Use Disorders Identification Test-Consumption (AUDIT-C), had a genetic correlation of only 0.52 with AUD diagnosis. Similarly, Johnson et al. [16] reported a genetic correlation of 0.50 between CUD and lifetime cannabis use. These findings suggest that the genetic factors influencing substance use initiation and frequency are not identical to those influencing the transition to dependence and problematic use.

Furthermore, substance dependence tends to have higher genetic correlations with other psychiatric disorders compared to the level of use traits. For example, PAU shows strong genetic correlations with depression ($rg = 0.61$), attention-deficit/hyperactivity disorder (ADHD) ($rg = 0.54$), and schizophrenia (SCZ) ($rg = 0.36$), while AUDIT-C scores have much weaker correlations with these disorders [17]. This pattern has also been observed for cannabis, with CUD showing stronger genetic overlap with major depression and SCZ compared to cannabis use frequency [16]. These findings underscore the genetic distinction between substance use and dependence and suggest that the latter may share more common genetic vulnerabilities with other psychiatric conditions.

While most of the genetic risk for SUDs is attributable to many variants of small effect, a few large-effect risk loci have been identified for certain substances. For alcohol, variants in the alcohol dehydrogenase (ADH1B) and aldehyde dehydrogenase (ALDH2) genes, which are involved in alcohol metabolism, have been robustly associated with alcohol dependence, particularly in East Asian populations where the risk alleles are more common [17]. Similarly, variants in the nicotinic acetylcholine receptor genes (CHRNA5–CHRNA3–CHRNB4) have been consistently linked to nicotine dependence and heavy smoking [49]. However, even these large-effect loci explain only a small portion of the overall genetic risk for alcohol and nicotine use disorders.

Furthermore, in a recent GWAS, 11 genomic loci were associated with both AUD and BD, and 10 loci with both AUD and SCZ, suggesting shared biological pathways [48], although most of the genetic risk for BD and SUDs remains unexplained by currently identified variants, and the causal nature of the relationships between these disorders is still unclear. Pleiotropy, where a genetic variant influences multiple traits, is widespread in psychiatry and complicates efforts to disentangle cause from consequence [20].

Additional statistical methods, such as genomic structural equation modeling (genomic SEM), have been employed to further dissect the genetic relationships between SUDs and BD. Genomic SEM can model the multivariate genetic architecture across traits and identify shared genetic factors [10]. This approach utilizes GWAS summary statistics rather than individual level data, thereby facilitating the study of genetic relationships across traits while maintaining participant privacy. Furthermore, unlike traditional GWASs that examine one trait at a time, genomic SEM can model multiple traits simultaneously, which allows for identifying genetic factors that are shared across traits (pleiotropy) as well as those that are specific to individual traits. When applied to SUDs, genomic SEM has identified potential substance-specific genetic factors as well as factors shared across all SUDs [13]. Similarly, genomic SEM has been used to examine the genetic relationships between BD, SCZ, and MDD, revealing that BD symptoms such as mania, psychosis, and depression are associated with disorder-specific genetic components [38].

Furthermore, Mendelian randomization (MR) is a method that uses genetic variants as instrumental variables to test for causal relationships between an exposure (e.g., substance use) and an outcome (e.g., BD). By using genetic variants that are associated with the exposure but not directly associated with the outcome, this approach can mitigate confounding and reverse causation that often plague observational studies. Among available studies focusing on mental health, smoking has been the most investigated in an MR framework, and there is robust evidence that smoking causally increases the odds of several mental disorders, more so than the reverse relationship, which aligns with findings from longitudinal cohort studies and animal models demonstrating neuropsychiatric impacts of smoking [43]. However, MR is subject to several challenges that can affect the validity of its conclusions. One of the core challenges is horizontal pleiotropy, which occurs when a genetic variant influences the outcome through pathways other than the exposure of interest [46]. For example, a genetic variant associated with alcohol consumption may also influence BD risk through its effects on sleep patterns or impulsivity, rather than solely through alcohol use. Moreover, if the genetic variants used as instruments explain only a small fraction of the variance in the exposure, the MR estimates may be biased and imprecise [1]. These challenges highlight the need for careful instrument selection and sensitivity analyses in MR studies of BD and SUDs.

Another key challenge is the lack of diversity in psychiatric genomics. The vast majority of large-scale GWASs have been conducted in populations of European ancestry, limiting the generalizability of findings to other ancestral groups[23]. Effect sizes of PRSs derived from European samples are significantly attenuated in non-European populations, underscoring the need for more inclusive research [6]. Increasing diversity in psychiatric genomics is crucial for ensuring equitable progress and realizing the full potential of precision medicine approaches.

In conclusion, recent genomic studies have provided valuable insights into the shared genetic architecture of BD and SUDs, revealing a complex interplay of common and rare variants, as well as substance-specific and disorder-specific genetic factors. The substantial genetic overlap between these disorders suggests that common biological pathways may underlie their comorbidity, offering potential targets for intervention and treatment. However, much work remains to be done to translate these genetic findings into a mechanistic understanding and clinical applications. Future research should prioritize increasing the diversity of study populations to ensure equitable representation and generalizability of findings. Integration of genetic data with other omics approaches, such as epigenomics and transcriptomics, may provide a more comprehensive understanding of the biological processes linking BD and SUDs. Furthermore, the development of more sophisticated statistical methods, such as those that can model the dynamic interplay between genetic and environmental factors across the lifespan, will be crucial for disentangling the complex etiologies of these disorders.

12.5 Strategies to Mitigate Substance Use in At-Risk Individuals for BD

The prevalence of SUD among individuals diagnosed with BD is high, affecting more than half of this population [36]. Similarly, individuals diagnosed with SUD frequently exhibit comorbid mental disorders, with BD being one of the most commonly linked conditions [9]. These data are alarming, as SUD tends to complicate the treatment of BD. An experimental study that compared participants diagnosed with BD and comorbid SUD to those with BD alone found that individuals with both conditions were less likely to adhere to mood stabilizers (65.5% vs. 82.5%, $p < 0.05$) and lithium (65.9% vs. 85.0%, $p < 0.05$) [22].

The bidirectionality of these disorders is well-established in the literature. However, effectively identifying individuals at risk of developing BD poses a significant challenge [37]. It is widely recognized that, before implementing any preventive intervention, it is imperative to identify this high-risk population. Although early identification remains a complex and evolving field, certain studies have started to provide preliminary data that could contribute to enhancing this detection process. In a recent study that evaluated perinatal factors involved in the development of BD, based on a birth cohort, the results showed that maternal smoking and passive smoking increased the risk of developing BD by approximately 1.43 (95% confidence interval (CI): 1.091–1.841; 95% CI: 1.086–1.875, respectively) [7]. Moreover, a study investigating clinical predictors of transition from MDD to BD in a birth cohort identified SUD as one of the primary predictors ($p = 0.024$) [34].

Considering the complexity of identifying individuals at risk of developing BD, along with the impact of SUD on this diagnosis, shifting the focus toward preventive strategies to mitigate SUD becomes essential. Given this context, a randomized clinical trial was conducted to assess the effectiveness of behavioral contingencies in reducing SUD [25]. The participants included were diagnosed with SCZ, Schizoaffective disorder, or some mood disorder (BD I, BD II, or Major Depression), and met the criteria for substance dependence through the Mini International Neuropsychiatric Interview . The recruitment occurred through a multisite community mental health and addiction treatment agency. They were divided into two groups, one being the Contingent Group and the other the Control Group. Both received Treatment as Usual (TAU), which consisted of support for mental health, dependence, housing, and employment. However, only one of the groups received tokens that were either written "good job" or associated with a cash prize ranging from $1 to $80 as a positive reinforcement when presenting negative results for drug tests in urine collections. Meanwhile, the Control Group received random, non-contingent drawings, only to match the drawings between groups and not to reinforce abstinence. At the end of the study, participants allocated to the Contingent Group were 2.4 times more likely to present negative urine tests, indicating non-use of substances. Additionally, the same group also had a decrease in psychiatric symptoms, indicated by the Brief Symptom Inventory $\beta = 0.25$ (CI = 0.08–0.43), $p < 0.05$. Overall, the study showed that applying contingency techniques can positively impact the reduction of substance use.

Cognitive behavioral techniques (CBTs) are also an option for managing substance and alcohol use. Data from an experimental study comparing three types of treatments showed that CBT had good results in reducing alcohol and other drug use [2]. The participants in this study were allocated to standard treatment, Mindfulness-Based Relapse Prevention (MBRP), or Relapse Prevention (RP). The standard treatment involved group sessions focused on recovery, following the 12 steps of Narcotics Anonymous. Participants attended 1.5-hour meetings once or twice a week. Both the MBRP and RP groups underwent eight weekly sessions, each lasting 2 h. MBRP members received psychoeducation on physical, emotional, cognitive, and mindfulness topics, practiced guided meditations for 20–30 min, and were assigned tasks to track cravings and mood. On the other hand, the RP group focused on identifying situations posing a risk of relapse, acquiring and applying cognitive and behavioral skills, setting goals, and monitoring cravings and mood. Results indicated that, although there were no differences between the groups at the 3-month follow-up, both RP and MBRP showed more favorable outcomes in reducing drug and alcohol relapses compared to standard treatment by the 6-month mark. Moreover, at 12 months, MBRP participants demonstrated fewer days of drug use and greater alcohol abstinence. In addition to CBT as potential means to reduce or prevent SUD, some authors also advocate for the public health model as a pathway to prevention. The following model considers three stages of prevention (Fig. 12.1) [31].

The model encompasses preventive strategies for different levels of involvement with substances. This approach is founded on the premise that public policies and programs play a critical role in reducing exposure to substances, given their potential to make access more difficult and consequently prevent SUD. Therefore, public policies should incorporate regulations on advertising, taxation, and educational programs across different contexts. Additionally, screening for SUD through scales is fundamental for an objective assessment of the patient. By utilizing validated scales, healthcare providers can acquire objective and reliable information about the

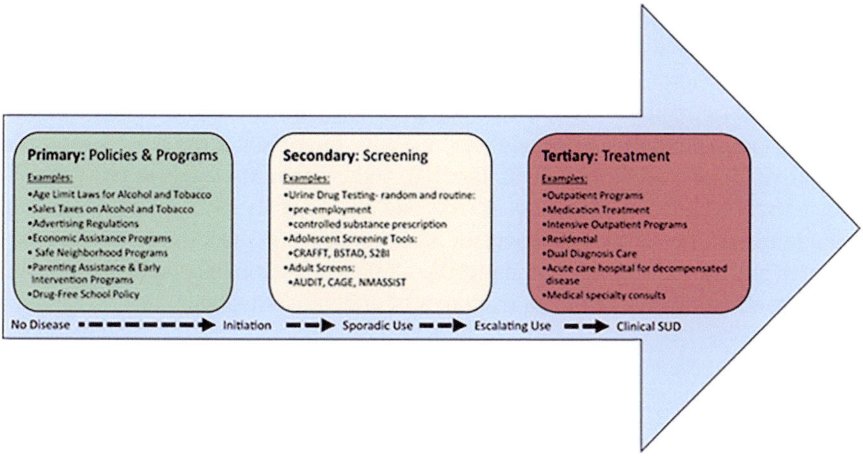

Fig. 12.1 Flow chart illustrating the stages of substance use disorder prevention and treatment. The chart is divided into three sections: Primary (policies and programs), Secondary (screening), and Tertiary (treatment). The arrow's base represents the progression from "No Disease" to "Clinical SUD" through initiation, sporadic use, and escalating use

patient's substance use. These screening tools may encompass questionnaires or interviews assessing various aspects, such as frequency, quantity, and consequences of use, thereby facilitating appropriate guidance based on the results obtained. The third and final aspect of the public health model addresses treatment options for individuals who already have some substance use. As previously mentioned, there is currently a range of effective strategies for reducing substance use. Psychosocial interventions form an integral part of treatment and may include individual counseling or group therapy. Generally, these interventions assist individuals in addressing underlying issues contributing to their substance use and in developing coping strategies to prevent relapse.

Considering protective factors related to substance use is also fundamental. A systematic review, synthesizing data from 13 studies, identified protective factors for SUD across three domains: individual, familial, and community [30]. Within the individual domain, traits such as optimism, high levels of mindfulness, anti-substance use beliefs, and a strong desire to maintain health were observed as protective factors. Family environment also played a pivotal role in protection, with families possessing extensive knowledge about drug use and providing support, counseling, and awareness being more effective in preventing drug use among their children. Another significant protective factor is the community context, where the positive influence of strong religious convictions was associated with a reduced likelihood of drug use. Additionally, maintaining a positive connection with school and receiving support from adults were also identified as important variables in preventing drug use.

Overall, the detrimental effects of SUD and BD comorbidity underscore the importance of interventions aimed at mitigating SUD to prevent the onset of BD in high-risk populations. Effective strategies such as behavioral contingencies and CBT techniques have demonstrated efficacy in reducing both SUD and associated psychiatric symptoms. Moreover, public health initiatives, including prevention policies and screening efforts, are pivotal in limiting access to substances and providing support to high-risk populations. Equally important is the consideration of protective factors at the individual, familial, and community levels to prevent substance use. Heightened awareness of risks and bolstered social support systems can help mitigate the adverse impacts of these concurrent conditions. Continuous research and the development of innovative strategies remain imperative for enhancing the well-being and treatment outcomes of affected individuals.

12.6 Clinical Considerations

- Men exhibit a higher lifetime susceptibility to SUD compared to women, a trend also observed in BD.
- Factors such as BD type I diagnosis, mixed features, and familial history of BD significantly contribute to the comorbidity of SUD in individuals with BD, highlighting the role of genetic predisposition and clinical characteristics in the overlap between the two disorders.
- SUD complicates the course of BD, leading to more mood episodes, hospitalizations, medical issues, and reduced treatment effectiveness.
- BD individuals with SUD have a higher likelihood of suicide attempts, highlighting a significant risk factor for suicidality in this population.
- SUD may predict the development of BD, with evidence suggesting its association with the transition from MDD to BD and its emergence preceding initial mood episodes in genetically predisposed individuals.
- Evidence suggests a correlation between SUD and earlier onset of BD, with studies indicating a decline in age at onset of BD type I alongside an increasing prevalence of SUD across successive birth cohorts.
- Recent genomic studies have provided valuable insights into the shared genetic architecture of BD and SUDs, revealing a complex interplay of common and rare variants, as well as substance-specific and disorder-specific genetic factors.
- Providing contingent rewards for negative drug tests has been effective in reducing substance use in individuals with BD.
- CBTs, including MBRP and RP, have shown promise in reducing drug and alcohol relapses in individuals with psychiatric disorders, including BD.
- Policies targeting advertising, taxation, and education are pivotal in curbing substance use by reducing exposure and access.
- The combination of objective screening tools for substance use assessment and the implementation of psychosocial interventions presents a multifaceted approach to addressing SUDs in individuals with BD.

12.7 Future Perspectives

Considering the complexities of SUD and BD and their bidirectional relationship, future clinical considerations must prioritize strategies to mitigate substance use as a preventive measure against the development of BD in at-risk individuals. Common markers between these disorders, such as genetic predisposition and clinical characteristics, underscore the need for targeted interventions. Behavioral contingencies and CBT have shown effectiveness in reducing substance use and associated psychiatric symptoms. Furthermore, public health approaches, including prevention policies and screening tools, are crucial in limiting access to substances and supporting vulnerable individuals. Protective factors at the individual, familial, and community levels also play a pivotal role in preventing substance use. Overall, continued research and the development of innovative strategies are essential for enhancing the quality of life and treatment outcomes for individuals affected by these comorbid conditions.

References

1. Bowden J, Fabiola Del Greco M, Minelli C, Smith GD, Sheehan NA, Thompson JR. Assessing the suitability of summary data for two-sample Mendelian randomization analyses using MR-Egger regression: the role of the I2 statistic. Int J Epidemiol. 2016;45(6):1961–74.
2. Bowen S, Witkiewitz K, Clifasefi SL, Grow J, Chawla N, Hsu SH, Carroll HA, et al. Relative efficacy of mindfulness-based relapse prevention, standard relapse prevention, and treatment as usual for substance use disorders: a randomized clinical trial. JAMA Psychiatry. 2014;71(5):547–56.
3. Carrà G, Bartoli F, Crocamo C, Brady KT, Clerici M. Attempted suicide in people with co-occurring bipolar and substance use disorders: systematic review and meta-analysis. J Affect Disord. 2014;167(June):125–35.
4. Duffy A, Alda M, Hajek T, Sherry SB, Grof P. Early stages in the development of bipolar disorder. J Affect Disord. 2010;121(1-2):127–35.
5. Duffy A, Horrocks J, Milin R, Doucette S, Persson G, Grof P. Adolescent substance use disorder during the early stages of bipolar disorder: a prospective high-risk study. J Affect Disord. 2012;142(1-3):57–64.
6. Duncan L, Shen H, Gelaye B, Meijsen J, Ressler K, Feldman M, Peterson R, Domingue B. Analysis of polygenic risk score usage and performance in diverse human populations. Nat Commun. 2019;10(1):3328.
7. Gnielka V, Montezano BB, Baldez DP, Shintani AO, Rabelo-da-Ponte FD, Menezes AMB, Wehrmeister FC, et al. Perinatal factors as risk factors of bipolar disorder onset in young adulthood: a 22-year birth cohort. Rev Bras Psiquiatr. 2024. https://doi.org/10.47626/1516-4446-2023-3338.
8. Gogia M, Shah AQ, Kapczinski F, de Azevedo CT. The impact of substance use disorder comorbidity on cognition of individuals with bipolar disorder: a systematic review. Psychiatry Res. 2022;311:114525. https://doi.org/10.1016/j.psychres.2022.114525.
9. Grant BF, Saha TD, June Ruan W, Goldstein RB, Patricia Chou S, Jung J, Zhang H, et al. Epidemiology of DSM-5 drug use disorder: results from the National Epidemiologic Survey on alcohol and related conditions-III. JAMA Psychiatry. 2016;73(1):39–47.

10. Grotzinger AD, Rhemtulla M, de Vlaming R, Ritchie SJ, Mallard TT, David Hill W, Ip HF, et al. Genomic structural equation modelling provides insights into the multivariate genetic architecture of complex traits. Nat Hum Behav. 2019;3(5):513–25.
11. Grunebaum MF, Galfalvy HC, Matthew Nichols C, Caldeira NA, Sher L, Dervic K, Burke AK, John Mann J, Oquendo MA. Aggression and substance abuse in bipolar disorder. Bipolar Disord. 2006;8(5 Pt 1):496–502.
12. Hatoum AS, Colbert SMC, Johnson EC, Huggett SB, Deak JD, Pathak G, Jennings MV, et al. Multivariate genome-wide association meta-analysis of over 1 million subjects identifies loci underlying multiple substance use disorders. Nat Ment Health. 2023;1(3):210–23.
13. Hatoum AS, Johnson EC, Colbert SMC, Polimanti R, Zhou H, Walters RK, Gelernter J, Edenberg HJ, Bogdan R, Agrawal A. The addiction risk factor: a unitary genetic vulnerability characterizes substance use disorders and their associations with common correlates. Neuropsychopharmacology. 2022;47(10):1739–45.
14. Hjorthøj C, Østergaard MLD, Benros ME, Toftdahl NG, Erlangsen A, Andersen JT, Nordentoft M. Association between alcohol and substance use disorders and all-cause and cause-specific mortality in schizophrenia, bipolar disorder, and unipolar depression: a nationwide, prospective, register-based study. Lancet Psychiatry. 2015;2(9):801–8.
15. Hunt GE, Malhi GS, Cleary M, Lai HMX, Sitharthan T. Prevalence of comorbid bipolar and substance use disorders in clinical settings, 1990–2015: systematic review and meta-analysis. J Affect Disord. 2016;206(December):331–49.
16. Johnson EC, Demontis D, Thorgeirsson TE, et al. Psychiatric Genomics Consortium Substance Use Disorders Workgroup. A large-scale genome-wide association study meta-analysis of cannabis use disorder. Lancet Psychiatry. 2020;7(12):1032–45.
17. Kranzler HR, Zhou H, Kember RL, Smith RV, Justice AC, Damrauer S, Tsao PS, et al. Genome-wide association study of alcohol consumption and use disorder in 274,424 individuals from multiple populations. Nat Commun. 2019;10(1):1499.
18. Lagerberg TV, Icick R, Aminoff SR, Nerhus M, Barrett EA, Bjella TD, Olsen SH, Høegh MC, Melle I. Substance misuse trajectories and risk of relapse in the early course of bipolar disorder. Front Psychiatry. 2021;12(May):656912.
19. Lalli M, Brouillette K, Kapczinski F, de Azevedo CT. Substance use as a risk factor for bipolar disorder: a systematic review. J Psychiatr Res. 2021;144:285–95. https://doi.org/10.1016/j.jpsychires.2021.10.012.
20. Lee PH, Feng Y-CA, Smoller JW. Pleiotropy and cross-disorder genetics among psychiatric disorders. Biol Psychiatry. 2021;89(1):20–31.
21. Lichtenstein P, Yip BH, Björk C, Pawitan Y, Cannon TD, Sullivan PF, Hultman CM. Common genetic determinants of schizophrenia and bipolar disorder in Swedish families: a population-based study. Lancet. 2009;373(9659):234–9.
22. Manwani SG, Szilagyi KA, Zablotsky B, Hennen J, Griffin ML, Weiss RD. Adherence to pharmacotherapy in bipolar disorder patients with and without co-occurring substance use disorders. J Clin Psychiatry. 2007;68(8):1172–6.
23. Martin AR, Kanai M, Kamatani Y, Okada Y, Neale BM, Daly MJ. Clinical use of current polygenic risk scores may exacerbate health disparities. Nat Genet. 2019;51(4):584–91.
24. Mazza M, Mandelli L, Di Nicola M, Harnic D, Catalano V, Tedeschi D, Martinotti G, et al. Clinical features, response to treatment and functional outcome of bipolar disorder patients with and without co-occurring substance use disorder: 1-year follow-up. J Affect Disord. 2009;115(1–2):27–35.
25. McDonell MG, Srebnik D, Angelo F, McPherson S, Lowe JM, Sugar A, Short RA, Roll JM, Ries RK. Randomized controlled trial of contingency management for stimulant use in community mental health patients with serious mental illness. Am J Psychiatry. 2013;170(1):94–101.
26. McGuffin P, Rijsdijk F, Andrew M, Sham P, Katz R, Cardno A. The heritability of bipolar affective disorder and the genetic relationship to unipolar depression. Arch Gen Psychiatry. 2003;60(5):497–502.

27. McIntyre RS, Nguyen HT, Soczynska JK, Maria TC, Lourenco HO, Woldeyohannes, and Jakub Z. Konarski. Medical and substance-related comorbidity in bipolar disorder: translational research and treatment opportunities. Dialogues Clin Neurosci. 2008;10(2):203–13.
28. Menculini G, Steardo L Jr, Verdolini N, Cirimbilli F, Moretti P, Tortorella A. Substance use disorders in bipolar disorders: clinical correlates and treatment response to mood stabilizers. J Affect Disord. 2022;300(March):326–33.
29. Mullins N, Forstner AJ, O'Connell KS, Coombes B, Coleman JRI, Qiao Z, Als TD, et al. Genome-wide association study of more than 40,000 bipolar disorder cases provides new insights into the underlying biology. Nat Genet. 2021;53(6):817–29.
30. Nawi AM, Ismail R, Ibrahim F, Hassan MR, Manaf MRA, Amit N, Ibrahim N, Shafurdin NS. Risk and protective factors of drug abuse among adolescents: a systematic review. BMC Public Health. 2021;21(1):2088.
31. Nelson LF, Weitzman ER, Levy S. Prevention of substance use disorders. Med Clin North Am. 2022;106(1):153–68.
32. Nestsiarovich A, Reps JM, Matheny ME, DuVall SL, Lynch KE, Beaton M, Jiang X, et al. Predictors of diagnostic transition from major depressive disorder to bipolar disorder: a retrospective observational network study. Transl Psychiatry. 2021;11(1):642.
33. Oliva V, De Prisco M, Pons-Cabrera MT, Guzmán P, Anmella G, Hidalgo-Mazzei D, Grande I, et al. Machine learning prediction of comorbid substance use disorders among people with bipolar disorder. J Clin Med Res. 2022;11(14). https://doi.org/10.3390/jcm11143935.
34. de Oliveira JP, Jansen K, de Azevedo Cardoso T, Mondin TC, de Mattos Souza LD, da Silva RA, Moreira FP. Predictors of conversion from major depressive disorder to bipolar disorder. Psychiatry Res. 2021;297(March):113740.
35. Palk AC, Dalvie S, de Vries J, Martin AR, Stein DJ. Potential use of clinical polygenic risk scores in psychiatry – ethical implications and communicating high polygenic risk. Philos Ethics Humanities Med (PEHM). 2019;14(1):4.
36. Preuss UW, Schaefer M, Born C, Grunze H. Bipolar disorder and comorbid use of illicit substances. Medicina. 2021;57(11). https://doi.org/10.3390/medicina57111256.
37. Rabelo-da-Ponte FD, Feiten JG, Mwangi B, Barros FC, Wehrmeister FC, Menezes AM, Kapczinski F, Passos IC, Kunz M. Early identification of bipolar disorder among young adults – a 22-year community birth cohort. Acta Psychiatr Scand. 2020;142(6):476–85.
38. Richards AL, Cardno A, Harold G, Craddock NJ, Di Florio A, Jones L, Gordon-Smith K, et al. Genetic liabilities differentiating bipolar disorder, schizophrenia, and major depressive disorder, and phenotypic heterogeneity in bipolar disorder. JAMA Psychiatry. 2022;79(10):1032–9.
39. Schaffer A, Isometsä ET, Tondo L, Moreno DH, Turecki G, Reis C, Cassidy F, et al. International society for bipolar disorders task force on suicide: meta-analyses and meta-regression of correlates of suicide attempts and suicide deaths in bipolar disorder. Bipolar Disord. 2015;17(1):1–16.
40. Scott J, Etain B, Azorin JM, Bellivier F. Secular trends in the age at onset of bipolar I disorder – support for birth cohort effects from interational, multi-centre clinical observational studies. Eur Psychiatry. 2018;52(August):61–7.
41. Strakowski SM, McElroy SL, Keck PE Jr, West SA. The effects of antecedent substance abuse on the development of first-episode psychotic mania. J Psychiatr Res. 1996;30(1):59–68.
42. Surace T, Capuzzi E, Caldiroli A, Ceresa A, Esposito CM, Auxilia AM, Tagliabue I, et al. Which clinical and biochemical parameters are associated with lifetime suicide attempts in bipolar disorder? Diagnostics (Basel, Switzerland). 2022;12(9). https://doi.org/10.3390/diagnostics12092215.
43. Treur JL, Munafò MR, Logtenberg E, Wiers RW, Verweij KJH. Using Mendelian randomization analysis to better understand the relationship between mental health and substance use: a systematic review. Psychol Med. 2021;51(10):1593–624.
44. Tsuboi T, Suzuki T, Azekawa T, Adachi N, Ueda H, Edagawa K, Katsumoto E, et al. Factors associated with non-remission in bipolar disorder: the multicenter treatment survey for

bipolar disorder in psychiatric outpatient clinics (MUSUBI). Neuropsychiatr Dis Treat. 2020;16(March):881–90.
45. Turkheimer E, D'Onofrio BM, Maes HH, Eaves LJ. Analysis and interpretation of twin studies including measures of the shared environment. Child Dev. 2005;76(6):1217–33.
46. Verbanck M, Chen C-Y, Neale B, Do R. Detection of widespread horizontal pleiotropy in causal relationships inferred from Mendelian randomization between complex traits and diseases. Nat Genet. 2018;50(5):693–8.
47. Verhulst B, Neale MC, Kendler KS. The heritability of alcohol use disorders: a meta-analysis of twin and adoption studies. Psychol Med. 2015;45(5):1061–72.
48. Wiström ED, O'Connell KS, Karadag N, Bahrami S, Hindley GFL, Lin A, Cheng W, et al. Genome-wide analysis reveals genetic overlap between alcohol use behaviours, schizophrenia and bipolar disorder and identifies novel shared risk loci. Addiction. 2022;117(3):600–10.
49. Zhang H, Kranzler HR, Poling J, Gelernter J. Variation in the nicotinic acetylcholine receptor gene cluster CHRNA5–CHRNA3–CHRNB4 and its interaction with recent tobacco use influence cognitive flexibility. Neuropsychopharmacology. 2010;35(11):2211–24.
50. Zhou H, Sealock JM, Sanchez-Roige S, Clarke T-K, Levey DF, Cheng Z, Li B, et al. Genome-wide meta-analysis of problematic alcohol use in 435,563 individuals yields insights into biology and relationships with other traits. Nat Neurosci. 2020;23(7):809–18.

Chapter 13
Suicidality and Latent Bipolar Disorder

Luciano Dias de Mattos Souza, Gessyka Wanglon Veleda, and Karen Jansen

13.1 Introduction

For centuries, suicide has been a subject of study across various scientific disciplines, yet it remains one of the most complex phenomena in humanity [1]. The ability to predict and prevent such an outcome is still minimal. The annual occurrence of suicides worldwide reaches alarming numbers [2]. Nonetheless, the quantity and quality of interactions among significant factors throughout human development that lead to suicide remain imprecisely delineated due to the low incidence rates of the phenomenon, its dynamic nature, and even lapses in its identification [2, 3].

Paradoxically, when we limit the analysis of this phenomenon to the equally complex development of mood disorders, certain factors appear to stand out clinically and, eventually, contribute to therapeutic management with the potential capability to prevent suicide [4]. Thus, the following chapter aims to detail this analysis by integrating definitions of suicidal behavior (SB), depressive disorders (DDs), and bipolar disorders (BDs); presenting relationships between models of understanding these conditions; and highlighting knowledge about SBs in mood disorders for better clinical management. Finally, possibilities for future scientific investigations will be explored.

L. D. de Mattos Souza (✉) · K. Jansen
Department of Health and Behavior, Catholic University of Pelotas, Pelotas, Brazil

G. W. Veleda
Postgraduate Program in Epidemiology, Federal University of Pelotas, Pelotas, Brazil

T. de Azevedo Cardoso et al. (eds.), *Latent Bipolar Disorder*,
https://doi.org/10.1007/978-3-032-01297-5_13

13.2 Definitions and Characteristics of Suicidality

Higher incidences of mortality are typically observed in mood disorders [5], with scientific literature indicating a reduced life expectancy in these individuals [6]. A substantial portion of these deaths is explained by the increased occurrence of suicidal behaviors.

The scientific definitions of SB encompass a range of activities from suicidal ideation to completed suicide. These behaviors exist on a spectrum that reflects varying degrees of intent and lethality [7, 8]. According to the American Foundation for Suicide Prevention [9], suicide is defined as death caused by an act of self-harm that is intended to be lethal. The same institution classifies SB as any behavior from suicide attempt and preparatory behaviors to completed suicide, while suicidal ideation refers to the cognitive processes of suicide (thinking, considering, or planning suicide). Thereby, the act of taking one's own life; non-fatal, self-directed, potentially injurious behavior with an intent to die and thoughts of causing one's own death are obviously interrelated. However, it is noteworthy that each involves unique pathways and requires tailored prevention strategies [10].

Recent critiques of the term "suicidality" in scientific literature highlight significant issues regarding its broad and often ambiguous use. Used in a similar way to SB, the term "suicidality" is frequently employed to encompass a wide range of suicidal thoughts and behaviors, including ideation, planning, attempts, and completed suicide [11]. However, this all-encompassing term can obscure important distinctions between these different phenomena, leading to potential misinterpretations and inadequate clinical responses. Its lack of specificity may hinder its clinical use. By grouping distinct phenomena under one term, researchers and clinicians might overlook the unique risk factors and treatment needs. Recent literature calls for more precise definitions and tailored approaches to address the various stages of SB. A systematic review of suicide interventions highlights the importance of distinguishing between different forms of SB to enhance the effectiveness of psychosocial interventions [12]. This review points out that interventions should be specifically designed to address the unique characteristics and needs of individuals at different stages of "suicidality," such as ideation, planning, and attempts, rather than relying on a one-size-fits-all approach [12].

Even though possible different underlying mechanisms occur in each definition that encompasses suicidality, we will use this term as a theoretical framework to group individuals who exhibit suicide ideation and suicide attempt to highlight its proximity to complete suicide in mood disorders. Most of the specific literature, especially on mood and BDs, uses suicide attempt as an outcome.

13.3 Broad Understanding of Suicidality

Different theories on understanding suicide are presented in the scientific literature. The traditional epidemiological approach, together with the comprehensive model of suicide proposed by Turecki and Brent [13], presents contributions to the analysis of the development of suicidality [7]. Additionally, theoretical frameworks positioned within the ideation-to-action perspective also need to be considered for a broad understanding of the problem. Among these, the interpersonal theory of suicide (ITS) [14], the integrated motivational-volitional (IMV) model of suicide behavior [15], and the three-step theory of suicide (3ST) [16] stand out. It is worth noting that these theories are not necessarily antagonistic or exclusive and, from the authors' point of view, they should be considered as complementary.

SB is typically understood through multi-etiological perspectives that integrate genetic, biological, psychological, and environmental factors. The SB model based on epidemiological data often focuses on the interaction between long-term (distal) factors, such as family history of suicide or mental disorders, and more immediate factors linked to SB stressors (proximal), like financial hardship or recent personal losses. Between these distal and proximal factors, there are developmental factors that increase the chances of engaging in suicidal ideation, suicidal attempt, and complete suicide. In addition to individual characteristics, this model also considers social contexts that are part of the individual's development and suicidality. Lack of cohesion and disruptions in the social structure or values, social isolation, economic turmoil, intense media reporting, easy access to lethal means, and poor access to mental health services are important social features to interact with individuals' suicidality features. Notably, this prominent paradigm posits that suicide results from the interaction of an individual's biopsychosocial vulnerabilities with environmental stressors [7, 13].

The risk factors presented by this model are supported by decades of epidemiological research on SB. Epidemiological statistical models still fail to indicate the specificity of each risk factor for suicide; however, they suggest that the greater quantity and intensity of certain factors effectively contribute to predicting this set of behaviors. Even though such evidence presents considerable methodological limitations [3], its usefulness is recognized in clinical practice, especially in the field of depressive and BDs. For the same reason, the focus on distinct mechanisms of suicide ideation and attempts in people living with bipolar or depressive disorder, as well as the need to detail these transitions, highlights the integration of theoretical frameworks.

13.3.1 Interpersonal Theory of Suicide

This theory is built on the premise that suicidal ideation arises from the interplay of two main factors: perceived burdensomeness and thwarted belongingness [14]. The theory also introduces a third critical component, the acquired capability for suicide, which explains why some individuals progress from suicidal desire to making an attempt. It is based on the idea that SB is not solely the result of an individual's mental health or psychological state but is also influenced by their social and interpersonal relationships.

The theory identifies key elements that contribute to the development of SB. The desire to die is a fundamental component of the theory. This desire is not necessarily a reflection of an individual's mental health but rather a manifestation of their own life perceptions as being without purpose or meaning. Individuals who think and feel that their lives are without purpose or meaning are more likely to experience a desire to die, which can be a precursor to SB.

In this sense, perceived burdensomeness refers to an individual's perception that they are a burden to others. This perception is often distorted and not aligned with reality, yet it is a powerful driver of suicidal ideation. Individuals who think and feel they are a burden may believe that their death would relieve others of a significant hardship, thus justifying their suicidal thoughts. Thwarted belongingness refers to an individual's cognition of not belonging or being disconnected from others. These feelings can lead to a sense of hopelessness and despair, which can increase the likelihood of SB. Humans have an intrinsic need to belong and form connections with others. When these needs are unmet, individuals experience profound loneliness and social isolation. The absence of reciprocal care and support significantly contributes to the desire for suicide. Thwarted belongingness can result from various life circumstances, such as the loss of loved ones, social rejection, or chronic loneliness.

The capability for suicide refers to an individual's ability to engage in SB. This capability is influenced by a range of factors, including the individual's mental health, their access to lethal means, and their ability to overcome the fear of death. Individuals who have the capability for suicide are more likely to engage in SB, as they have the means and the motivation to do so.

The theory suggests that SB is strongly influenced by the individual social and interpersonal relationships. Lethal or near-lethal suicide attempts occur when an individual has both the desire and the capability for suicide. The desire arises from perceived burdensomeness and thwarted belongingness, while the capability is acquired through habituation to pain and fear. Importantly, the authors suggest that, while many people may experience one or both components of the suicidal desire, it is the addition of the acquired capability that elevates the risk to a critical level.

ITS has garnered significant empirical support and has been influential in both clinical and research settings. Studies have shown that perceived burdensomeness and thwarted belongingness are strong predictors of suicidal ideation [17]. Additionally, individuals with a history of painful and challenging experiences are more likely to report a higher acquired capability for suicide [18].

The ITS has significant implications for clinical actions. Interventions that include fostering social connections, enhancing social support networks, and addressing cognitive distortions that contribute to feelings of burdensomeness might reduce it, as discussed later in this chapter.

13.3.2 IMV Model of Suicide Behavior

The IMV model of SB, developed by Rory C. O'Connor and Olivia J. Kirtley [15], is particularly valuable as it distinguishes between the emergence of suicidal ideation and the transition from ideation to SB, addressing a significant gap in previous theoretical models. The IMV model is structured into three distinct phases: pre-motivational, motivational, and volitional. Each phase encompasses specific factors that contribute to the development and enactment of SB.

The pre-motivational phase involves the biopsychosocial context within which suicidal thoughts and behaviors may develop. This phase is similar to models already presented and includes various vulnerability factors such as genetic predispositions, personality traits, and early life adversities, which increase an individual's sensitivity to stress. Environmental and social factors, such as socioeconomic status, cultural influences, and exposure to traumatic events, also play a critical role in this phase.

The motivational phase focuses on the psychological processes that lead to the development of suicidal ideation. Central to this phase are the concepts of defeat and entrapment. Defeat refers to feelings of failure and humiliation, while entrapment describes a perceived lack of escape from these negative emotions. According to the IMV model, these feelings of defeat and entrapment are primary drivers of suicidal ideation. Several moderators influence the relationship between defeat/entrapment and suicidal ideation. These include individual coping strategies, social support, and cognitive processes such as rumination and problem-solving abilities. For instance, individuals who are better at solving problems and who have strong social support networks are less likely to transition from feelings of defeat and entrapment to suicidal ideation.

The volitional phase addresses the factors that facilitate the transition from suicidal thoughts to actual SBs. Key components in this phase include the acquired capability for suicide, which involves an increased pain tolerance and a reduced fear of death. This capability is often developed through repeated exposure to painful or fear-inducing experiences, such as self-harm or witnessing the SB of others. Volitional moderators (VMs) play a crucial role in this phase. These factors include access to means of suicide, exposure to suicide, impulsivity, and detailed planning. For example, individuals with easy access to lethal means or who have a history of impulsive behaviors are at a higher risk of attempting suicide. Mental imagery and rehearsing suicidal acts mentally also increase the likelihood of transitioning from ideation to behavior.

The IMV model has presented substantial empirical support since its inception. Studies have consistently shown that defeat and entrapment are strong predictors of suicidal ideation, while volitional factors such as access to means and impulsivity significantly increase the risk of suicide attempts [19–21]. This model has been validated across different populations and settings, providing a robust framework for both research and clinical practice. By distinguishing between the emergence of suicidal thoughts and the transition to suicidal acts, the IMV model offers valuable insights into the psychological processes underlying suicide.

This model has significant implications for both research and clinical practice, highlighting the importance of targeted interventions to reduce SB. As our understanding of these complex processes continues to evolve, the IMV model will remain a critical tool in the ongoing efforts to prevent suicide and improve mental health outcomes.

13.3.3 *Three-Step Theory of Suicide*

The 3ST, developed by Klonsky and May, is a significant advancement in the understanding and prediction of SB [16]. It is also rooted in the "ideation-to-action" framework; the 3ST posits that the factors leading to suicidal ideation are distinct from those that facilitate the transition from ideation to attempts. This theory is predicated on three core components: pain and hopelessness, connectedness, and the capacity for suicide.

The first step in the 3ST involves the onset of suicidal ideation, which is primarily driven by psychological or emotional pain. The theory does not limit the type of pain, acknowledging that various forms of distress, including physical suffering, social isolation, burdensomeness, defeat, entrapment, and negative self-perceptions, can contribute to suicidal thoughts. However, pain alone is insufficient to cause suicidal ideation; hopelessness must also be present. This combination of pain and hopelessness decreases an individual's desire to live, making the prospect of suicide more appealing. Thus, the interplay of these two factors is crucial for the emergence of suicidal ideation.

The second step in the 3ST differentiates between moderate and strong suicidal ideation based on the individual's sense of connectedness. Connectedness encompasses relationships with people, roles, projects, or any purpose that gives life meaning. According to the 3ST, pain and hopelessness lead to moderate ideation if the person's sense of connectedness remains strong. However, if pain exceeds connectedness, ideation becomes strong, increasing the risk of SB. For instance, a parent experiencing daily pain and hopelessness may still refrain from strong suicidal ideation if their connection to their children outweighs their pain. Conversely, if pain surpasses any form of connectedness, the individual is likely to progress to strong suicidal ideation.

The third step finally addresses the transition from suicidal ideation to attempts. The 3ST posits that the key determinant is the individual's capacity for suicide, which comprises dispositional, acquired, and practical factors. Dispositional factors are inherent traits such as pain sensitivity, which may be influenced by genetics. Acquired factors involve habituation to painful or fear-inducing experiences, increasing one's tolerance for pain and injury. Practical factors include access to means and knowledge of methods, which can significantly ease the transition from ideation to attempts. This step highlights that individuals will only attempt suicide if they possess the capacity to overcome the instinctual fear of death and pain.

Even though the 3ST does not introduce any innovative elements in its structure, it synthesizes certain factors in understanding the individual's decision-making mechanism and highlights the difference between those with suicidal ideation and those who actually attempt suicide. By clearly delineating the transitional steps from ideation to action, the 3ST provides a more nuanced and actionable framework for understanding and preventing suicide. This perspective is also crucial to inform the development of targeted interventions to prevent suicide.

13.3.4 Diathesis-Stress Framework in the Etiologies of Mood Disorders, Latent Bipolar Disorder, and Suicidality

Similar to the understanding of suicidality, mood disorders can also be comprehended within this diathesis-stress framework. After the release of the DSM-5 [22] and the nosological division between the two group categories of BDs and DDs, the term "mood disorders" fell out of use. However, from a clinical perspective, the predominant logic of observing specific criteria for these disorders based on the occurrence of mood oscillation episodes still results in the longitudinal evaluation of periods of elevated and reduced mood functioning. The inclusion of the mixed features as a diagnostic specifier of depressive episodes brought controversy but also attention to the symptoms' overlapping. Mixed features in individuals with a diagnosis of DD occur in approximately 11% of cases, whereas around one-quarter of individuals with BD present with mixed features. Both conditions are associated with the manifestation of more intense clinical symptoms, a poorer prognosis, and a higher risk of suicidality. Due to its severity, medication treatment for mixed features appears to be beneficial but differs for cases of DDs or BDs [23].

The etiology of BD involves a complex interplay of genetic, neurobiological, and environmental factors. Genetic predisposition plays a crucial role, with multiple studies identifying specific gene variants associated with BD [24]. These include genes involved in neurotransmitter regulation, neurodevelopment, and intracellular signaling pathways [25]. Dysfunctions in neurotransmitter systems, additional abnormalities in neuroendocrine functions, and inflammatory pathways highlight the multifaceted biological disruptions in BD [26]. These genetic factors create a vulnerability that can be triggered or exacerbated by environmental stressors, leading to the onset of BD or mood symptoms [27, 28]. Adverse childhood experiences, especially maltreatments, predict not only later mental disorders [29] but also unfavorable clinical features and course of illness in people with BD [30]. Consequently, epigenetic responses reported in BD are commonly associated with an acceleration of aging (DNA methylation, myelination, and neuronal maturation) [31]. All these neurobiological systemic dysfunctions are correlated and mutually reinforce mood symptoms, behavioral pattern disruptions, and psychosocial impairments.

The diathesis-stress model of the etiology of DD posits that depression arises from the interaction between underlying vulnerabilities and environmental stressors. Genetic predispositions and early life experiences form the diathesis, or vulnerability, which can be activated by subsequent stress. These interactions affect neurobiological systems, leading to dysregulation in neurotransmitter pathways and neuroendocrine functions, thereby increasing the individual's vulnerability to stressors [32]. All these changes contribute to the development of cognitive vulnerabilities, such as negative cognitive biases and maladaptive schemas, which predispose individuals to depressive reactions when faced with stress. This cognitive-emotional response triggers or worsens biological processes, such as inflammatory responses and dysregulation of neurochemical systems. Thus, the diathesis-stress model underscores the complex interplay between genetic, neurobiological, cognitive, and environmental factors in the etiology of DDs [33, 34].

In this scenario, the concept of latent BD emerges, often referring to a subthreshold BD, involving depressive episodes with subtle signs of mania or hypomania. These individuals do not fully meet the criteria for bipolar I or II disorders but are at high risk for transitioning to these conditions. This subclinical stage often leads to a delay in accurate diagnosis and appropriate treatment, and this might correlate, besides other factors, with suicidality.

13.3.5 Impact of Suicidality on BD

It is estimated that one-third of individuals with BD have attempted suicide at some point in their lives [35, 36]. The rates of suicide attempts are at least 20 times higher in BD than in the adult general population and over 50 times higher in juvenile samples. Similar to the general population, women exhibit a higher occurrence of suicide attempts compared to men, although men have a higher number of deaths by suicide [37, 38]. Self-poisoning is the most common method of suicide attempt in BD [39], making it highly probable that the differences observed between attempts and completed suicides among men and women occur due to the choice of method. The lethality of the attempts is considered significant. It is estimated that, in BD, there is one death for every 56 suicide attempts [40].

Due to epigenetic and sociocultural characteristics, females with mood disorders experience a heightened vulnerability to stressors throughout their lives [41–45], rendering them particularly susceptible to suicidal ideation and attempts according to the suicidality theoretical framework already mentioned. Sex might be considered a distal factor to suicide behavior, while its impact on lifespan a developmental factor. Women often face unique stressors, including gender discrimination, domestic violence, and caregiving responsibilities, which can increase their psychological burden. In contrast, males may be more prone to completing suicide due to a convergence of cultural and genetic factors that influence dispositional, practical, and learned aspects of SB indicated at the third step of Klonsky and May's theory. Culturally, men are often socialized to suppress emotional expression and avoid seeking help for mental health issues, which can lead to a buildup of untreated psychological distress. Furthermore, men are more likely to choose more aggressive methods when attempting suicide, such as firearms or hanging, which contributes to the higher lethality. Scientific studies support these gender differences in SB and also discuss how cultural scripts and norms around masculinity and femininity shape SBs differently in men and women [46]. The interplay of these genetic, sociocultural, and behavioral factors underscores the need for gender-specific understanding, prevention, and intervention strategies to effectively address suicide risk in both men and women with mood disorders [47–50].

Among sociodemographic factors, it is important to highlight that individuals with a diagnosis of BD who have higher incomes, as well as those in developed countries, exhibit higher prevalence rates of suicide attempts according to a meta-analysis [35]. The authors mention that the small number of studies in low- and middle-income countries and different methods of measuring income may have biased the results. Although greater stigmatization and social disadvantages are more common among individuals with low-income [51], the impact of impoverishment or unemployment can be perceived in an amplified manner among high-income individuals with BD. This suggests a higher likelihood of experiencing feelings of social disconnection, defeat, and entrapment. High-income individuals with BD may face intense social and professional pressures, leading to greater psychological distress when confronted with financial instability or job loss. For instance, research has shown that the stigma associated with mental health issues can be particularly detrimental to individuals in higher socioeconomic positions, as they may fear judgment and social exclusion more acutely [52]. Furthermore, the heightened expectations and responsibilities often associated with high-income roles can exacerbate feelings of failure and isolation when these individuals face economic downturns [53]. The disparity between their previous status and their current situation can lead to profound thoughts and feelings of defeat and entrapment presented in the motivational phase of IMV theory, which operates as a trigger to a volitional phase and is also a critical proximal risk factor for suicidal attempts in Tureck and Brent's model.

In the same direction, living alone, being divorced, having no children, and the lack of religious affiliation are risk factors for suicidality in BD [39, 54] and are clearly features that increase conditions theoretically related to suicide ideation, as disconnection, less sense of meaning, and social isolation. These social developmental characteristics are not only risk factors but also exacerbate BD and SB by creating environments where individuals are more likely to feel unsupported and hopeless. Individuals with BD who lacked social support were more likely to experience functional impairment [55], and it might have an impact on suicidal ideation and attempts [56]. Similarly, living alone and being divorced have been linked to higher rates of mood instability and depressive episodes, which are critical components of BD and can precipitate SB [57]. The absence of religious affiliation may also reduce an individual's sense of meaning and purpose, which are protective factors against suicide. Religious involvement is inversely related to suicide rates, suggesting that spiritual beliefs and community can provide critical emotional and psychological support [58]. These factors create a cycle where the presence of BD leads to social withdrawal, which, in turn, exacerbates the symptoms of the disorder and increases the risk of suicide, making the comorbidity of these conditions particularly challenging. We highlight that this development profile is consistent with the incidence of suicidal ideation and behaviors, which, in turn, constitute strong proximal stressors for the occurrence of a mood episode in BD. Research indicates that the presence of suicidal thoughts and attempts can significantly increase the likelihood of a subsequent mood episode in individuals with BD [59–61]. Studies have shown that the presence of suicidal thoughts and behaviors is a significant predictor of the later development of BD [60, 61]. It is important to note that meta-analytically pooled suicide attempter rates indicated a greater proportion in BD versus DD observed under the same conditions [62].

A family history of suicide and early maltreatment are commonly associated with the development of BD [39, 63]. This characteristic warrants significant clinical attention in understanding suicide in the context of BD. Evidently, among the negative psychosocial consequences related to a family history of suicide and early maltreatment is the increased likelihood of developing suicidal, aggressive, and impulsive behaviors through social modeling [64, 65]. Additionally, epigenetic factors related to both BD and SB also contribute to the impairment of neurobiological mechanisms, leading to poorer cognitive functioning and behavioral maladjustment. Thus, individuals with BD and SB may present accelerated biological aging, which provides putative biological mechanisms for morbidity and premature mortality in this population [66]. The literature also indicates that other developmental features such as impulsivity and comorbidity with substance use disorders may play important roles in the development of suicidal ideation and suicide attempts in mood disorders [67]. Adverse childhood experiences, along with early maladaptive schemas [68] such as entitlement, social isolation, and defectiveness, are associated with suicidality in BD inpatients [69, 70], as well as impulsivity and drug use in mood disorders [71]. Social isolation and defectiveness exhibit cognitive processing similar to that of individuals who have attempted suicide, according to the ITS and IMV. Entitlement is correlated with recurrent SBs [72], shares characteristics with cluster B personality disorders, and is linked to manic and hypomanic symptoms, such as impulsivity and drug use, increasing the likelihood of developing BD [73, 74]. These schemas may elevate suicidal risk by exacerbating comorbid mood disorders, personality traits, disruptive behaviors, and dysfunctional interpersonal relationships. We particularly highlight these scenarios in mixed presentations of mood disorders. Cannabis use as well as alcohol abuse increases the likelihood of a suicide attempt in BD [75] and DD [76]. In this manner, they represent particularly significant mediational and proximal characteristics in the risk of suicidality. While the chronic use of substances contributes to the deterioration of the individual's general clinical condition and mental health in mood disorders, alcohol abuse, through greater tolerance to pain and reduction of fear responses related to death, enhances the transition from ideation to SB. Abuse of more than one substance is also correlated to suicidality in BD [67]. It is important to note that, in addition to resistance to the use of antidepressants, substance use is associated with cases of diagnostic conversion from DD to BD [77, 78].

Some clinical features associated with suicide attempts in BD are also frequently expressed in cases of DD that convert to BD, age at onset of unipolar disorder, number of depressive episodes, the occurrence of psychotic symptoms, the prevalence of chronic depression, and severity of depression [35, 36, 67, 79]. Together with treatment resistance to antidepressants and a family history of BD, this profile is also present in the development of latent BD.

As a significant proportion of young individuals with depression, who lack a history of hypomanic or manic episodes, may eventually convert to BD in the future, a condition that can be termed as latent bipolar depression [80], it seems important to address this issue to understand the clinical characteristics of young patients with mood complaints. Unipolar polarity of first episode, depressive polarity of current/

recent episode, and depressive predominance polarity of episodes are quite frequent in suicide attempters with BD, just as a more physically and emotionally exhausting expression of symptoms during mood episodes is associated with these clinical conditions [38, 81]. The history of hospitalization, mixed-agitated-dysphoric moods, rapid mood shifts, mixed features, and rapid cycling are common in suicide attempts in BD and also are predictors of conversion to BD [35, 39, 82]. It is worth emphasizing that people who converted to BD during treatment with antidepressants, when compared to those who converted to BD spontaneously, more often convert to BD type 2 and have more suicide attempts.

Similar to other settings, a history of suicide attempts in BDs is the strongest risk factor for a subsequent attempt [36, 67, 83]. It is concluded that the risk of suicide attempts remains elevated in cases of BD, resulting in completed suicide occurring in 5–20% of adults with this diagnosis, along with the use of violent methods [40, 84]. This alarming progression underscores the importance of vigilant monitoring and early intervention in depressive youth to identify suicide risk and manage potential latent BD promptly.

13.3.6 Clinical Implications of These Findings

In light of these findings, considering the significant risk of suicide in mood disorders and their associated characteristics, certain priorities should be emphasized. First, efforts should be made to increase detection and prevention. Hence, population-level suicide prevention programs can, in addition to raising awareness and promoting help-seeking behavior, also restrict access to lethal means. This condition is associated with an increased capability for suicide, which, in turn, may impact engagement in SB [13, 45].

Therefore, identifying subgroups of patients at higher risk of suicide, such as individuals with psychiatric comorbidities and a history of suicide attempts, should also be emphasized. A national study [85] found that more than one-third of suicides occurred within 4 months following discharge, with the highest risk among patients admitted for depressive and mixed episodes. The same relationship was identified in a study involving 1673 Italian patients with BD [86]. Primary healthcare services can be crucial allies in identifying these individuals and facilitating their access to appropriate treatment.

Regarding the choice of treatments, the combination of mood stabilizing medications, such as lithium, along with psychosocial therapies, remains the most recommended option. Evidence favoring lithium treatment is stronger than for other measures, although encouraging findings are emerging for other treatments [67]. Lithium is the only treatment that has shown anti-suicide potential that goes beyond its mood-stabilizing capacity, making it a preferred choice for patients with BD at high risk of suicide. Despite this, the findings suggest a potential protective effect of antiepileptics against the risk of suicide, highlighting the need for further investigation [36, 87].

Regarding psychosocial interventions, cognitive-behavioral therapy (CBT) is widely recognized as an effective approach for treating suicidality. This therapy helps patients develop coping strategies to manage suicidal thoughts and self-harm behaviors by modifying dysfunctional thought patterns and promoting problem-solving skills. It is worth noting that problem-solving skills and increased social support, which can be developed through psychosocial interventions, are important moderators in the process of suicidal ideation according to the ITS [34, 88–90].

Other focal psychosocial interventions, such as interpersonal and social rhythm therapy (IPSRT), show promise. In a preliminary randomized clinical trial, social rhythm therapy , a component of IPSRT focused on teaching behavioral strategies to maintain healthy routines, significantly improved social rhythm regularity, reduced mood symptoms, and decreased suicide propensity. The regularization of social rhythms was associated with a reduction in suicide propensity, even after controlling for reductions in mood symptoms. The intervention was conducted via telehealth, highlighting the potential of synchronous interventions. Indeed, interventions that combine psychoeducation about BD with structured changes in individuals' routines should be prioritized [91].

These results show that iCBT interventions (CBT delivered online) are associated with significant reductions in suicidal ideation compared with control conditions. Considering their high scalability, iCBT interventions have the potential to reduce suicide mortality. Future research should assess the effect of these digital health interventions on SB and identify moderators and mediators to advance understanding of the mechanisms of effectiveness of these interventions [92].

Early psychosocial interventions appear to promote the best possible developmental trajectory. CBT-based treatments are associated with improved outcomes for children and adolescents with major mood disorders (BD and DD). Even though the results of clinical trials show considerable variability and heterogeneity, there is a slight reduction in the manifestation of mood symptoms and behavioral problems, with clear acceptance and satisfaction with the treatments. This is associated with improvements in psychosocial functioning in adolescents and enhanced skills and knowledge about BD in both adolescents and their parents [93–95].

Regarding suicide prevention in youths, interventions located in post-primary school-based settings, targeting suicidal thoughts and behaviors as the primary outcome and other health and well-being outcomes, show great potential in reducing the incidence of suicide attempts and suicidal ideation in adolescents. The stable maintenance of this outcome over a year and larger effect sizes for fewer suicide attempts support the effectiveness of interventions lasting more than 1 week [96]. School life characteristics, such as schooling status and total years of education, along with loneliness, are highly relevant in predicting suicide attempts in adolescents with mental disorders [97]. Youths experiencing acute life stressors are more likely to feel defeated and trapped, leading to suicidal ideation. It seems beneficial for psychosocial intervention strategies to include both family and school environments. Supportive and connective approach of these two fundamental social institutions might mitigate the volitional potential to attempt suicide, in addition to inhibiting the willingness to learn about the capacity for suicide. Integrating these elements can enhance the effectiveness of interventions aimed at reducing the risk of SB in this vulnerable population.

13.4 Clinical Considerations

- Implement regular screening for suicidality in patients with mood disorders, particularly focusing on those with mixed features, a family history of suicide, or early maltreatment.
- Address social support information (social isolation, lack of social support, and loneliness), which are significant risk factors for suicidality in patients with mood disorders.
- Consider the impact of socioeconomic status as an important feature in coping with stressful life events on the evaluation of patients with mood disorders.
- Tailor interventions to account for gender differences, with targeted support for women facing gender-specific stressors and men who may be more prone to using lethal methods of suicide.
- Monitor for substance use in the treatment of mood disorders to choose the best clinical management.
- Implement pharmacological treatments, including mood stabilizers like lithium, which have demonstrated anti-suicidal properties beyond mood stabilization.
- Utilize evidence-based psychotherapeutic interventions, such as CBT and IPSRT, to manage mood symptoms and reduce suicidal ideation.
- Involve family members in treatment plans to enhance social support and reduce feelings of burdensomeness and thwarted belongingness in patients.
- Educate families about the importance of maintaining supportive and stable environments to improve patient outcomes.

13.5 Future Perspectives

The definition of clear operational clinical criteria for latent BD that collaborate with the practice of mental health professionals is necessary [98, 99]. Consequently, risk calculators that include clinical, social, and biological variables developed, replicated, and validated in large samples that generate accurate predictive models can be useful tools to prevent premature deaths and clinical improvement in these patients [99].

It is important to integrate mental health research with technological advancements that enable the cost-effective and large-scale measurement of physiological stress markers, particularly inflammatory markers associated with suicide attempts in individuals with mental disorders and the occurrence of the mental disorders themselves [100, 101]. In this regard, advancements in technological tools that accurately measure cognitive processes—such as attention, memory, and executive functions [102, 103]—in everyday contexts hold significant potential for better understanding the role of SB in mental disorders and latent BD. By providing more precise and contextually relevant data, these technologies can enhance our comprehension of cognitive dysfunctions associated with SB, leading to more effective prevention and intervention strategies for individuals at risk. This integration can enhance the understanding and prevention of these complex phenomena, contributing to more effective and targeted interventions.

To this end, longitudinal research tracking young individuals with mood disorders who are at risk of developing suicidal behavior and/or BD is essential. While incorporating clinical history variables of mental health is necessary, augmenting this data with real-time information from wearable electronic devices can significantly enhance the objective prediction and precise uunderstanding of these complex phenomena.

References

1. Rosen G. History in the study of suicide. Psychol Med. 1971;1(4):267–85. https://doi.org/10.1017/S0033291700042239.
2. Lovero KL, Dos Santos PF, Come AX, Wainberg ML, Oquendo MA. Suicide in global mental health. Curr Psychiatry Rep. 2023;25(6):255–62. https://doi.org/10.1007/s11920-023-01423-x.
3. Franklin JC, Ribeiro JD, Fox KR, Bentley KH, Kleiman EM, Huang X, et al. Risk factors for suicidal thoughts and behaviors: a meta-analysis of 50 years of research. Psychol Bull. 2017;143(2):187–232. https://doi.org/10.1037/bul0000084.
4. Fox KR, Huang X, Guzmán EM, Funsch KM, Cha CB, Ribeiro JD, Franklin JC. Interventions for suicide and self-injury: a meta-analysis of randomized controlled trials across nearly 50 years of research. Psychol Bull. 2020;146(12):1117–45. https://doi.org/10.1037/bul0000305.
5. Baldessarini RJ. Epidemiology of suicide: recent developments. Epidemiol Psychiatr Sci. 2019;29:e71. https://doi.org/10.1017/S2045796019000672.
6. Dome P, Rihmer Z, Gonda X. Suicide risk in bipolar disorder: a brief review. Medicina (Kaunas). 2019;55(8):403. https://doi.org/10.3390/medicina55080403.
7. Turecki G, Brent DA, Gunnell D, O'Connor RC, Oquendo MA, Pirkis J, Stanley BH. Suicide and suicide risk. Nat Rev Dis Primers. 2019;5(1):74. https://doi.org/10.1038/s41572-019-0121-0.
8. Huang X, Ribeiro JD, Franklin JC. The differences between suicide ideators and suicide attempters: simple, complicated, or complex? J Consult Clin Psychol. 2020;88(6):554–69. https://doi.org/10.1037/ccp0000498.
9. MSD Manuals. Suicidal behavior. In: The MSD manuals: professional edition. Available from: https://www.msdmanuals.com/en-gb/professional/psychiatric-disorders/suicidal-behavior-and-self-injury/suicidal-behavior. Accessed 6 June 2024.
10. Harmer B, Lee S, Rizvi A, Pal S, Jackson D, Saadabadi A. Suicidal ideation. In: StatPearls [Internet]. Treasure Island (FL): StatPearls Publishing; 2024. [Updated 2024 Apr 20; cited 2024 Jun 5]. Available from: https://www.ncbi.nlm.nih.gov/books/NBK565877/.
11. Keefner TP, Stenvig T. Suicidality: an evolutionary concept analysis. Issues Ment Health Nurs. 2020;42(3):227–38. https://doi.org/10.1080/01612840.2020.1793243.
12. Martínez-Rives NL, Martín Chaparro MDP, Dhungel B, Gilmour S, Colman RD, Kotera Y. Suicide interventions in Spain and Japan: a comparative systematic review. Healthcare (Basel). 2024;12(7):792. https://doi.org/10.3390/healthcare12070792.

13. Turecki G, Brent DA. Suicide and suicidal behaviour. Lancet. 2016;387(10024):1227–39. https://doi.org/10.1016/S0140-6736(15)00234-2.
14. Joiner TE, Van Orden KA, Witte TK, Rudd MD. The interpersonal theory of suicide: guidance for working with suicidal clients. Washington, DC: American Psychological Association; 2009.
15. O'Connor RC, Kirtley OJ. The integrated motivational–volitional model of suicidal behaviour. Philos Trans R Soc B. 2018;373:20170268. https://doi.org/10.1098/rstb.2017.0268.
16. Klonsky ED, May AM. The three-step theory (3ST): a new theory of suicide rooted in the "ideation-to-action" framework. Int J Cogn Ther. 2015;8(2):114–29. https://doi.org/10.1521/ijct.2015.8.2.114.
17. Ma J, Batterham PJ, Calear AL, Han J. A systematic review of the predictions of the interpersonal-psychological theory of suicidal behavior. Clin Psychol Rev. 2016 Jun;46:34–45. https://doi.org/10.1016/j.cpr.2016.04.008.
18. Smith PN, Cukrowicz KC. Capable of suicide: a functional model of the acquired capability component of the interpersonal-psychological theory of suicide. Suicide Life Threat Behav. 2010;40(3):266–75. https://doi.org/10.1521/suli.2010.40.3.266.
19. Teismann T, Brailovskaia J. Entrapment, positive psychological functioning and suicide ideation: a moderation analysis. Clin Psychol Psychother. 2020;27(1):34–41. https://doi.org/10.1002/cpp.2403.
20. Klonsky ED, May AM, Saffer BY. Suicide, suicide attempts, and suicidal ideation. Annu Rev Clin Psychol. 2016;12:307–30. https://doi.org/10.1146/annurev-clinpsy-021815-093204.
21. da Silva AG, Malloy-Diniz LF, Garcia MS, Figueiredo CGS, Figueiredo RN, Diaz AP, Palha AP. Cognition as a therapeutic target in the suicidal patient approach. Front Psych. 2018;9:31. https://doi.org/10.3389/fpsyt.2018.00031.
22. American Psychiatric Association. Diagnostic and statistical manual of mental disorders. 5th ed. Arlington: American Psychiatric Association; 2013.
23. Na KS, Kang JM, Cho SE. Prevalence of DSM-5 mixed features: a meta-analysis and systematic review. J Affect Disord. 2021;282:203–10. https://doi.org/10.1016/j.jad.2020.12.149.
24. Mullins N, Forstner AJ, O'Connell KS, Coombes B, Coleman JRI, Qiao Z, et al. Genome-wide association study of more than 40,000 bipolar disorder cases provides new insights into the underlying biology. Nat Genet. 2021;53(6):817–29. https://doi.org/10.1038/s41588-021-00857-4.
25. Calabrò M, Mandelli L, Crisafulli C, Sidoti A, Jun TY, Lee SJ, et al. Genes involved in neurodevelopment, neuroplasticity, and bipolar disorder: CACNA1C, CHRNA1, and MAPK1. Neuropsychobiology. 2016;74(3):159–68. https://doi.org/10.1159/000468543.
26. Juruena MF, Cleare AJ, Young AH. Neuroendocrine and stress pathways in bipolar disorders. In: Biomarkers in bipolar disorders. Academic; 2022. p. 313–30. https://doi.org/10.1016/B978-0-12-821398-8.00018-7.
27. Ejiohuo O, Bilska K, Narożna B, Skibińska M, Kapelski P, Dmitrzak-Węglarz M, Szczepankiewicz A, Pawlak J. The implication of ADRA2A and AVPRIB gene variants in the aetiology of stress-related bipolar disorder. J Affect Disord. 2024;S0165-0327(24):01562–3. https://doi.org/10.1016/j.jad.2024.09.072.
28. Akram S, Ali M, Mutahir Z, Ibad N, Sarmad S, Mehboob S, Saleem M. Role of TNF-α -308G/A polymorphism in bipolar disorder and its relationship with clinical and demographic variables. Innov. Clin Neurosci. 2023;20(1–3):60–71. PMID: 37122575; PMCID: PMC10132278
29. McKay MT, Cannon M, Chambers D, Conroy RM, Coughlan H, Dodd P, et al. Childhood trauma and adult mental disorder: a systematic review and meta-analysis of longitudinal cohort studies. Acta Psychiatr Scand. 2021;143(3):189–205. https://doi.org/10.1111/acps.13268.
30. Agnew-Blais J, Danese A. Childhood maltreatment and unfavorable clinical outcomes in bipolar disorder: a systematic review and meta-analysis. Lancet Psychiatry. 2016;3(4):342–9. https://doi.org/10.1016/S2215-0366(15)00544-1.

31. Bourdon C, Etain B, Spano L, Belzeaux R, Leboyer M, Delahaye-Duriez A, et al. Accelerated aging in bipolar disorders: an exploratory study of six epigenetic clocks. Psychiatry Res. 2023;327:115373. https://doi.org/10.1016/j.psychres.2023.115373.
32. Kouba BR, de Araujo BL, Borges de Souza P, Gil-Mohapel J, ALS R. Role of inflammatory mechanisms in major depressive disorder: From etiology to potential pharmacological targets. Cells. 2024;13(5):423. https://doi.org/10.3390/cells13050423.
33. Su YY, D'Arcy C, Li M, O'Donnell KJ, Caron J, Meaney MJ, Meng X. Specific and cumulative lifetime stressors in the aetiology of major depression: a longitudinal community-based population study. Epidemiol Psychiatr Sci. 2022;31:e3. https://doi.org/10.1017/S2045796021000779.
34. Beck AT, Bredemeier K. A unified model of depression: integrating clinical, cognitive, biological, and evolutionary perspectives. Clin Psychol Sci. 2016;4(4):596–619. https://doi.org/10.1177/2167702616628523.
35. Dong M, Lu L, Zhang L, Zhang Q, Ungvari GS, Ng CH, Yuan Z, Xiang Y, Wang G, Xiang YT. Prevalence of suicide attempts in bipolar disorder: a systematic review and meta-analysis of observational studies. Epidemiol Psychiatr Sci. 2019;29:e63. https://doi.org/10.1017/S2045796019000593.
36. Plans L, Barrot C, Nieto E, Rios J, Schulze TG, Papiol S, et al. Association between completed suicide and bipolar disorder: a systematic review of the literature. J Affect Disord. 2019;242:111–22. https://doi.org/10.1016/j.jad.2018.08.054.
37. Hu FH, Jia YJ, Zhao DY, Fu XL, Zhang WQ, Tang W, et al. Gender differences in suicide among patients with bipolar disorder: a systematic review and meta-analysis. J Affect Disord. 2023;339:601–14. https://doi.org/10.1016/j.jad.2023.07.060.
38. Tondo L, Pompili M, Forte A, Baldessarini RJ. Suicide attempts in bipolar disorders: comprehensive review of 101 reports. Acta Psychiatr Scand. 2016;133(3):174–86. https://doi.org/10.1111/acps.12517.
39. Schaffer A, Isometsä ET, Tondo L, Moreno DH, Sinyor M, Kessing LV, et al. Epidemiology, neurobiology and pharmacological interventions related to suicide deaths and suicide attempts in bipolar disorder: part I of a report of the International Society for Bipolar Disorders Task Force on suicide in bipolar disorder. Aust N Z J Psychiatry. 2015;49(9):785–802. https://doi.org/10.1177/0004867415594427.
40. Glenn CR, Kleiman EM, Kellerman J, Pollak O, Cha CB, Esposito EC, et al. Annual research review: a meta-analytic review of worldwide suicide rates in adolescents. J Child Psychol Psychiatry. 2020;61(3):294–308. https://doi.org/10.1111/jcpp.13106.
41. Slavich GM, Sacher J. Stress, sex hormones, inflammation, and major depressive disorder: extending social signal transduction theory of depression to account for sex differences in mood disorders. Psychopharmacology. 2019;236(10):3063–79. https://doi.org/10.1007/s00213-019-05326-9.
42. Mengelkoch S, Slavich GM. Sex differences in stress susceptibility as a key mechanism underlying depression risk. Curr Psychiatry Rep. 2024;26(4):157–65. https://doi.org/10.1007/s11920-024-01490-8.
43. Aas M, Henry C, Andreassen OA, Bellivier F, Melle I, Etain B. The role of childhood trauma in bipolar disorders. Int J Bipolar Disord. 2016;4:2. https://doi.org/10.1186/s40345-015-0042-0.
44. Dell'Osso B, Cafaro R, Ketter TA. Has bipolar disorder become a predominantly female gender related condition? Analysis of recently published large sample studies. Int J Bipolar Disord. 2021;9:3. https://doi.org/10.1186/s40345-020-00207-z.
45. Arnone D, Karmegam SR, Östlundh L, Alkhyeli F, Alhammadi L, Alhammadi S, et al. Risk of suicidal behavior in patients with major depression and bipolar disorder – a systematic review and meta-analysis of registry-based studies. Neurosci Biobehav Rev. 2024;159:105594. https://doi.org/10.1016/j.neubiorev.2024.105594.
46. Canetto SS, Sakinofsky I. The gender paradox in suicide. Suicide Life Threat Behav. 1998;28(1):1–23.

47. Nock MK, Borges G, Bromet EJ, Cha CB, Kessler RC, Lee S. Suicide and suicidal behavior. Epidemiol Rev. 2008;30(1):133–54. https://doi.org/10.1093/epirev/mxn002.
48. Arowosegbe A, Oyelade T. Suicide risk assessment and prevention tools in the UK: current landscape and future directions. Psychiatry Int. 2023;4:354–69. https://doi.org/10.3390/psychiatryint4040032.
49. Mitchell RHB, Hower H, Birmaher B, Strober M, Merranko J, Rooks B, et al. Sex differences in the longitudinal course and outcome of bipolar disorder in youth. J Clin Psychiatry. 2020;81(6):19m13159. https://doi.org/10.4088/JCP.19m13159.
50. Polidori L, Sarli G, Berardelli I, Pompili M, Baldessarini RJ. Risk of suicide attempt with gender diversity and neurodiversity. Psychiatry Res. 2024;333:115632. https://doi.org/10.1016/j.psychres.2023.115632.
51. Grover S, Hazari N, Aneja J, Chakrabarti S, Avasthi A. Stigma and its correlates among patients with bipolar disorder: a study from a tertiary care hospital of North India. Psychiatry Res. 2016;244:109–16. https://doi.org/10.1016/j.psychres.2016.07.012.
52. Levy B, Tsoy E, Brodt M, Petrosyan K, Malloy M. Stigma, social anxiety, and illness severity in bipolar disorder: implications for treatment. Ann Clin Psychiatry. 2015;27(1):55–64. https://doi.org/10.12788/acp.0007.
53. Elbogen EB, Lanier M, Montgomery AE, Strickland S, Wagner HR, Tsai J. Financial strain and suicide attempts in a nationally representative sample of US adults. Am J Epidemiol. 2020;189(11):1266–74. https://doi.org/10.1093/aje/kwaa146.
54. Schaffer A, Isometsä ET, Azorin JM, Cassidy F, Goldstein T, Rihmer Z, et al. A review of factors associated with greater likelihood of suicide attempts and suicide deaths in bipolar disorder: part II of a report of the International Society for Bipolar Disorders Task Force on suicide in bipolar disorder. Aust N Z J Psychiatry. 2015;49(11):1006–20. https://doi.org/10.1177/0004867415594428.
55. Sylvia LG, Montana RE, Deckersbach T, Thase ME, Tohen M, Reilly-Harrington N, et al. Poor quality of life and functioning in bipolar disorder. Int J Bipolar Disord. 2017;5(1):10. https://doi.org/10.1186/s40345-017-0078-4.
56. Almeida VF, Bezerra-Filho S, Studart-Bottó P, Léda-Rego G, Silva ITF, Kapczinski F, et al. History of suicide attempts in patients with bipolar disorder type I: socio-demographic and clinical factors, quality of life and functioning. Nord J Psychiatry. 2021;75(4):306–13. https://doi.org/10.1080/08039488.2020.1853230.
57. Wang J, Mann F, Lloyd-Evans B, Ma R, Johnson S. Associations between loneliness and perceived social support and outcomes of mental health problems: a systematic review. BMC Psychiatry. 2018;18(1):156. https://doi.org/10.1186/s12888-018-1736-5.
58. Koenig HG. Religion, spirituality, and health: the research and clinical implications. ISRN Psychiatry. 2012;2012:278730. https://doi.org/10.5402/2012/278730.
59. Du N, Zhou YL, Zhang X, Guo J, Sun XL. Do some anxiety disorders belong to the prodrome of bipolar disorder? A clinical study combining retrospective and prospective methods to analyse the relationship between anxiety disorder and bipolar disorder from the perspective of biorhythms. BMC Psychiatry. 2017;17:351. https://doi.org/10.1186/s12888-017-1509-6.
60. Rabelo-da-Ponte FD, Feiten JG, Mwangi B, Barros FC, Wehrmeister FC, Menezes AM, et al. Early identification of bipolar disorder among young adults – a 22-year community birth cohort. Acta Psychiatr Scand. 2020;142(6):476–85. https://doi.org/10.1111/acps.13233.
61. Cardoso TA, Mondin TC, Azevedo LB, Toralles LMD, de Mattos Souza LD. Is suicide risk a predictor of diagnosis conversion to bipolar disorder? Psychiatry Res. 2018;268:473–7. https://doi.org/10.1016/j.psychres.2018.08.026.
62. Serra G, De Crescenzo F, Maisto F, Galante JR, Iannoni ME, Trasolini M, et al. Suicidal behavior in juvenile bipolar disorder and major depressive disorder patients: systematic review and meta-analysis. J Affect Disord. 2022;311:572–81. https://doi.org/10.1016/j.jad.2022.05.063.

63. Duarte D, Belzeaux R, Etain B, Greenway KT, Rancourt E, Correa H, et al. Childhood-maltreatment subtypes in bipolar patients with suicidal behavior: systematic review and meta-analysis. Braz J Psychiatry. 2020;42(5):558–67. https://doi.org/10.1590/1516-4446-2019-0592.
64. Melhem NM, Brent DA, Ziegler M, Iyengar S, Kolko D, Oquendo M, et al. Familial pathways to early-onset suicidal behavior: familial and individual antecedents of suicidal behavior. Am J Psychiatry. 2007;164(9):1364–70. https://doi.org/10.1176/appi.ajp.2007.06091522.
65. Brent DA, Melhem N. Familial transmission of suicidal behavior. Psychiatr Clin North Am. 2008;31(2):157–77. https://doi.org/10.1016/j.psc.2008.02.001.
66. Lima CNC, Suchting R, Scaini G, Cuellar VA, Favero-Campbell AD, Walss-Bass C, et al. Epigenetic GrimAge acceleration and cognitive impairment in bipolar disorder. Eur Neuropsychopharmacol. 2022;62:10–21. https://doi.org/10.1016/j.euroneuro.2022.06.007.
67. Tondo L, Vázquez GH, Baldessarini RJ. Prevention of suicidal behavior in bipolar disorder. Bipolar Disord. 2021;23(1):14–23. https://doi.org/10.1111/bdi.13017.
68. Young JE. Cognitive therapy for personality disorders: a schema-focusedapproach. Sarasota, FL: Professional Resource Press/Professional Resource Exchange; 1999.
69. Khosravani V, Mohammadzadeh A, Sharifi Bastan F, Amirinezhad A, Amini M. Early maladaptive schemas and suicidal risk in inpatients with bipolar disorder. Psychiatry Res. 2019;271:351–9. https://doi.org/10.1016/j.psychres.2018.11.067.
70. Hawke LD, Provencher MD. Early maladaptive schemas among patients diagnosed with bipolar disorder. J Affect Disord. 2012;136(3):803–11. https://doi.org/10.1016/j.jad.2011.09.036.
71. Yatham LN, Chakrabarty T, Bond DJ, Schaffer A, Beaulieu S, Parikh SV, et al. Canadian Network for Mood and Anxiety Treatments (CANMAT) and International Society for Bipolar Disorders (ISBD) recommendations for the management of patients with bipolar disorder with mixed presentations. Bipolar Disord. 2021;23(8):767–88. https://doi.org/10.1111/bdi.13135.
72. Dale R, Power K, Kane S, Stewart AM, Murray L. The role of parental bonding and early maladaptive schemas in the risk of suicidal behavior repetition. Arch Suicide Res. 2010;14(4):311–28. https://doi.org/10.1080/13811118.2010.524066.
73. Smith LM, Johns LC, Mitchell R. Characterizing the experience of auditory verbal hallucinations and accompanying delusions in individuals with a diagnosis of bipolar disorder: a systematic review. Bipolar Disord. 2017;19(6):417–33. https://doi.org/10.1111/bdi.12520.
74. Mansell W, Jones SH. The brief-HAPPI: a questionnaire to assess cognitions that distinguish between individuals with a diagnosis of bipolar disorder and non-clinical controls. J Affect Disord. 2006;93(1–3):29–34. https://doi.org/10.1016/j.jad.2006.04.004.
75. Bartoli F, Crocamo C, Carrà G. Cannabis use disorder and suicide attempts in bipolar disorder: a meta-analysis. Neurosci Biobehav Rev. 2019;103:14–20. https://doi.org/10.1016/j.neubiorev.2019.05.017.
76. O'Connor EA, Perdue LA, Coppola EL, Henninger ML, Thomas RG, Gaynes BN. Depression and suicide risk screening: updated evidence report and systematic review for the US preventive services task force. JAMA. 2023;329(23):2068–85. https://doi.org/10.1001/jama.2023.7787.
77. Kung FH, Tsai CK, Cheng CM, Tsai SJ, Su TP, Chen TJ, et al. Diagnostic conversion to bipolar disorder among adolescents and young adults with major depressive disorder: a nationwide longitudinal study. Eur Child Adolesc Psychiatry. 2024; https://doi.org/10.1007/s00787-024-02401-1.
78. de Azevedo CT, Jansen K, Mondin TC, Pedrotti Moreira F, de Lima BS, da Silva RA, et al. Lifetime cocaine use is a potential predictor for conversion from major depressive disorder to bipolar disorder: a prospective study. Psychiatry Clin Neurosci. 2020;74(8):418–23. https://doi.org/10.1111/pcn.13012.
79. Kessing LV, Willer I, Andersen PK, Bukh JD. Rate and predictors of conversion from unipolar to bipolar disorder: a systematic review and meta-analysis. Bipolar Disord. 2017;19(5):324–35. https://doi.org/10.1111/bdi.12513.

80. Terao T. Latent bipolar depression. Lancet. 2023;401(10372):191. https://doi.org/10.1016/S0140-6736(22)02608-3.
81. Schaffer A, Isometsä ET, Tondo L, Moreno DH, Turecki G, Reis C, et al. International Society for Bipolar Disorders Task Force on suicide: meta-analyses and meta-regression of correlates of suicide attempts and suicide deaths in bipolar disorder. Bipolar Disord. 2015;17(1):1–16. https://doi.org/10.1111/bdi.12271.
82. Tondo L, Miola A, Pinna M, Contu M, Baldessarini RJ. Antidepressant-associated diagnostic change from major depressive to bipolar disorder. Acta Psychiatr Scand. 2024; https://doi.org/10.1111/acps.13721.
83. Pemau A, Marin-Martin C, Diaz-Marsa M, de la Torre-Luque A, Ayad-Ahmed W, Gonzalez-Pinto A, et al. Risk factors for suicide reattempt: a systematic review and meta-analysis. Psychol Med. 2024;54:1897–904. https://doi.org/10.1017/S0033291724000904.
84. Lengvenyte A, Aouizerate B, Aubin V, Loftus J, Marlinge E, Belzeaux R, et al. Violent suicide attempt history in elderly patients with bipolar disorder: the role of sex, abdominal obesity, and verbal memory: results from the FACE-BD cohort (FondaMental Advanced center of Expertise for Bipolar Disorders). J Affect Disord. 2022;296:265–76. https://doi.org/10.1016/j.jad.2021.09.097.
85. Iliachenko EK, Bengtsson M, Jonsson U, Joas E, Pålsson E, Pivina L, et al. Suicide mortality after discharge from inpatient care for bipolar disorder: a 14-year Swedish national registry study. J Psychiatr Res. 2020;127:20–7. https://doi.org/10.1016/j.jpsychires.2020.05.008.
86. Buoli M, Cesana BM, Bolognesi S, Caldiroli A, Cumerlato Melter C, Camurri C, et al. Factors associated with lifetime suicide attempts in bipolar disorder: results from an Italian nationwide study. Eur Arch Psychiatry Clin Neurosci. 2022;272:359–70. https://doi.org/10.1007/s00406-021-01343-y.
87. Ng VW, Leung MT, Chan EW, Lee EH, Hayes JF, Osborn DP, et al. Association between the mood stabilizing treatment of bipolar disorder and risk of suicide attempts: a self-controlled case series study. Psychiatry Res. 2023;325:115236. https://doi.org/10.1016/j.psychres.2023.115236.
88. Stanley B, Brown G, Brent D, Wells K, Poling K, Curry J, et al. Cognitive-behavioral therapy for suicide prevention (CBT-SP): treatment model, feasibility, and acceptability. J Am Acad Child Adolesc Psychiatry. 2009;48:1005–13. https://doi.org/10.1097/CHI.0b013e3181b5dbfe.
89. Wood A, Trainor G, Rothwell J, Moore A, Harrington R. Randomized trial of group therapy for repeated deliberate self-harm in adolescents. J Am Acad Child Adolesc Psychiatry. 2001;40:1246–53. https://doi.org/10.1097/00004583-200111000-00003.
90. Rudd M, Williams B, Trotter D. The psychological and behavioural treatment of suicidal behaviour: what are the common elements of treatment that work? In: Wasserman D, Wasserman C, editors. Oxford textbook of suicidology and suicide prevention: a global perspective. Oxford: Oxford University Press; 2009. p. 427–47.
91. Sankar A, Schenkel LS, Parente MK, Hilimire MR, Zarate M, Shankman SA, et al. Telehealth social rhythm therapy to reduce mood symptoms and suicide risk among adolescents and young adults with bipolar disorder. Am J Psychother. 2021;74(4):172–7. https://doi.org/10.1176/appi.psychotherapy.20210011.
92. Büscher R, Torok M, Terhorst Y, Sander L. Internet-based cognitive behavioral therapy to reduce suicidal ideation: a systematic review and meta-analysis. JAMA Netw Open. 2020;3(4) https://doi.org/10.1001/jamanetworkopen.2020.3933.
93. Fristad MA, Verducci JS, Walters K, Young ME. Impact of multifamily psychoeducational psychotherapy in treating children aged 8 to 12 years with mood disorders. Arch Gen Psychiatry. 2009 Sep;66(9):1013–21. https://doi.org/10.1001/archgenpsychiatry.2009.112.
94. Bäckström B, Rask O, Knutsson J. Adolescent and family-focused cognitive-behavioral therapy for pediatric bipolar disorders: an open trial and individual trajectories study in routine psychiatric care. Child Psychiatry Hum Dev. 2023; https://doi.org/10.1007/s10578-023-01504-1.

95. van Es CM, El Khoury B, van Dis EAM, Te Brake H, van Ee E, Boelen PA, Mooren T. The effect of multiple family therapy on mental health problems and family functioning: a systematic review and meta-analysis. Fam Process. 2023;62(2):499–514. https://doi.org/10.1111/famp.12876.
96. Walsh EH, McMahon J, Herring MP. Research review: the effect of school-based suicide prevention on suicidal ideation and suicide attempts and the role of intervention and contextual factors among adolescents: a meta-analysis and meta-regression. J Child Psychol Psychiatry. 2022;63(8):836–45. https://doi.org/10.1111/jcpp.13598.
97. Wang Y, Liu J, Chen S, Zheng C, Zou X, Zhou Y. Exploring risk factors and their differences on suicidal ideation and suicide attempts among depressed adolescents based on decision tree model. J Affect Disord. 2024;352:87–100. https://doi.org/10.1016/j.jad.2024.02.035.
98. Kapczinski F, Montezano BB, de Azevedo CT. Latent bipolar disorder. Lancet. 2023;401(10394):2109. https://doi.org/10.1016/S0140-6736(23)00402-6.
99. Silva Ribeiro J, Pereira D, Salagre E, Coroa M, Santos Oliveira P, Santos V, et al. Risk calculators in bipolar disorder: a systematic review. Brain Sci. 2020;10(8):525. https://doi.org/10.3390/brainsci10080525.
100. Wiebenga JXM, Heering HD, Eikelenboom M, van Hemert AM, van Oppen P, Penninx BWJH. Associations of three major physiological stress systems with suicidal ideation and suicide attempts in patients with a depressive and/or anxiety disorder. Brain Behav Immun. 2022;102:195–205. https://doi.org/10.1016/j.bbi.2022.02.021.
101. Kuring JK, Mathias JL, Ward L, Tachas G. Inflammatory markers in persons with clinically-significant depression, anxiety or PTSD: a systematic review and meta-analysis. J Psychiatr Res. 2023;168:279–92. https://doi.org/10.1016/j.jpsychires.2023.10.009.
102. Keilp JG, Gorlyn M, Russell M, Oquendo MA, Burke AK, Harkavy-Friedman J, Mann JJ. Neuropsychological function and suicidal behavior: attention control, memory and executive dysfunction in suicide attempt. Psychol Med. 2013;43(3):539–51. https://doi.org/10.1017/S0033291712001419.
103. Escobar LE, Liew M, Yirdong F, Mandelos KP, Ferraro-Diglio SR, Abraham BM, Polanco-Roman L, Benau EM. Reduced attentional control in individuals with a history of suicide attempts compared to those with suicidal ideation: results from a systematic review and meta-analysis. J Affect Disord. 2024;349:8–20. https://doi.org/10.1016/j.jad.2023.12.082.

Chapter 14
Intelligence Quotient and Latent Bipolar Disorder

Mateus Frizzo Messinger, Mirela Paiva Vasconcelos-Moreno, Rochele Paz Fonseca, and Flávio Pereira Kapczinski

14.1 Introduction

The potential connection between intelligence and bipolar disorder (BD) has been explored since Plato's studies of "mania" (or "madness") in Classical Antiquity. Plato perceived the epistemological aspect of the term as relating to a "divine" origin, describing it as a means of attaining complete knowledge—specifically, the journey from the sensible world to the ideal or intelligible realm [1].

Associations between the symptoms of BD and intelligence, contemporaneously defined as a set of abilities to learn from diverse experiences and adapt to a wide range of environments, remain a subject of ongoing discussion [2, 3]. The g factor, also referred to as the general cognitive factor and a primary focus of assessment in

M. F. Messinger (✉)
Laboratory of Molecular Psychiatry, Hospital de Clínicas de Porto Alegre (HCPA), Porto Alegre, Brazil

Universidade Federal do Rio Grande do Sul, School of Medicine, PhD Program in Psychiatry and Behavioral Sciences, Department of Psychiatry, Porto Alegre, Brazil
e-mail: mateus.messinger@ufrgs.br

M. P. Vasconcelos-Moreno · F. P. Kapczinski
Laboratory of Molecular Psychiatry, Hospital de Clínicas de Porto Alegre (HCPA), Porto Alegre, Brazil

Universidade Federal do Rio Grande do Sul, School of Medicine, PhD Program in Psychiatry and Behavioral Sciences, Department of Psychiatry, Porto Alegre, RS, Brazil

Instituto Nacional de Ciência e Tecnologia Translacional em Medicina (INCT-TM), Porto Alegre, Brazil

R. P. Fonseca
Universidade Federal de Minas Gerais (UFMG), Medicine Department, Post-Graduate Program in Child and Adolescent Health, Belo Horizonte, Brazil

Conectare NeuroPsi, Porto Alegre, Brazil

T. de Azevedo Cardoso et al. (eds.), *Latent Bipolar Disorder*,
https://doi.org/10.1007/978-3-032-01297-5_14

Intelligence Quotient (IQ) tests, is highly heritable [4] and is one of the most predictive genetic factors for significant life outcomes, including education, occupation, and both physical and mental health. Research has established a correlation between intelligence and BD, indicating a higher prevalence of BD among individuals with both high and low intelligence [5, 6].

Young individuals with a familial predisposition to BD who exhibit nonspecific symptoms but have not yet developed hypomania or mania may demonstrate a latent form of the disorder [7]. Thus, cognitive features observed in healthy family members of those with BD may offer valuable insights into the comprehension of latent BD.

This chapter aims to present and discuss evidence from this expanding field of research, integrating theoretical and psychometric advancements in intelligence and a latent phase of BD derived from studies on childhood and adolescent neurodevelopment.

14.2 Part 1: Theories of Intelligence and Cognitive Neurodevelopment

14.2.1 Intelligence and Mental Health

David Wechsler (1958), the architect of one of the primary psychometric tools for assessing intelligence, defined intelligence as "the individual's global capacity to act purposefully, to think rationally, and to deal effectively with his environment" [8]. This definition characterizes intelligence as a dimensional construct of mental functioning that continues to evolve across the fields of psychology, medicine, and pedagogy [9].

In its early development during the nineteenth century, a biological theory of intelligence was introduced by geneticist Francis Galton, who investigated the heritability of talents across generations. Galton posited that giftedness was negatively correlated with certain physical and psychological traits, suggesting that exceptional performance might be linked to emotional dysregulation. This concept, known as Divergence Theory, bore similarities to metaphysical approaches by relying on the myth of the "mad genius." Galton later advanced the notion that individual differences in intelligence could and should be quantifiable [10].

During the nineteenth century, the study of intelligence as a neurodevelopmental phenomenon evolved through various descriptive models, with the most significant being the single-factor and multifactor models. The single-factor general intelligence model originated from correlation studies conducted by psychologist Charles E. Spearman (1863–1945), who identified a general factor known as "general intelligence" or the g factor [11].

In contrast, the multiple intelligences model conceptualizes intelligence in a multifactorial or multidimensional framework. This approach was primarily developed in the latter half of the twentieth century by researchers such as Cattell [12], Gardner [13], Goleman [14], and Sternberg [15]. Moreover, the constructs of emotional and social intelligence have been integrated into the broader term "social cognition" within the contemporary scientific community [16], encompassing skills such as emotional self-awareness, empathy, recognition of others' emotions, the ability to utilize information for decision-making, conflict management, and teamwork [17].

The most widely accepted model of intelligence is the Cattell-Horn-Carroll (CHC) model—CHC theory of cognitive abilities—developed by Cattell, Horn, and Carroll, who synthesized key theories under this framework. This model comprises three tiers [18, 19]:

I. The lowest tier, which includes narrow abilities such as processing speed, psychomotor skills, and short-term memory;
II. The middle tier, which represents crystallized intelligence (associated with language and memory) and fluid intelligence (associated with executive functions and adaptability to novel situations);
III. The highest tier, the g factor, or general intelligence.

Working memory, which involves the integration of information from various memory systems to manage concurrent tasks, and attentional control, essential for tasks requiring cognitive effort, are critical components associated with intelligence [18].

The investigation of intelligence in the neurodevelopment of children and adolescents is guided by a central theoretical framework that tracks intellectual milestones and developmental stages. A key reference is Piaget's conceptualization of these stages, which continues to be highly relevant in contemporary clinical practice [20]. According to Piaget, intelligence is not solely inherited or learned; it develops through the replacement of previous cognitive schemas with new ones, rather than merely adding cognitive skills. He outlined four stages of cognitive development, each characterized by distinct mental and behavioral structures that vary in quantity and quality, occurring in a sequential and gradually enriching manner, as illustrated in Table 14.1.

14.2.2 Psychometric Theories and Main IQ Tests

The first quantitative intelligence test was developed by Alfred Binet (1857–1911) and Théodore Simon (1873–1961) in 1904, aimed at addressing the challenge of distinguishing intellectually healthy children from those with cognitive deficits in French public schools, thereby defining the scope of special education. The test's evaluation criteria focused on the comprehension of words, concepts, phrases, and images, considered key indicators of cognitive ability. The reference measure was the ratio of mental age (determined by passing at least half of the tasks typical for children of a specific age) to chronological age, used as an index of developmental delay [21].

In 1916, Lewis M. Terman (1877–1956) of Stanford University revised the Binet-Simon test, creating a broader and more refined version known as the Stanford-Binet Intelligence Scale, which remains widely used today. In the late 1930s and early 1940s, David Wechsler (1896–1981), questioning the Binet test's reliance on "mental age" as a measure of developmental delay, introduced his own system incorporating a mathematical-statistical approach. He set the average and median intelligence at a value of 100, with a standard deviation of 15 points [8]. The previously proposed Spearman "g" factor was reinterpreted as two distinct groups: a verbal scale (measuring linguistic and arithmetic abilities) and a performance scale (measuring visuospatial abilities) [8]. Currently, the most well-known, researched, and widely used intelligence tests globally are the Stanford-Binet Intelligence Scale and the tests initially developed by Wechsler, available in various revised editions [9].

The results of IQ tests in the general population typically follow a bell-shaped distribution curve, a parametric measure that defines intellectual disability as an IQ score of ≤70 (second percentile, or 2 standard deviations below the mean) and high intelligence as an IQ score of ≥130 (98th percentile, or 2 standard deviations above the mean) [8]. IQ assessment has traditionally focused on conditions involving intellectual developmental disorders, as outlined by diagnostic manuals. However, recent updates in the fifth edition of the Wechsler Adult Intelligence Scale Fifth Edition (WAIS-5) include modifications for better identification of high intelligence and giftedness [22], reflecting a shift in clinical practice toward recognizing the importance of this profile. WAIS-5 also introduces the option of telepractice [23].

Table 14.1 Phases of the development of intelligence by Piaget [20]

Phase	Age (years)	Main domains	Mental operations
Sensorimotor period	0–2	Congenital reflex acts; thoughtless sensorimotor activities; imitation	Gradual perception of "permanent objects"; concepts of things, space, time, and causality
Preoperative period	2–7	Mastery of symbols, language, interpersonal feelings, and social relationships	Development of representative capacity; "half-logic" (no notion of reversibility); development of drawing, playing, language; inner language (basis of thought)
Concrete operational period	7–12	Classes, relations, and numbers; logical thinking in concrete operations	Operability following logic; awareness of the implications and consequences of your ideas and thoughts
Formal operational period	12–16	Fully abstract thinking, with symbolic systems	Establish complex and abstract relationships; forecasting ability; inverse, negative, reciprocal, and contrary operations

According to Diagnostic and statistical manual of mental disorders, fifth edition, text revision (DSM-5-TR) and international classification of diseases, 11th revision (ICD-11), the assessment of intelligence requires the use of psychometrically validated instruments to measure cognitive functions and adaptive behaviors. When standardized instruments are unavailable or impractical, assessments should rely on specialized clinical judgment [24]. Table 14.2 lists the instruments commonly used in neuropsychological assessments within psychiatric clinics to evaluate intellectual and adaptive functioning.

14.2.3 Updates on Intellectual Developmental Disorder: DSM-5-TR and ICD-11

According to the DSM-5-TR, the diagnosis of intellectual developmental disorder (Intellectual Disability) requires deficits in both intellectual and adaptive functioning across conceptual, social, and practical domains. The diagnostic criteria include (A) confirmation through both clinical assessment and standardized, individualized intelligence testing, (B) failure to meet developmental and sociocultural standards for personal independence and social responsibility, and (C) onset of symptoms during the developmental period (childhood or adolescence). Severity is specified as mild, moderate, severe, or profound, based not on IQ but on the level of adaptive functioning [25]. Borderline intellectual functioning, though challenging to assess in neuropsychological evaluations for mental health, is an important intermediate clinical presentation, characterized by limited intellectual capacity for complex daily cognitive tasks and reduced neuroprotection [26].

The classification adopted by the ICD-11 uses the same terminology as the DSM-5-TR: Intellectual Developmental Disorder. In both systems, neurodevelopmental disorders are characterized by behavioral and cognitive impairments that arise during the developmental period (childhood and adolescence, or before age 18), including significant difficulties in the acquisition and execution of intellectual, motor, language, or other functions, as well as specific social challenges [27]. The ICD-11 includes seven categories, with Intellectual Developmental Disorder (6A00) categorized alongside speech or language developmental disorders (6A01), autism spectrum disorder (6A02), developmental learning disorder (6A03), developmental motor coordination disorder (6A04), attention deficit hyperactivity disorder (6A05), and stereotypic movement disorder (6A06) [28].

The revisions in the DSM-5-TR and ICD-11 diagnostic manuals are particularly important for guiding research and clinical practice in the field of intelligence. Both systems replaced the term "mental" with "intellectual" and "retardation" with "developmental disorder." Additionally, the ICD-11 removed the feature of "behavioral impairment" from the severity definitions..

These changes emphasize intellectual development as the central feature of the diagnosis and align the terminology with theoretical models of intelligence, such as

Table 14.2 Common measures of intellectual functioning and adaptive functioning in children and adolescents

Instrument and current version	Age range	Description
Measures of intellectual functioning		
Stanford L Binet Intelligence Scale (SB5)	2–85 years	Full Scale Intelligence score Subtests: verbal reasoning, abstract/visual reasoning, quantitative memory, and short-term memory
Wechsler Preschool and Primary Scale of Intelligence-Revised (WPPSI-R)	2 years and 6 months to 7 years and 3 months	Full Scale Intelligence Score Subtests: verbal, processing, performance, and general language
Wechsler Intelligence Scale for Children-V (WISC-V)	6–16 years	Full Scale Intelligence: four core areas: verbal comprehension, perceptual reasoning, working memory, and processing speed
WAIS-5	16–89 years	Full scale Intelligence: four core areas: verbal comprehension, perceptual reasoning, working memory, and processing speed
Leiter International Performance Scale-3 (Leiter-3)	3–75+ years	Nonverbal Intelligence Quotient; two groupings of subtests, cognitive and attention/memory, ten subtests total. Measures fluid reasoning, visualization, memory, attention, and cognitive interference
Raven's Colored Progressive Matrices (CPM)	5 years to 11 years and 11 months	Nonverbal fluid intelligence; one of the most heavily used cognitive assessments in published research studies
Wechsler Abbreviated Scale of Intelligence—Second Edition (WASI-II)	6–89 years	Screening measure of verbal, performance, and general intellectual ability
Measures of adaptative functioning		
Bayley Scales of Infant and Toddler Development (BSID-III)	2–49 months	Subtests: language, receptive and expressive, gross motor, fine motor, cognitive problem-solving ability, and sustained attention
Vineland Adaptive Behavior Scales-Third Edition (Vineland-3)	Birth to adulthood	Survey Interview, Parent/Caregiver Rating Forms, Expanded Interview Form, Teacher Rating Form. Assesses communication, daily living skills, socialization, motor skills, and maladaptive behaviors
Scales of Independent Behavior -Revised	Infancy to 80+ years	Interview or checklist. Assesses 14 areas of adaptive behavior and 8 areas of problem behavior.

(continued)

Table 14.2 (continued)

Instrument and current version	Age range	Description
AAIDD's Diagnostic Adaptive Behavior Scale (DABS)	4–21 years	Under development. Standardized assessment including three domains: conceptual skills, social skills, and practical skills.
Adaptive Behavior Assessment Scale - Third Edition (ABAS-3)	Birth to 89 years	Parent/Primary Caregiver form or Teacher/daycare provider form. Assesses three domains of adaptive behavior: conceptual, social, and practical

Adapted and updated from Siegel et al. [24]

the CHC three-stratum theory, as previously discussed [26]. Furthermore, the ICD-11 conceptualizes intellectual developmental disorder as a health condition or disorder, shifting the focus from a disability-centered perspective to one that highlights the importance of considering commonly associated mental disorders, thereby allowing for dual diagnoses [28].

14.2.4 High Intelligence and Giftedness

Conceptually, the measurement of intelligence using standardized instruments produces a normal distribution curve in the population, with a mean of 100 points, as shown in Fig. 14.1. Individuals scoring 2 standard deviations above the mean (IQ ≥130), corresponding to the 98th percentile, are often categorized as having "high intelligence" or being "gifted." Only recently has this group received attention in mental health research as a form of atypical neurodevelopment, characterized by distinct patterns of experience, resilience, vulnerability, and sensitivity. Changes in concepts and terms, such as "giftedness," have emerged in response to the expansion of intelligence theories, which propose broader criteria than those defined solely by IQ tests. This shift aims to integrate new multidimensional models of intelligence, recognizing neurodevelopmental characteristics in giftedness as independent of the rigid "Procrustean" criteria imposed by traditional IQ assessments [29].

In the field of pragmatic movements, two of them mainly spearhead the multidimensional approach: the first is Study of Mathematically Precocious Youth at Johns Hopkins University which gave rise to the Talent Search model across the United States; the second is Renzulli's (1977) "triad model," which considers giftedness to be a dynamic state in which a triad of common rings generates a stable concept for individual differences as shown in Fig. 14.2. The Renzulli model connects high ability, creativity, and commitment to the task, with particular goal orientation in educational programs [10, 30].

Gifted individuals are often characterized by the potential to develop overexcitabilities in sensory, emotional, imaginative, intellectual, and psychomotor domains.

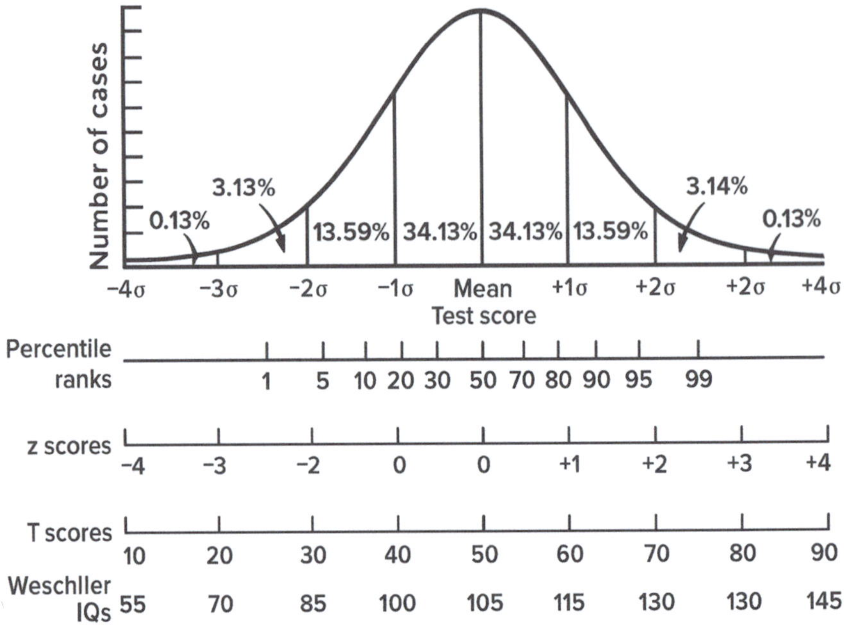

Fig. 14.1 Representation of the population distribution curve following a mean of 100 points and an SD of 15 points, used for IQ tests such as Wechsler's

Fig. 14.2 Renzulli's three-ring conception of giftedness [30]

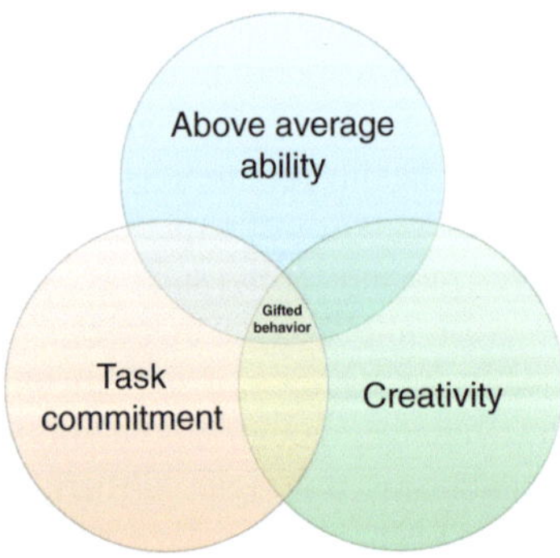

These traits are measurable using the Overexcitability Questionnaire-Two (OEQ-II), which is also described in K. Dabrowski's Positive Disintegration Theory , a developmental model [10]. The OEQ-II has potential clinical utility in assessing overexcitabilities and may be valuable in clinical research, particularly in studying correlations with psychiatric symptoms [31]. For instance, under emotional stress, psychomotor overexcitability may manifest as nervous tics, nail-biting, workaholism, acting out, compulsive talking, or impulsive actions, while sensual overexcitability could lead to behaviors such as hyperphagia, sexual disinhibition, or excessive spending [32].

14.3 Part 2: Neurodevelopment of Intelligence and Latent BD

14.3.1 Latent BD and Intellectual Neurodevelopment

14.3.1.1 Low IQ and BD

Rabelo-da-Ponte et al. [33] conducted a cohort study demonstrating that a low or borderline intelligence quotient (IQ) at 18 years of age was a predictor for the diagnosis of BD by 22 years of age. Additionally, individuals diagnosed with BD exhibited a higher frequency of prior academic failures compared to those without mood disorders. The study further identified the number of school failures as a risk factor specifically associated with BD type I, whereas the absence of school dropout emerged as a protective factor against the development of BD.

Francisco et al. [34] investigated a sample of children and adolescents in an outpatient setting and found that individuals with pediatric BD who had attempted suicide exhibited lower estimated IQ scores compared to those without a history of suicide attempts. The study further emphasized the uncertainty regarding whether a lower IQ predisposes individuals with pediatric BD to a more severe course associated with suicide attempts or whether the observed lower IQ is a consequence of the severity of the disorder itself.

The meta-analysis by Kloiber et al. [35] identified low cognitive ability as a predictor of adult affective disorders, with endocrinological factors serving as potential neurodevelopmental risk factors for BD associated with cognitive impairment. A U.S. cohort study found that perinatal oxytocin exposure was associated with an increased risk of BD and impaired cognitive performance in adolescence [36]. In the evaluated sample, a reduction in executive function and prefrontal cortical activity was suggested as an explanation for the observed results, which were measured using the Raven's Progressive Matrices scale.

MacCabe et al. [5] conducted a whole-population cohort study to investigate the associations between scholastic achievement at ages 15–16 and subsequent BD from ages 17 to 31. Their findings revealed that individuals with the lowest grades were found to be at a moderately elevated risk for BD.

14.3.1.2 High IQ and BD

Research into the association between high intelligence and psychiatric symptoms reveals both protective and risk effects [37] though studies remain limited for a comprehensive understanding. Population-based studies by Kyaga et al. [38, 39] in Sweden demonstrated a higher prevalence of creativity and leadership traits among individuals with BD, while another study found that emotional dysregulation and a greater propensity for mental disorders were linked to increased overexcitability in gifted Mensa volunteers [40]; in contrast, individuals of average intelligence in the control group exhibited a mitigated or even protective effect against such symptoms. Mac Cabe et al. [5] cohort study also stated that individuals with exceptional academic performance exhibited nearly a fourfold increased risk of developing BD compared to those with average grades.

Individuals at familial risk for BD may exhibit characteristics that begin in childhood, including symptoms such as anxiety and sleep disturbances. During adolescence, mood disturbances and suicidal behaviors may emerge, often preceding the diagnosis of manic or hypomanic episodes in adulthood [41]. On the other hand, Boschi et al. [41] and Karpinski [42] highlighted the frequent occurrence of perfectionism, rumination, and excessive worry in individuals with high intelligence, traits often linked to high intensity and overexcitabilities. These characteristics can lead to diagnostic challenges due to their overlap with symptoms of anxiety and depression [43].

A meta-analysis by Tourreix [44] on non-cognitive characteristics associated with gifted individuals indicated that, based on longitudinal studies, individuals with high intelligence may be at greater risk of developing BD in adulthood compared to those with average intelligence. This pattern contrasts with other mental disorders, such as schizophrenia, depression, and anxiety disorders, where high intelligence appears to exert a protective effect. The study cautions, however, that the data should be interpreted carefully, as some cohorts did not exclusively focus on gifted individuals, and in one population, high intelligence was defined by performance on a national exam rather than by IQ. This caution may involve distinguishing executive function from IQ measures, as an observational study on occupational status in patients with BD by Drakopoulos et al. [45] demonstrated that executive functioning was a stronger predictor of occupational status than IQ and other clinical factors, including illness severity.

14.3.2 Association Between IQ and Clinical Features in BD

A meta-analysis by Halac et al. [46] in pediatric patients with BD found no association between IQ scores and social cognition, but, in this population, social cognition did not fully recover between interepisodic periods likewise evidence concerning adults with BD, and theory of mind (ToM) evaluation could have trait-marker properties of the illness [47]. Adult patients with BD presented higher ToM impairment in manic episodes and in those with subsyndromal BD than in euthymic individuals [41].

A meta-analysis by Zwarte et al. [48] found that IQ measures in first-degree relatives of patients with BD were slightly lower or borderline compared to those of control groups. Another study compared cognitive abilities in young first-degree relatives (ages 10–25) of patients with BD (types I and II) with healthy controls. The results demonstrated that the relatives performed significantly worse in visual and verbal memory, processing speed, and sustained attention, but not in executive functions or working memory. Specifically, significant impairments were observed in tasks involving list learning, delayed recall, and Stroop performance [49].

Similarly, Kulkarni [50] reported that unaffected siblings of patients with BD performed worse than healthy controls on tasks such as the Tower of London, Rey's Auditory Verbal Learning Test, and Rey's Complex Figure Test. Bellia et al. [51] further highlighted a strong association between BD and other disorders, using dimensional measures of verbal and non-verbal IQ, as well as adaptive functioning.

An increasingly relevant area for studying mental disorders in association with intelligence is the field of genetic heritability. It is well established that IQ is influenced by both genetic and environmental factors. Willoughby et al. [52] reported a correlation of approximately 65% between the IQ of parents and their biological children, as well as between midparent IQ and offspring IQ. Additionally, Zabaneh et al. [4] demonstrated high heritability of the general intelligence (g) factor, ranging from 40% in childhood to 80% in adulthood. Although IQ is a highly stable quantitative trait, it can be enhanced through early, intensive psychoeducational interventions and may decline with age due to illness [53]. BD, in turn, is considered a highly heritable condition, with estimates from twin studies indicating a heritability range of 60–90%. These studies assess the concordance of the disorder between monozygotic and dizygotic twins [53, 54].

A genome-wide association (GWA) study on heritability revealed that the genetic correlation between intelligence and BD is near zero. Conversely, positive genetic correlations were observed between intelligence and anorexia nervosa and autism spectrum disorder, while negative correlations were identified with schizophrenia, attention-deficit/hyperactivity disorder, major depressive disorder (MDD), and neuroticism [37]. In a Mendelian randomization analysis, Ohi et al. [55] did not identify a bidirectional causal association between intelligence and risk for BD, as was observed for schizophrenia. The study highlighted that lower intelligence shared a notable risk association with both schizophrenia and BD, with a stronger effect in this direction than the inverse, suggesting a potential causal link between intelligence and susceptibility to BD types I and II. Interestingly, using another GWA summary dataset, higher intelligence was unexpectedly associated with an increased risk for BD type I (odds ratio 0.98).

14.3.3 The Cognitive Reserve Model

The cognitive reserve model is an active framework used to explain how the brain, affected by psychiatric conditions, may demonstrate compensatory mechanisms over time. In this model, crystallized intelligence and premorbid education levels act as moderators of cognitive outcomes in debilitating conditions such as BD [56, 57].

Cognitive reserve or resilience have among its proxies intelligence [58]. A meta-analysis by Camprodon-Boadas [59] indicated a positive relationship, both qualitative and quantitative, between cognitive domains and measures of cognitive reserve in individuals with mood disorders. Cognitive reserve thus appears to be a protective factor that helps mitigate cognitive impairments associated with BD and MDD. Additionally, longitudinal studies suggest that cognitive reserve may influence the variability in cognitive profiles during the progression of BD. For instance, a 5-year follow-up study found that individuals with lower IQ scores experienced a significant decline in verbal memory [60], whereas engagement in leisure activities was significantly correlated with improvements in verbal memory, verbal fluency, and story memory in BD patients [61].

The relationship between premorbid adjustment and bipolar BD remains debated, with evidence indicating an association between poor premorbid functioning and more severe manifestations of the disorder. Evidence points that high IQ increases the risk of developing BD, while high IQ is associated with fewer bipolar episodes and protects against cognitive impairment, and high levels of education and stable employment also appear to protect against cognitive impairment [62]. According to Arango et al. [63], late-onset BD is linked to higher scholastic achievement and better-preserved neurodevelopmental profiles, while lower cognitive functioning may be a significant risk factor for the earlier onset of BD, though it may not substantially affect the overall incidence of the disorder. Specifically, the negative association between hypo/manic episodes and executive function impairments was attenuated in individuals with higher premorbid IQ [64] However, when executive function deficits remain stable, this may suggest the presence of subgroups with distinct pathophysiological characteristics [64].

14.4 Part 3: Future Perspectives

Evidence suggests that both low and high levels of intelligence and academic performance during youth are associated with an increased risk of developing BD [37, 64]. High IQ may also act as a protective factor for some individuals, similar to other mental illnesses [64]. While IQ assessments predominantly provide clinical data on intellectual developmental disorders, growing evidence highlights the importance of assessing high IQ in its interplay to BD. In this framework, overexcitabilities linked to high intelligence may offer deeper insights into the symptomatology and aid in the differential diagnosis of BD [40].

A potential biochemical approach to linking intelligence and BD is suggested by evidence showing an increased urinary concentration of the neuronal membrane glycoprotein disintegrin and metalloprotease 12 (ADAM12), particularly its 92 kDa form, in patients with BD undergoing lithium treatment compared to both non-lithium-treated patients and healthy controls [65]. ADAM12 is implicated in multiple central nervous system diseases, including brain tumors, multiple sclerosis, amyotrophic lateral sclerosis, Alzheimer's disease, schizophrenia, autism, and BD. It has also been observed at elevated gene expression levels in GWA analyses of individuals with very high intelligence [66].

Another future direction for research is the investigation of common genetic signatures between BD and intelligence. In a study by Shang et al. [67], substantial polygenic overlap between intelligence and BD was identified, revealing multiple loci associated with both conditions, although no genetic correlation was found. Cotrena et al. [68] emphasized that further studies, particularly those incorporating control groups, could provide greater clarity on this issue.

A cognitive rehabilitation program may benefit patients with BD who exhibit low premorbid IQ, limited educational attainment, and insecure employment status, as these factors are associated with a poorer prognosis, characterized by a higher frequency of bipolar episodes and/or cognitive decline [62].

14.5 Conclusion

A more comprehensive assessment could provide valuable insights for clinical practice in managing individuals at risk of developing BD or monitoring the course of the disorder. The construct of intelligence itself is still an evolving concept that requires further investigation into measurement tools for all associated abilities. Thus, its correlation with the emergence of latent BD may become clearer as additional studies bridge intelligence and IQ testing with mental health research, particularly regarding risk factors for BD.

Clinical Considerations:

- Intelligence is contemporaneously defined as a set of abilities to learn from diverse experiences and adapt to a wide range of environments.
- The most widely accepted model of intelligence is the Cattell-Horn-Carroll (CHC) model, which comprises three tiers: narrow abilities, crystallized/fluid intelligence, and the g-factor.
- Traits of perfectionism, rumination, and excessive worry in individuals with high intelligence are often linked to high intensity and overexcitabilities.
- Research into the association between high intelligence and psychiatric symptoms reveals both protective and risk effects.
- Cognitive reserve appears to be a protective factor that helps mitigate cognitive impairments associated with BD and major depressive disorder.
- Future research directions include the interplay between high IQ and BD, biochemical approaches, and the exploration of shared genetic signatures.

References

1. Berrios GE. Of mania: introduction. Hist Psychiatry (SAGE Publications Ltd). 2004;15:105–24.
2. Smith DJ, Anderson J, Zammit S, Meyer TD, Pell JP, Mackay D. Childhood IQ and risk of bipolar disorder in adulthood: prospective birth cohort study. BJPsych Open. 2015 Jun 2;1(1):74–80.
3. Flaaten CB, Melle I, Gardsjord E, Bjella T, Engen MJ, Vaskinn A, et al. Course of intellectual functioning in schizophrenia and bipolar disorder: a 10-year follow-up study. Psychol Med. 2023 Apr 8;53(6):2662–70.
4. Zabaneh D, Krapohl E, Gaspar HA, Curtis C, Lee SH, Patel H, et al. A genome-wide association study for extremely high intelligence. Mol Psychiatry. 2018 May 1;23(5):1226–32.
5. MacCabe JH, Lambe MP, Cnattingius S, Sham PC, David AS, Reichenberg A, et al. Excellent school performance at age 16 and risk of adult bipolar disorder: national cohort study. Br J Psychiatry. 2010 Feb 2;196(2):109–15.
6. Kendler KS, Ohlsson H, Mezuk B, Sundquist K, Sundquist J. A swedish national prospective and co-relative study of school achievement at age 16, and risk for schizophrenia, other nonaffective psychosis, and bipolar illness. Schizophr Bull. 2015;42:77–86.
7. Gitlin MJ. Diagnosing latent bipolar disorder: a clinical dilemma. Bipolar Disord. 2018 Jun 10;20(4):300–2.
8. Wechsler D. Wechsler abbreviated scale of intelligence. Baltimore: Williams & Wilkins; 1958.
9. Dalgalarrondo P. In: Bispo de Lima L, editor. Psicopatologia e Semiologia dos Transtornos Mentais, vol. 1. 3rd ed. Porto Alegre: Artmed; 2019.
10. Shavinina LV. International handbook on giftedness. Dordrecht: Springer Netherlands; 2009.
11. Spearman CE. General intelligence, objectively determined and measured. Am J Psychol. 1904;15:201–99.
12. Cattel R. Abilities: their structure, grouth and action. Boston: Houghton Miffl; 1971.
13. Gardner H. Estruturas da mente: a teoria das inteligências múltiplas. Porto Alegre: Artmed; 1994.
14. Goleman D. Emotional intelligence: why it can matter more than IQ. New York: Bantam; 1994.
15. Sternberg R. The concept of intelligence and its role in lifelong learning and success. Am Psychol. 1997;52:1030–7.
16. Mecca T, Martins Dias N, Berberian A. Cognição Social: teoria, pesquisa e aplicação. 1st ed. São Paulo: Mennon Edições Científicas; 2016.
17. Bar-On R, Parker J. Manual de inteligência emocional. Porto Alegre: Artmed; 2002.
18. McGrew KS, Schneider WJ, Decker SL, Bulut O. A psychometric network analysis of CHC intelligence measures: implications for research, theory, and interpretation of broad CHC scores "Beyond g". J Intelligence. 2023;11(1):19.
19. Intelligence SJ. Dialogues Clin Neurosci. 2012;14(1):19–27.
20. Piaget J, Inhelder B. A psicologia da criança. São Paulo: Difusão Européia do Livro; 1973.
21. Richardson K. Compreender a inteligência. Lisboa: Instituto Piaget; 1999.
22. Pearson Assessments. Wechsler adult intelligence scale fifth edition – WAIS 5 [Internet]. 2024 [cited 2024 Oct 8]. Available from: https://www.pearsonassessments.com/store/usassessments/en/Store/Professional-Assessments/Cognition-%26-Neuro/Wechsler-Adult-Intelligence-Scale-%7C-Fifth-Edition/p/P100071002.html?tab=product-details.
23. Pearson Assessments. Telepractice and the WAIS-5 [Internet]. [cited 2024 Oct 8]. Available from: https://www.pearsonassessments.com/content/dam/school/global/clinical/us/assets/telepractice/guidance-documents/telepractice-and-the-wais-5.pdf.
24. Siegel M, McGuire K, Veenstra-VanderWeele J, Stratigos K, King B, Bellonci C, et al. Practice parameter for the assessment and treatment of psychiatric disorders in children and adolescents with intellectual disability (intellectual developmental disorder). J Am Acad Child Adolesc Psychiatry. 2020 Apr 1;59(4):468–96.
25. American Psychiatric Association. Diagnostic and statistical manual of mental disorders. American Psychiatric Association Publishing; 2022.
26. Barrea C, Leroy P, Debray F, Alkan S, Rousselle L. Un trouble du développement intellectuel chez l'enfant. Rev Med Liege. 2020;75(10):686–91.

27. de Oliveira SES, Trentini CM. In: de Lima LB, editor. Avanços em Psicopatologia, vol. 1. 1st ed. Porto Alegre: Artmed; 2023.
28. World Health Organization (WHO). International classification of diseases, eleventh revision (ICD-11), vol. 1. Geneva: WHO; 2022.
29. Tasca I, Guidi M, Turriziani P, Mento G, Tarantino V. Behavioral and socio-emotional disorders in intellectual giftedness: a systematic review. Child Psychiatry Hum Dev. 2024 Jun 1;55(3):768–89.
30. Renzulli JS, Reis SM. The three-ring conception of giftedness: a developmental approach for promoting creative productivity in young people. In: APA handbook of giftedness and talent. Washington: American Psychological Association; 2018. p. 185–99.
31. De Bondt N, Van Petegem P. Psychometric evaluation of the overexcitability questionnaire-two applying Bayesian structural equation modeling (BSEM) and multiple-group BSEM-based alignment with approximate measurement invariance. Front Psychol. 2015;6:1963.
32. Piechowski MM. Co Jest Normaline? Psychologia Wychowawcza. 2015;NR8:122127.
33. Rabelo-da-Ponte FD, Marchionatti LE, Watts D, Roza TH, Amoretti S, Barros FC, et al. Premorbid intelligence quotient and school failure as risk markers for bipolar disorder and major depressive disorder. J Psychiatr Res. 2024;169:160–5.
34. Francisco AP, Motta GLCL, Zortea F, Mugnol FE, Acosta J, Kohmann AM, et al. Lower estimated intelligence quotient is associated with suicide attempts in pediatric bipolar disorder. J Affect Disord. 2020 Jan;15(261):103–9.
35. Kloiber S, Rosenblat JD, Husain MI, Ortiz A, Berk M, Quevedo J, et al. Neurodevelopmental pathways in bipolar disorder. Neurosci Biobehav Rev (Elsevier Ltd). 2020;112:213–26.
36. Freedman D, Brown AS, Shen L, Schaefer CA. Perinatal oxytocin increases the risk of offspring bipolar disorder and childhood cognitive impairment. J Affect Disord. 2015 Mar;1(173):65–72.
37. Hill WD, Arslan RC, Xia C, Luciano M, Amador C, Navarro P, et al. Genomic analysis of family data reveals additional genetic effects on intelligence and personality. Mol Psychiatry. 2018 Dec 1;23(12):2347–62.
38. Kyaga S, Lichtenstein P, Boman M, Hultman C, Långström N, Landén M. Creativity and mental disorder: family study of 300 000 people with severe mental disorder. Br J Psychiatry. 2011 Nov;199(5):373–9.
39. Kyaga S, Lichtenstein P, Boman M, Landén M. Bipolar disorder and leadership – a total population study. Acta Psychiatr Scand. 2015 Feb 1;131(2):111–9.
40. Alker L. "Living beyond limits": neurogenic influences of overexcitabilities on the mental health of the highly gifted. ASEAN J Psychiatry. 2024;25:1–3.
41. Boschi A, Planche P, Hemimou C, Demily C, Vaivre-Douret L. From high intellectual potential to asperger syndrome: evidence for differences and a fundamental overlap-A systematic review. Front Psychol (Frontiers Media SA). 2016;7:1605.
42. Karpinski RI, Kinase Kolb AM, Tetreault NA, Borowski TB. High intelligence: a risk factor for psychological and physiological overexcitabilities. Intelligence. 2018 Jan;1(66):8–23.
43. Nolen-Hoeksema S. The role of rumination in depressive disorders and mixed anxiety/depressive symptoms. J Abnorm Psychol. 2000 Aug;109(3):504–11.
44. Tourreix E, Besançon M, Gonthier C. Non-cognitive specificities of intellectually gifted children and adolescents: a systematic review of the literature. J Intell Multidisciplinary Digital Publishing Institute (MDPI). 2023;11:141.
45. Drakopoulos J, Sparding T, Clements C, Pålsson E, Landén M. Executive functioning but not IQ or illness severity predicts occupational status in bipolar disorder. Int J Bipolar Disord. 2020;8(1):7.
46. Halac E, Ciray RO, Turan S, Tuncturk M, Agac N, Elmas FN, et al. Impaired theory of mind and emotion recognition in pediatric bipolar disorder: a systematic review and meta-analysis. J Psychiatr Res. 2021 Jun;138:246–55.
47. Bora E, Pantelis C. Meta-analysis of social cognition in attention-deficit/hyperactivity disorder (ADHD): comparison with healthy controls and autistic spectrum disorder. Psychol Med. 2016 Mar 28;46(4):699–716.

48. de Zwarte SMC, Brouwer RM, Agartz I, Alda M, Alonso-Lana S, Bearden CE, et al. Intelligence, educational attainment, and brain structure in those at familial high-risk for schizophrenia or bipolar disorder. Hum Brain Mapp. 2022 Jan 7;43(1):414–30.
49. Bora E, Özerdem A. A meta-analysis of neurocognition in youth with familial high risk for bipolar disorder. Eur Psychiatry (Elsevier Masson SAS). 2017;44:17–23.
50. Kulkarni S, Jain S, Janardhan Reddy Y, Kumar KJ, Kandavel T. Impairment of verbal learning and memory and executive function in unaffected siblings of probands with bipolar disorder. Bipolar Disord. 2010 Sep 27;12(6):647–56.
51. Bellia G, Chang J, Liew Z, Vernetti A, Macari S, Powell K, et al. Family history of psychiatric conditions and development of siblings of children with autism. Autism Res. 2024 Aug 1;17(8):1665–76.
52. Willoughby EA, McGue M, Iacono WG, Lee JJ. Genetic and environmental contributions to IQ in adoptive and biological families with 30-year-old offspring. Intelligence. 2021 Sep;1:88.
53. Salthouse T. The processing-speed theory of adult age diferences in cognition. Psychol Rev. 1996;103:403–28.
54. Smoller JW, Finn CT. Family, twin, and adoption studies of bipolar disorder. Am J Med Genet C Semin Med Genet. 2003 Nov 15;123C(1):48–58.
55. Ohi K, Takai K, Kuramitsu A, Sugiyama S, Soda M, Kitaichi K, et al. Causal associations of intelligence with schizophrenia and bipolar disorder: a Mendelian randomization analysis. Eur Psychiatry. 2021;64(1):e61.
56. Satz P, Cole MA, Hardy DJ, Rassovsky Y. Brain and cognitive reserve: mediator(s) and construct validity, a critique. J Clin Exp Neuropsychol. 2011 Jan 5;33(1):121–30.
57. Stern Y. What is cognitive reserve? Theory and research application of the reserve concept. J Int Neuropsychol Soc. 2002 Mar;8(3):448–60.
58. Hommel B, Kochhann R. Editorial: cognitive reserve and resilience in aging [Internet]. Available from: https://reserveandresilience.com/.
59. Camprodon-Boadas P, De Prisco M, Rabelo-da-Ponte FD, Sugranyes G, Clougher D, Baeza I, et al. Cognitive reserve and cognition in mood disorders: a systematic review and meta-analysis. Psychiatry Res. 2024 Sep;1:339.
60. Hinrichs KH, Easter RE, Angers K, Pester B, Lai Z, Marshall DF, et al. Influence of cognitive reserve on neuropsychological functioning in bipolar disorder: findings from a 5-year longitudinal study. Bipolar Disord. 2017 Feb 6;19(1):50–9.
61. Sato K, Matsui M, Ono Y, Miyagishi Y, Tsubomoto M, Naito N, et al. The relationship between cognitive reserve focused on leisure experiences and cognitive functions in bipolar patients. Heliyon. 2023;9(11):e21661.
62. Matsumoto K, Hamatani S. Impact of cognitive reserve on bipolar disorder: a systematic review. Front Psych. 2024 Feb;2:14.
63. Arango C, Fraguas D, Parellada M. Differential neurodevelopmental trajectories in patients with early-onset bipolar and schizophrenia disorders. Schizophr Bull. 2014 Mar 1;40(Suppl 2):S138–46.
64. Martino DJ, Valerio MP, Szmulewicz AG, Strejilevich SA. The effect of premorbid intelligence on neurocognitive and psychosocial functioning in bipolar disorder. J Affect Disord. 2017 Mar;1(210):226–9.
65. Nadri C, Bersudsky Y, Belmaker RH, Agam G. Elevated urinary ADAM12 protein levels in lithium-treated bipolar patients. J Neural Transm. 2007 Apr;114(4):473–7.
66. Bernstein HG, Keilhoff G, Dobrowolny H, Lendeckel U, Steiner J. From putative brain tumor marker to high cognitive abilities: emerging roles of a disintegrin and metalloprotease (ADAM) 12 in the brain. J Chem Neuroanat (Elsevier BV). 2020;109:101846.
67. Shang MY, Wu Y, Zhang CY, Qi HX, Zhang Q, Huo JH, et al. Bidirectional genetic overlap between bipolar disorder and intelligence. BMC Med. 2022;20(1):464.
68. Cotrena C, Branco LD, Ponsoni A, Shansis FM, Fonseca RP. Cognitive reserve may outperform age, mood and psychiatric comorbidities as a predictor of executive functioning in bipolar disorder and healthy adults. J Clin Exp Neuropsychol. 2021 Jul 3;43(6):611–22.

Chapter 15
Childhood Trauma and Latent Bipolar Disorder

Joana Bücker, Dayane Santos Martins, and Mathias Hasse-Sousa

15.1 Introduction

Childhood trauma is a prevalent phenomenon that affects numerous children worldwide. It encompasses physical and sexual abuse, as well as psychological (or emotional or mental) abuse, neglect, or dysfunction within the home environment of individuals under 18 years of age. Adversity in childhood has emerged as a key transdiagnostic risk factor for mental disorders, particularly bipolar disorder (BD) [1, 2]. It is widely acknowledged that BD exhibits a higher frequency of childhood trauma compared to both community samples and other psychiatric disorders. Prevalence rates stand at 30% for emotional abuse, 18% for physical abuse, 22% for sexual abuse, 31% for emotional neglect, and 30% for physical neglect [3, 4].

Moreover, childhood maltreatment correlates with adverse outcomes such as cognitive impairment, dysfunction in psychosocial functioning, alterations in brain structure and biological markers, as well as earlier onset and increased severity of BD. There exists a recognized challenge among clinicians in accurately diagnosing BD early in its course, which heightens the risk of prescribing antidepressants without accompanying mood stabilizers and misdiagnosing patients with unipolar depression rather than latent BD [5]. Identifying potential risk factors, including a

J. Bücker (✉)
Programa de Pós-Graduação em Ciências Médicas, Universidade do Vale do Taquari (UNIVATES), Lajeado, RS, Brazil

D. S. Martins
Programa de Pós Graduação em Psiquiatria e Ciências do Comportamento, Universidade Federal do Rio Grande do Sul, Porto Alegre, Brazil

M. Hasse-Sousa
Programa de Pós-Graduação em Psicologia, Departamento de Psicologia do Desenvolvimento e da Personalidade, Instituto de Psicologia, Universidade Federal do Rio Grande do Sul, Porto Alegre, Brazil

T. de Azevedo Cardoso et al. (eds.), *Latent Bipolar Disorder*,
https://doi.org/10.1007/978-3-032-01297-5_15

history of adverse childhood experiences, among individuals who later develop BD, may aid clinicians in identifying those most susceptible to the disorder.

On the other hand, the mechanism leading to the development of BD is still not entirely clear, and there is a need for greater understanding of the role of childhood trauma as a risk factor. Therefore, it is crucial to elucidate the impact of childhood trauma on neurobiological development, as it is hypothesized that early adverse experiences, in interaction with a vulnerable genetic background, may precipitate the first mood episode, potentially resulting in an earlier onset of the disorder (Fig. 15.1).

Furthermore, resilience might serve as a protective factor for individuals who have experienced traumatic events during childhood. Therefore, recognizing childhood trauma as a significant neurodevelopmental marker associated with adverse outcomes in adulthood may aid in identifying latent BD, particularly in young individuals. In this chapter, we examine the role of childhood trauma as a potential marker of latent BD and discuss its impact on the course of BD and its associated poorer outcomes. Additionally, we underscore the importance of resilience as a protective factor in BD and advocate for the inclusion of intervention strategies aimed at enhancing psychological resilience within medical contexts.

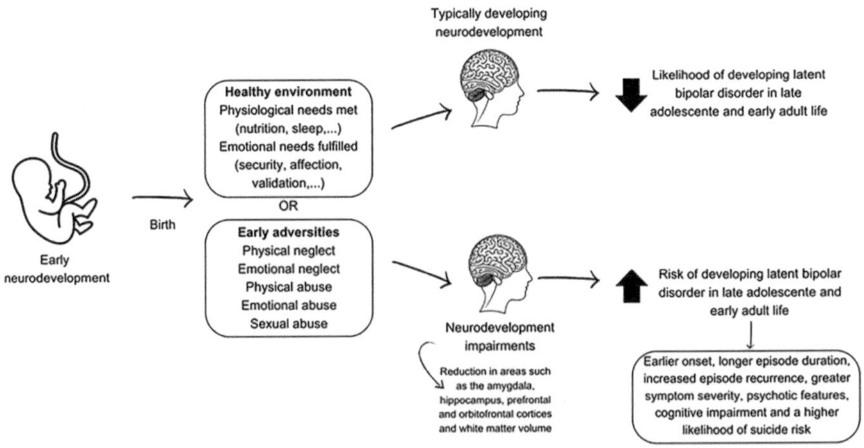

Fig. 15.1 Illustrates the impact of different types of experiences and environments on neurodevelopment. Individuals who have experienced traumatic events are more vulnerable to the development of latent BD

15.2 Theories from a Developmental and Vulnerability Perspective

Multiple theories about the developmental and vulnerability perspective have been studied over time to explain how early adversities impact individuals throughout life. The diathesis-stress model is broadly used to explain how the combination of genetic factors (diathesis) and early life adversities (stress) can contribute to the development of mental disorders. According to this model, the interaction between genetic vulnerability and any type of childhood trauma makes individuals more susceptible. In summary, individuals with genetic risk are more likely to develop BD following exposure to childhood trauma compared to those without such an experience. Another model of susceptibility focuses attention on the idea of differential susceptibility. That means that individuals who are more susceptible will respond directly according to their environment: in more stressful and/or resource-limited environments, they will have greater difficulty in developing coping mechanisms for adversities; conversely, in safe and encouraging environments, they will thrive and develop more compared to less susceptible individuals [6, 7].

From the moment they are born, individuals have a series of evolutionary tasks that follow a normal course as they develop. For example, babies learn to support their heads, then to sit, chew food, stand, and so on. Furthermore, developmental theories understand that we have basic needs, such as hunger and security, which also emerge from birth. Physiological needs are essential for the physical survival of individuals, encompassing hunger, regulation of the sleep-wake cycle, breathing, and waste elimination. Basic psychological needs are crucial for emotional survival and consist of the need for a secure attachment, a sense of autonomy and competence, leisure, realistic boundaries, and freedom of expression [8]. Individuals whose basic needs are minimally met tend to develop stronger internal resources that foster resilience. Conversely, when basic needs are not met or when individuals experience persistent frustration or exposure to adverse and stressful situations, it can lead to heightened vulnerability and the development of psychopathological traits. Those who face adversity in childhood often receive inadequate support to meet their essential needs [9].

Childhood trauma can be characterized by five types:

- Physical neglect: Lack of adequate care for the health, safety, and physical well-being of a person (e.g., absence of provision of food, water, clean clothes, shelter, and medical care).
- Physical abuse: Intentional use of physical force that can cause harm to the physical integrity of the individual (e.g., kicking, punching, and slapping).
- Emotional neglect: Absence of support to meet basic emotional needs (e.g., lack of affection, attention, and emotional validation).
- Emotional abuse: Use of behaviors or words that can cause emotional harm (e.g., humiliation, manipulation, intimidation, and/or disrespecting a person).
- Sexual abuse: Any type of non-consensual, forced, or coercive sexual activity.

The five most commonly studied subtypes of childhood trauma indicate that, when at least one of them occurs, some basic need will not be met—whether it is physical or emotional. Consequently, individuals who have experienced any type of childhood trauma may have physical and emotional scars that can last a lifetime. The hypothesis of stress sensitization suggests that the interplay between genetic risk and a stressful environment could result in abnormal brain development [7]. For example, severe exposure to stress during this period can lead to brain alterations in different structures and impair neuroplasticity [10, 11]. A systematic review of different studies aimed to identify potential biomarkers associated with childhood trauma and psychiatric disorders showed that the interaction between brain-derived neurotrophic factor (BDNF), which is a neurotrophin involved in brain plasticity, and environmental factors could be a predictor of mood disorders [10]. In the same line, other studies found a similar association between childhood trauma and BDNF [12–14] and pointed out that it could influence the emotional regulation ability [13, 14]. Considering the response model of prolonged stress, the hyperarousal state continues even when the stressor has dissipated and affect three circuits: the hypothalamic–pituitary–adrenal (HPA) axis, the limbic system, and the prefrontal cortex [15, 16]. Childhood trauma can dysregulate the HPA axis, leading to abnormal and persistent stress responses that can negatively impact development [7, 16]. Studies show that individuals with BD who were exposed to trauma during childhood have neurostructural changes, such as a reduction in areas such as the hippocampus and amygdala, and increase the level of cortisol [16–18].

15.3 Prevalence

Considering the categories of childhood trauma, large population studies have revealed that the prevalence of having experienced at least one adverse event in childhood can reach up to around 60% of adult individuals and 20–30% three or more traumatic experiences [19, 20]. When analyzing studies involving clinical samples (including individuals with mental health conditions), the numbers are very similar [21, 22].

As previously observed, childhood trauma exposure is associated with the development of BD in adulthood. BD is a serious mental health condition that could significantly impact the functioning and quality of life of individuals with this disorder. The course of the disorder and the recurrence of mood episodes cause damage to individuals' brains, and it is estimated that 1.5–2% of the world's population has the disorder [23, 24]. The first episode commonly occurs at the beginning of adulthood, and studies show that earlier onset is associated with more serious manifestations of the disease [23]. Furthermore, it is estimated that it may take up to 10 years for an individual to receive the correct diagnosis [24]. Among individuals with BD, there is a prevalence of 30% for emotional abuse and physical neglect, 18% for physical abuse, 22% for sexual abuse, and 31% for emotional neglect [3].

15.4 Earlier Onset and Greater Severity

Various biological pathways affected by trauma during development—such as the HPA axis, neuroplasticity, and circadian rhythm—are associated with an early onset of symptoms and an increased risk of suicide [25]. A recent magnetic resonance imaging (MRI) study comparing individuals with BD with and without cognitive impairment, individuals with depression and cognitive impairment, and healthy controls revealed a relationship between lower cerebral white matter (WM) volume and higher severity of childhood trauma in BD individuals [26]. These findings, combined with the literature on brain abnormalities and childhood trauma in BD, underscore the impact of trauma on neurodevelopment and its role in exacerbating the disorder's severity. Considering that childhood trauma alters developmental trajectories in these brain regions, the occurrence of traumatic events in childhood is a significant risk factor for BD in adulthood [17, 25, 27].

Individuals with BD with a history of childhood trauma tend to exhibit an earlier onset age of the disorder, longer episode duration, increased episode recurrence, greater symptom severity, heightened risk of developing psychotic features, cognitive decline, and a higher likelihood of suicide risk when compared to those without a history of childhood trauma [25, 28–32]. Thus, childhood trauma not only impacts the course of the illness, making it more severe, but also serves as a marker for identifying latent BD.

15.5 Risk Factors for the Development of BD

As seen thus far, the risk factors for developing BD encompass biological, environmental, and psychological spheres. These factors cannot be understood separately, as the etiology of the disorder is multifactorial [24, 33]. Higher heritability interacts with environmental factors (such as pre- and perinatal factors, immigration, early life stress) and contributes to making individuals more vulnerable to developing the disorder in early adulthood [7, 23, 24, 33–35]. More specifically, an environmental factor strongly related to the development of BD is childhood trauma. The association between childhood trauma and BD is observed in various cultures and ethnicities, as demonstrated by population studies from China [32], Colombia [36], Brazil [28, 37], Iceland [38], and France [39].

The events occurring during the neurodevelopmental period, specifically in childhood and adolescence, merit substantial attention for a comprehensive understanding of the early manifestations of BD. For instance, a comprehensive twin study seeking to ascertain the etiology of hypomanic symptoms demonstrated that environmental factors, notably childhood trauma, exerted a significant influence on the variance of hypomanic symptoms [34]. The occurrence of subsyndromal hypomanic symptoms alongside depressive symptoms has also emerged as a risk factor for the development of BD in a systematic review of cohort studies involving high-risk youth [40]. These findings underscore the importance of early identification and intervention for these symptoms, aiming to reduce the impairments caused by BD.

15.6 Cognition

Cognition is commonly impaired in BD [41], even in youth [42] and older age [43]. The domains more frequently impaired are memory, executive functioning, and processing speed [42–44]. Psychotic symptoms are particularly associated with higher cognitive impairments [45, 46]. There are proposals of cognitive neuroprogression, positing further impairments along the lifespan. While there is evidence in favor of cognitive neuroprogression in BD [47], studies have also found either no evidence [48–50], selective impairments [51], or even improvements at follow-up [52].

Early exposure to traumatic experiences commonly leads to neurodevelopmental insults, as well as impaired cognition [53, 54]. Indeed, exposure to childhood trauma has been suggested as a moderator of cognitive impairment in both individuals with psychotic disorders and healthy controls alike [55]. Possible reasons for this involve dysfunctions of the HPA axis as a response to trauma, particularly repeated exposures [56, 57]. One of the primary functions of the HPA axis is the production of cortisol, which is posited to contribute to several negative health outcomes when dysregulated, particularly immune and inflammation ones [58]. Thus, trauma-induced prolonged hyperactivation of the HPA axis, when interacting with genetic vulnerabilities, may contribute to an increased risk for the development of both psychiatric disorders and cognitive impairment [7, 59].

In BD, trauma exposure in childhood is associated with impairments in cognition. This is evidenced by two systematic reviews that found general cognitive ability as the domain most associated with an increased history of childhood trauma [55, 60]. Regarding intelligence, physical abuse was negatively associated with IQ in one study [61]. Another study found a weak correlation between childhood trauma and IQ ($r = -0.19$), although childhood trauma was no longer associated with IQ when included in a model with brain volume, age, gender, and diagnosis as determinants [62]. In a study of schizophrenia, schizoaffective disorder, BD I with a history of psychosis, and healthy controls, a study found that increased childhood trauma was associated with worse performance in a working memory task (n-back) among all groups, with no behavioral differences between them [63]. Finally, one study of BD and schizophrenia found that physical abuse in childhood was associated with worse verbal ability (similarities and vocabulary tasks), working memory, executive functioning (verbal fluency and letter fluency tasks), and visuospatial ability, but not memory in BD [64]. In the same study, sexual abuse was associated with worse verbal ability, executive functioning, and visuospatial abilities in BD, while physical neglect was associated with verbal abilities, working memory, executive functioning, and visuospatial abilities across all groups [64].

Nevertheless, there is also evidence of cognitive heterogeneity in BD. Several studies have found three clusters of cognitive performance: a globally impaired group, a group with selective impairments, and a globally preserved one [65–67]. In another study, individuals with BD with a higher history of traumatic experiences were more likely to appear among the globally impaired group, in which processing speed and attention domains were the most impaired [29]. The same study found that physical negligence was the most associated event with impaired cognition [29].

15.7 Brain Alterations

Childhood trauma may also alter brain functioning and morphology. Evidence from meta-analyses points to several neurological abnormalities in individuals with a history of trauma: in adolescents, a whole-brain voxel-based morphometry study found increased left precentral gyrus volume and reduced bilateral cerebellum, bilateral middle temporal gyrus, left rostrum of corpus callosum, and bilateral supramarginal gyrus volume [68]. Another voxel-based morphometry meta-analysis of adults exposed to childhood trauma found reduced right dorsolateral prefrontal cortex, hippocampal, and amygdala gray matter [69]. An additional meta-analysis found abnormal cortical thickness and gray matter volume in individuals exposed to childhood maltreatment, as well as regional cortical thinning in the right anterior cingulate/paracingulate gyri and left frontal gyrus and reduced gray matter in the left supplementary motor area [70]. Finally, a meta-analysis of functional MRI studies found functional alterations in the left superior frontal gyrus, left centromedial amygdala, left precuneus, and left putamen of individuals exposed to prenatal or postnatal adverse childhood experiences [71].

In individuals with BD, childhood trauma is associated with several neurological alterations. A review of neuroimaging studies in individuals with BD with a history of childhood trauma found that the most consistent result was reduced hippocampal gray matter volume [18], although one study reported larger hippocampal volumes [72]. Other gray matter findings include abnormal volumes in the thalamus [73, 74], the amygdala [72, 75], and frontal regions such as the prefrontal and orbitofrontal cortices and the middle frontal gyrus [73, 74, 76, 77]. Finally, studies investigating WM found reduced volumes and fractional anisotropy in the corpus callosum, uncinate fasciculus, and corona radiata [75, 78, 79].

15.8 Biological Markers

Traumatic experiences may also alter several biological markers, such as inflammatory, metabolic, and cardiovascular conditions [80]. Inflammation, as measured by markers such as tumor necrosis factor-α (TNF-α), interleukin-6 (IL-6), and C-reactive protein (CRP), is an indicator of a potentially compromised or overworked immune system. A meta-analysis found that adults with a history of childhood trauma presented higher levels of TNF-α, IL-6, and CRP [81]. When investigated independently, different types of trauma accounted for specific elevated biological markers: childhood sexual abuse was associated with elevated TNF-α; physical abuse with TNF-α and IL-6; and parental absence with CRP (although analyses for the other markers were not possible for this subgroup) [81]. It is worth noting, however, that an updated review found predominantly non-significant associations between childhood trauma and TNF-α, IL-6, and CRP levels, although IL-6 and CRP displayed higher variations of significance status [82].

Additionally, BDNF is one of the most studied biomarkers. BDNF is the most abundant neurotrophin in the central nervous system and is responsible for mediating cellular growth and survival, as well as synaptic plasticity. A meta-analysis of individuals with post-traumatic stress disorder (PTSD) found increased levels of BDNF among those with a PTSD diagnosis [83]. Contrastingly, another meta-analysis of individuals with early childhood trauma found no significant differences in BDNF levels compared to unexposed groups [84].

Other altered biomarkers associated with a history of trauma include shorter telomere length and DNA methylation [85–87], which are associated with accelerated aging. Telomere length is time-dependent due to repetitive cycles of DNA replication, being commonly used as a biomarker of aging. Childhood separation, particularly, was the only type of individual trauma associated with telomere erosion in a meta-analysis of childhood trauma and telomere length in adulthood [87]. DNA methylation may interfere with DNA structure and inhibit its transcription, being commonly used as a measure of aging. Most genome-wide association studies of DNA methylation report differences between individuals with and without childhood trauma [85].

Individuals with BD frequently present altered biomarkers [88–90]. Meta-analytic results show that peripheral BDNF levels, for instance, are reduced in manic and depressive stages, although not during euthymia [91]. Additionally, BDNF levels are also negatively correlated with manic and depressive symptom severity [91]. Another meta-analysis found altered biomarkers according to mood episode in BD: during euthymia, IL-6 and CRP levels were elevated; during depression, BDNF was reduced and TNF-α elevated; during mania, IL-6, BDNF, and TNF-α were elevated and BDNF was reduced [92]. Overall, pro-inflammatory cytokines are elevated and anti-inflammatory cytokines are reduced in BD, particularly during mania and depression [89].

15.8.1 Biomarkers and Childhood Trauma in BD

Reduced BDNF levels have been proposed as a potential mediator of the onset of both BD and PTSD [93]. Similarly, individuals with BD with a history of trauma presented reduced levels of BDNF compared to those without trauma history, despite no other significant clinical differences [94]. When compared to healthy controls, however, individuals with BD I with a history of psychosis did not differ significantly in TNF-α, IL-6, and CRP levels [95]. Similarly, women with BD with a history of early trauma no longer presented significant differences in CRP levels from healthy controls after controlling for body mass index [96].

Such results suggest that the role of childhood trauma and biomarkers is far from established in BD. This unclear position reflects the current status of biomarkers in psychiatry, which are not yet sufficiently established for precise identification of a specific disorder or for clinical utility [97]. Nevertheless, biomarker abnormalities may warrant careful clinical investigation in order to identify individuals at risk of latent BD, particularly among those who have a history of early adversities and trauma. As both biomarkers and traumatic experiences may be risk factors for BD, their roles may interact and converge into clinical profiles such as latent BD.

15.9 Resilience and Treatment

The primary focus of research studies on psychiatric disorders is often directed toward identifying risk factors associated with their development or gathering clinical information regarding the progression of the illnesses. However, less attention has been given to protective factors against adverse consequences, such as resilience. Psychological resilience is defined as the ability to successfully adapt to adversity, trauma, tragedy, or significant threats, and individual responses to stressful situations may vary depending on their level of resilience [98]. It is widely recognized that resilience has a positive impact on an individual's mental health and is a crucial component for psychosocial adaptation, facilitating positive outcomes and adjustment when confronted with adverse circumstances. Thus, resilience extends beyond merely resisting the development of illness to encompass the ways in which individuals respond after illness has manifested.

On the other hand, current literature suggests that patients with BD who have a history of severe childhood trauma demonstrate lower levels of psychological resilience compared to healthy controls [99], particularly among those who experienced emotional abuse and neglect [100]. These patients also exhibit a low tolerance for stress and adversity in life, and higher levels of impulsivity and increased depressive symptoms [101]. Therefore, studying resilience in the context of latent BD is of paramount importance for enhancing understanding of the protective factors involved in the development and clinical improvement of the illness. It might also provide valuable insight into the heterogeneous outcomes associated with these disorders (Fig. 15.2).

Resilience may serve to modify and diminish the impact of early adversities on various aspects in patients with BD, including depressive symptoms, impulsivity, aggression, psychotic symptoms, rumination, and suicide attempts. It can also act as a mediator, explaining improvements in personal recovery from BD, better quality of life, and positive attitudes toward pharmacologic treatment [4, 102]. A recent meta-analysis has also demonstrated that psychological resilience acts as a

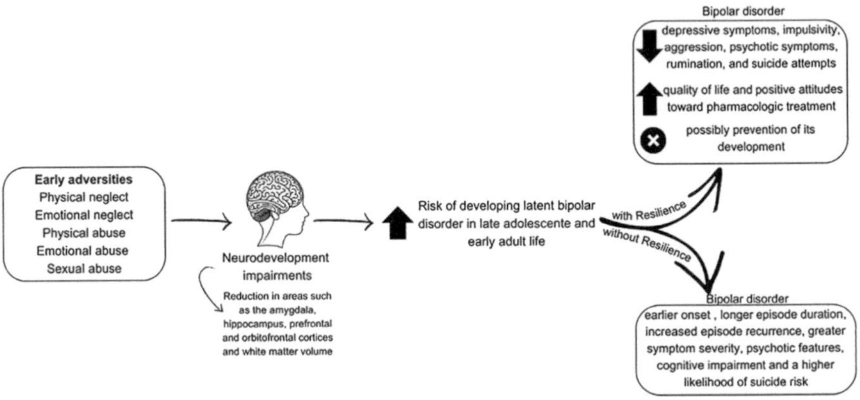

Fig. 15.2 Illustrates the role of resilience as a protective factor for individuals at risk of developing BD in adulthood. Resilience not only improves the prognosis for those already diagnosed but may also prevent the onset of the disorder. Conversely, individuals who lack resilience are at increased risk for a poorer prognosis

protective factor against the development of mood disorders, and psychotherapy interventions, particularly cognitive behavioral therapy, may play a pivotal role in enhancing resilience [99]. These interventions can assist patients in better managing stressful situations throughout the course of their illness and promote more adaptive and positive coping strategies during their recovery process. It is also important to emphasize the necessity of developing and monitoring the effectiveness of systematic resilience-enhancing programs tailored to prevent the recurrence of depressive episodes in patients with BD. Therefore, by elucidating the factors contributing to resilience and potentially developing interventions to enhance it, one could facilitate recovery and psychological well-being in patients with BD.

15.10 Clinical Considerations

- Childhood trauma is associated with adverse outcomes in patients with BD, including cognitive impairment, alterations in brain structure and function, dysfunction in psychosocial functioning, earlier onset, and greater severity of the illness.
- Childhood trauma might be recognized as a transdiagnostic risk factor for BD.
- Patients with BD exhibit higher rates of childhood trauma and lower levels of psychological resilience compared to healthy controls.
- The interaction between the genetic risk and the occurrence of childhood trauma may be a potential marker for latent BD.
- Psychological resilience serves as a protective factor against the development of mood disorders and may represent a crucial treatment target among individuals with BD.

- Childhood trauma may be considered a potential marker of latent BD.
- Childhood trauma significantly contributes to the neurobiological changes commonly observed in BD.

15.11 Future Perspectives

In summary, childhood trauma plays a significant role and could be considered a risk factor for the development of BD. This underscores the importance for clinicians to gather comprehensive trauma histories and to consider these risks in managing the disorder. Therefore, the evaluation of childhood maltreatment in individuals with BD should be systematically integrated into routine care.

The interaction between genetic background and early maltreatment might trigger the first episode, resulting in an early onset of the illness and poorer outcomes. Identifying and addressing childhood trauma early in life could potentially prevent the future development of BD and might be beneficial in identifying a subgroup of individuals who may continue to exhibit subthreshold symptoms even after receiving standard treatment.

Additionally, future research should assess programs aimed at stress management (e.g., trauma-focused therapies) with the objective of modifying the course of the illness and enhancing the quality of life for individuals with BD. Moreover, early interventions targeting the reduction of childhood trauma in vulnerable families at high risk of mood disorders could be fundamental in preventing adverse outcomes in future generations. Utilizing childhood trauma as a predictive factor for BD may lead to more precise treatment approaches for young adults experiencing their first episode of depression.

On the other hand, the protective factors associated with latent BD, such as psychological resilience, warrant further exploration. Future studies could focus on psychosocial interventions aimed at promoting these protective factors in mental health and underscore the importance of resilience-based interventions. For instance, psychotherapy interventions targeting high-risk individuals with a history of childhood maltreatment may help prevent adverse outcomes in the future. Furthermore, additional research is needed to investigate the impact of resilience on the clinical trajectory and treatment outcomes of patients with BD.

References

1. Hogg B, Gardoki-Souto I, Valiente-Gómez A, Rosa AR, Fortea L, Radua J, et al. Psychological trauma as a transdiagnostic risk factor for mental disorder: an umbrella meta-analysis. Eur Arch Psychiatry Clin Neurosci. 2023;273(2):397–410.
2. hello@interactivethings.com IT. Violence Info—Child maltreatment [Internet]. [citado 6 de mayo de 2024]. Disponible en: http://apps.who.int/violence-info/child-maltreatment

3. Zhang S, Lin X, Yang T, Zhang S, Pan Y, Lu J, et al. Prevalence of childhood trauma among adults with affective disorder using the Childhood Trauma Questionnaire: a meta-analysis. J Affect Disord. 2020;276:546–54.
4. Vieira IS, Pedrotti Moreira F, Mondin TC, de Azevedo Cardoso T, Branco JC, Kapczinski F, et al. Resilience as a mediator factor in the relationship between childhood trauma and mood disorder: a community sample of young adults. J Affect Disord. 2020;274:48–53.
5. Gitlin MJ. Diagnosing latent bipolar disorder: a clinical dilemma. Bipolar Disord. 2018;20(4):300–2.
6. Belsky J, Pluess M. Beyond diathesis stress: differential susceptibility to environmental influences. Psychol Bull. 2009;135(6):885–908.
7. Quidé Y, Tozzi L, Corcoran M, Cannon DM, Dauvermann MR. The impact of childhood trauma on developing bipolar disorder: current understanding and ensuring continued progress. Neuropsychiatr Dis Treat. 2020;16:3095–115.
8. Young JE, Klosko JS, Weishaar ME. Schema therapy: a practitioner's guide. New York: Guilford Press; 2003. xii, 436 p. (Schema therapy: A practitioner's guide).
9. Vansteenkiste M, Ryan RM. On psychological growth and vulnerability: basic psychological need satisfaction and need frustration as a unifying principle. J Psychother Integr. 2013;23(3):263–80.
10. Di Benedetto MG, Scassellati C, Cattane N, Riva MA, Cattaneo A. Neurotrophic factors, childhood trauma and psychiatric disorders: a systematic review of genetic, biochemical, cognitive and imaging studies to identify potential biomarkers. J Affect Disord. 2022;308:76–88.
11. McKay MT, Cannon M, Chambers D, Conroy RM, Coughlan H, Dodd P, et al. Childhood trauma and adult mental disorder: a systematic review and meta-analysis of longitudinal cohort studies. Acta Psychiatr Scand. 2021;143(3):189–205.
12. Bücker J, Fries GR, Kapczinski F, Post RM, Yatham LN, Vianna P, et al. Brain-derived neurotrophic factor and inflammatory markers in school-aged children with early trauma. Acta Psychiatr Scand. 2015;131(5):360–8.
13. Chauhan VS, Sharma M, Chatterjee K, Prakash J, Srivastava K, Chaudhury S. Childhood trauma and bipolar affective disorder: is there a linkage? Ind Psychiatry J. 2023;32(Suppl 1):S9–14.
14. Tian T, Li J, Zhang G, Wang J, Liu D, Wan C, et al. Effects of childhood trauma experience and BDNF Val66Met polymorphism on brain plasticity relate to emotion regulation. Behav Brain Res. 2021;398:112949.
15. Agorastos A, Pervanidou P, Chrousos GP, Baker DG. Developmental trajectories of early life stress and trauma: a narrative review on neurobiological aspects beyond stress system dysregulation. Front Psych. 2019;10:118.
16. Murphy F, Nasa A, Cullinane D, Raajakesary K, Gazzaz A, Sooknarine V, et al. Childhood trauma, the HPA Axis and psychiatric illnesses: a targeted literature synthesis. Front Psych. 2022;13:748372.
17. Brietzke E, Kauer Sant'anna M, Jackowski A, Grassi-Oliveira R, Bucker J, Zugman A, et al. Impact of childhood stress on psychopathology. Rev Bras Psiquiatr Sao Paulo Braz 1999. 2012;34(4):480–8.
18. Zovetti N, Perlini C, Brambilla P, Bellani M. Childhood adversities and bipolar disorder: a neuroimaging focus. Epidemiol Psychiatr Sci. 2022;31:e12.
19. Broekhof R, Nordahl HM, Bjørnelv S, Selvik SG. Prevalence of adverse childhood experiences and their co-occurrence in a large population of adolescents: a Young HUNT 3 study. Soc Psychiatry Psychiatr Epidemiol. 2022;57(12):2359–66.
20. Merrick MT, Ford DC, Ports KA, Guinn AS. Prevalence of adverse childhood experiences from the 2011–2014 behavioral risk factor surveillance system in 23 States. JAMA Pediatr. 2018;172(11):1038–44.
21. Knipschild R, Hein I, Pieters S, Lindauer R, Bicanic IAE, Staal W, et al. Childhood adversity in a youth psychiatric population: prevalence and associated mental health problems. Eur J Psychotraumatol. 2024;15(1):2330880.

22. Sucich J, Breitbart V, Williams S, Sanichar N, Candelaria-Arce E, Frankle WG, et al. Prevalence of childhood trauma in a community-based mental health clinic. Community Ment Health J. 2023;59(6):1136–49.
23. Carvalho AF, Firth J, Vieta E. Bipolar disorder. N Engl J Med. 2020;383(1):58–66.
24. Grande I, Berk M, Birmaher B, Vieta E. Bipolar disorder. Lancet Lond Engl. 2016;387(10027):1561–72.
25. Aas M, Henry C, Andreassen OA, Bellivier F, Melle I, Etain B. The role of childhood trauma in bipolar disorders. Int J Bipolar Disord. 2016;4(1):2.
26. Jørgensen JL, Macoveanu J, Petersen JZ, Knudsen GM, Kessing LV, Jørgensen MB, et al. Association of childhood trauma with cognitive impairment and structural brain alterations in remitted patients with bipolar disorder. J Affect Disord. 2023;337:75–85.
27. Bortolato B, Köhler CA, Evangelou E, León-Caballero J, Solmi M, Stubbs B, et al. Systematic assessment of environmental risk factors for bipolar disorder: an umbrella review of systematic reviews and meta-analyses. Bipolar Disord. 2017;19(2):84–96.
28. Farias C de A, Cardoso T de A, Mondin TC, Souza LD de M, da Silva RA, Kapczinski F, et al. Clinical outcomes and childhood trauma in bipolar disorder: a community sample of young adults. Psychiatry Res. 2019;275:228–32.
29. Jiménez E, Solé B, Arias B, Mitjans M, Varo C, Reinares M, et al. Impact of childhood trauma on cognitive profile in bipolar disorder. Bipolar Disord. 2017;19(5):363–74.
30. Marwaha S, Briley PM, Perry A, Rankin P, DiFlorio A, Craddock N, et al. Explaining why childhood abuse is a risk factor for poorer clinical course in bipolar disorder: a path analysis of 923 people with bipolar I disorder. Psychol Med. 2020;50(14):2346–54.
31. Rowe AL, Perich T, Meade T. Bipolar disorder and cumulative trauma: a systematic review of prevalence and illness outcomes. J Clin Psychol. 2024;80(3):692–713.
32. Xie P, Wu K, Zheng Y, Guo Y, Yang Y, He J, et al. Prevalence of childhood trauma and correlations between childhood trauma, suicidal ideation, and social support in patients with depression, bipolar disorder, and schizophrenia in southern China. J Affect Disord. 2018;228:41–8.
33. Shintani AO, Rabelo-da-Ponte FD, Marchionatti LE, Watts D, Ferreira de Souza F, Machado CDS, et al. Prenatal and perinatal risk factors for bipolar disorder: a systematic review and meta-analysis. Neurosci Biobehav Rev. 2023;144:104960.
34. Hosang GM, Martin J, Karlsson R, Lundström S, Larsson H, Ronald A, et al. Association of etiological factors for hypomanic symptoms, bipolar disorder, and other severe mental illnesses. JAMA Psychiatry. 2022;79(2):143–50.
35. Rabelo-da-Ponte FD, Feiten JG, Mwangi B, Barros FC, Wehrmeister FC, Menezes AM, et al. Early identification of bipolar disorder among young adults – a 22-year community birth cohort. Acta Psychiatr Scand. 2020;142(6):476–85.
36. Guillen-Burgos H, Moreno-Lopez S, Acevedo-Vergara K, Pérez-Florez M, Pachón-Garcia C, Gálvez-Flórez JF. Risk of childhood trauma exposure and severity of bipolar disorder in Colombia. Int J Bipolar Disord. 2023;11(1):7.
37. Bauer A, Fairchild G, Hammerton G, Murray J, Santos IS, Tovo Rodrigues L, et al. Associations between childhood trauma and childhood psychiatric disorders in Brazil: a population-based, prospective birth cohort study. Lancet Psychiatry. 2022;9(12):969–77.
38. Köhler-Forsberg O, Ge F, Hauksdóttir A, Thordardottir EB, Ásbjörnsdóttir K, Rúnarsdóttir H, et al. Adverse childhood experiences and psychological functioning among women with schizophrenia or bipolar disorder: population-based study. Br J Psychiatry J Ment Sci. 2024;224(1):6–12.
39. Etain B, Lajnef M, Henry C, Aubin V, Azorin JM, Bellivier F, et al. Childhood trauma, dimensions of psychopathology and the clinical expression of bipolar disorders: a pathway analysis. J Psychiatr Res. 2017;95:37–45.
40. Keramatian K, Chakrabarty T, Saraf G, Yatham LN. Transitioning to bipolar disorder: a systematic review of prospective high-risk studies. Curr Opin Psychiatry. 2022;35(1):10–21.

41. Bo Q, Mao Z, Li X, Wang Z, Wang C, Ma X. Use of the MATRICS consensus cognitive battery (MCCB) to evaluate cognitive deficits in bipolar disorder: a systematic review and meta-analysis. PLoS One. 2017;12(4):e0176212.
42. Elias LR, Miskowiak KW, Vale AMO, Köhler CA, Kjærstad HL, Stubbs B, et al. Cognitive impairment in euthymic pediatric bipolar disorder: a systematic review and meta-analysis. J Am Acad Child Adolesc Psychiatry. 2017;56(4):286–96.
43. Montejo L, Torrent C, Jiménez E, Martínez-Arán A, Blumberg HP, Burdick KE, et al. Cognition in older adults with bipolar disorder: an ISBD task force systematic review and meta-analysis based on a comprehensive neuropsychological assessment. Bipolar Disord. 2022;24(2):115–36.
44. Cotrena C, Damiani Branco L, Ponsoni A, Samamé C, Milman Shansis F, Paz FR. Executive functions and memory in bipolar disorders I and II: new insights from meta-analytic results. Acta Psychiatr Scand. 2020;141(2):110–30.
45. Bora E. Neurocognitive features in clinical subgroups of bipolar disorder: a meta-analysis. J Affect Disord. 2018;229:125–34.
46. Lynham AJ, Hubbard L, Tansey KE, Hamshere ML, Legge SE, Owen MJ, et al. Examining cognition across the bipolar/schizophrenia diagnostic spectrum. J Psychiatry Neurosci. 2018;43(3):170076.
47. Cardoso T, Bauer IE, Meyer TD, Kapczinski F, Soares JC. Neuroprogression and cognitive functioning in bipolar disorder: a systematic review. Curr Psychiatry Rep. 2015;17(9):75.
48. Bora E, Özerdem A. Meta-analysis of longitudinal studies of cognition in bipolar disorder: comparison with healthy controls and schizophrenia. Psychol Med. 2017;47(16):2753–66.
49. Martins DS, Hasse-Sousa M, de FX RR, de O LC, Petry-Perin C, Britto MJ, et al. A five-year follow-up of the verbal memory performance of individuals with bipolar disorder and schizophrenia: evidence of unchanging deficits under treatment. Cognit Neuropsychiatry. 2023;28(1):19–35.
50. Samamé C, Cattaneo BL, Richaud MC, Strejilevich S, Aprahamian I. The long-term course of cognition in bipolar disorder: a systematic review and meta-analysis of patient-control differences in test-score changes. Psychol Med. 2022;52(2):217–28.
51. Santos JL, Aparicio A, Bagney A, Sánchez-Morla EM, Rodríguez-Jiménez R, Mateo J, et al. A five-year follow-up study of neurocognitive functioning in bipolar disorder. Bipolar Disord. 2014;16(7):722–31.
52. Flaaten CB, Melle I, Bjella T, Engen MJ, Åsbø G, Wold KF, et al. Long-term course of cognitive functioning in bipolar disorder: a ten-year follow-up study. Bipolar Disord. 2024;26(2):136–47.
53. Rosa M, Scassellati C, Cattaneo A. Association of childhood trauma with cognitive domains in adult patients with mental disorders and in non-clinical populations: a systematic review. Front Psychol. 2023;14:1156415.
54. Vargas T, Lam PH, Azis M, Osborne KJ, Lieberman A, Mittal VA. Childhood trauma and neurocognition in adults with psychotic disorders: a systematic review and meta-analysis. Schizophr Bull. 2019;45(6):1195–208.
55. Dauvermann MR, Donohoe G. The role of childhood trauma in cognitive performance in schizophrenia and bipolar disorder – a systematic review. Schizophr Res Cogn. 2019;16:1–11.
56. Matte-Landry A, Grisé Bolduc MÈ, Tanguay-Garneau L, Collin-Vézina D, Ouellet-Morin I. Cognitive outcomes of children with complex trauma: a systematic review and meta-analyses of longitudinal studies. Trauma Violence Abuse. 2023;24(4):2743–57.
57. Raymond C, Marin MF, Majeur D, Lupien S. Early child adversity and psychopathology in adulthood: HPA axis and cognitive dysregulations as potential mechanisms. Prog Neuro-Psychopharmacol Biol Psychiatry. 2018;85:152–60.
58. Adam EK, Quinn ME, Tavernier R, McQuillan MT, Dahlke KA, Gilbert KE. Diurnal cortisol slopes and mental and physical health outcomes: a systematic review and meta-analysis. Psychoneuroendocrinology. 2017;83:25–41.

59. Holtzman CW, Trotman HD, Goulding SM, Ryan AT, Macdonald AN, Shapiro DI, et al. Stress and neurodevelopmental processes in the emergence of psychosis. Neuroscience. 2013;249:172–91.
60. Barczyk ZA, Foulds JA, Porter RJ, Douglas KM. Childhood trauma and cognitive functioning in mood disorders: a systematic review. Bipolar Disord. 2023;25(4):263–77.
61. Martins DS, Hasse-Sousa M, Petry-Perin C, Arrial-Cordeiro RT, Rabelo-da-Ponte FD, Lima FM, et al. Perceived childhood adversities: impact of childhood trauma to estimated intellectual functioning of individuals with bipolar disorder. Psychiatry Res. 2019;274:345–51.
62. Vreeker A, Abramovic L, Boks MPM, Verkooijen S, van Bergen AH, Ophoff RA, et al. The relationship between brain volumes and intelligence in bipolar disorder. J Affect Disord. 2017;223:59–64.
63. Quidé Y, O'Reilly N, Rowland JE, Carr VJ, Elzinga BM, Green MJ. Effects of childhood trauma on working memory in affective and non-affective psychotic disorders. Brain Imaging Behav. 2017;11(3):722–35.
64. Aas M, Steen NE, Agartz I, Aminoff SR, Lorentzen S, Sundet K, et al. Is cognitive impairment following early life stress in severe mental disorders based on specific or general cognitive functioning? Psychiatry Res. 2012;198(3):495–500.
65. Jensen JH, Knorr U, Vinberg M, Kessing LV, Miskowiak KW. Discrete neurocognitive subgroups in fully or partially remitted bipolar disorder: associations with functional abilities. J Affect Disord. 2016;205:378–86.
66. Lima F, Rabelo-da-Ponte FD, Bücker J, Czepielewski L, Hasse-Sousa M, Telesca R, et al. Identifying cognitive subgroups in bipolar disorder: A cluster analysis. J Affect Disord. 2019;246:252–61.
67. Miskowiak KW, Kjærstad HL, Lemvigh CK, Ambrosen KS, Thorvald MS, Kessing LV, et al. Neurocognitive subgroups among newly diagnosed patients with schizophrenia spectrum or bipolar disorders: a hierarchical cluster analysis. J Psychiatr Res. 2023;163:278–87.
68. Tymofiyeva O, Hu R, Kidambi R, Nguyen C, Max JE, Yang TT. A meta-analysis of brain morphometric aberrations in adolescents who experienced childhood trauma. Front Hum Neurosci. 2022;16:1022791.
69. Paquola C, Bennett MR, Lagopoulos J. Understanding heterogeneity in grey matter research of adults with childhood maltreatment-A meta-analysis and review. Neurosci Biobehav Rev. 2016;69:299–312.
70. Yang W, Jin S, Duan W, Yu H, Ping L, Shen Z, et al. The effects of childhood maltreatment on cortical thickness and gray matter volume: a coordinate-based meta-analysis. Psychol Med. 2023;53(5):1681–99.
71. Kraaijenvanger EJ, Pollok TM, Monninger M, Kaiser A, Brandeis D, Banaschewski T, et al. Impact of early life adversities on human brain functioning: a coordinate-based meta-analysis. Neurosci Biobehav Rev. 2020;113:62–76.
72. Janiri D, Sani G, Rossi PD, Piras F, Iorio M, Banaj N, et al. Amygdala and hippocampus volumes are differently affected by childhood trauma in patients with bipolar disorders and healthy controls. Bipolar Disord. 2017;19(5):353–62.
73. Duarte DGG, de Castro Lourenço Neves M, Albuquerque MR, de Souza-Duran FL, Busatto G, Corrêa H. Gray matter brain volumes in childhood-maltreated patients with bipolar disorder type I: a voxel-based morphometric study. J Affect Disord. 2016;197:74–80.
74. Poletti S, Vai B, Smeraldi E, Cavallaro R, Colombo C, Benedetti F. Adverse childhood experiences influence the detrimental effect of bipolar disorder and schizophrenia on corticolimbic grey matter volumes. J Affect Disord. 2016;189:290–7.
75. Souza-Queiroz J, Boisgontier J, Etain B, Poupon C, Duclap D, d'Albis MA, et al. Childhood trauma and the limbic network: a multimodal MRI study in patients with bipolar disorder and controls. J Affect Disord. 2016;200:159–64.
76. Begemann MJH, Schutte MJL, van Dellen E, Abramovic L, Boks MP, van Haren NEM, et al. Childhood trauma is associated with reduced frontal gray matter volume: a large transdiagnostic structural MRI study. Psychol Med. 2023;53(3):741–9.

77. Song H, Chon MW, Ryu V, Yu R, Lee DK, Lee H, et al. Cortical volumetric correlates of childhood trauma, anxiety, and impulsivity in bipolar disorder. Psychiatry Investig. 2020;17(7):627–35.
78. Bücker J, Muralidharan K, Torres IJ, Su W, Kozicky J, Silveira LE, et al. Childhood maltreatment and corpus callosum volume in recently diagnosed patients with bipolar I disorder: data from the systematic treatment optimization program for early mania (STOP-EM). J Psychiatr Res. 2014;48(1):65–72.
79. Stevelink R, Abramovic L, Verkooijen S, Begemann MJH, Sommer IEC, Boks MP, et al. Childhood abuse and white matter integrity in bipolar disorder patients and healthy controls. Eur Neuropsychopharmacol J Eur Coll Neuropsychopharmacol. 2018;28(7):807–17.
80. Cooke EM, Connolly EJ, Boisvert DL, Hayes BE. A systematic review of the biological correlates and consequences of childhood maltreatment and adverse childhood experiences. Trauma Violence Abuse. 2023;24(1):156–73.
81. Baumeister D, Akhtar R, Ciufolini S, Pariante CM, Mondelli V. Childhood trauma and adulthood inflammation: a meta-analysis of peripheral C-reactive protein, interleukin-6 and tumour necrosis factor-α. Mol Psychiatry. 2016;21(5):642–9.
82. Brown M, Worrell C, Pariante CM. Inflammation and early life stress: an updated review of childhood trauma and inflammatory markers in adulthood. Pharmacol Biochem Behav. 2021;211:173291.
83. Mojtabavi H, Saghazadeh A, van den Heuvel L, Bucker J, Rezaei N. Peripheral blood levels of brain-derived neurotrophic factor in patients with post-traumatic stress disorder (PTSD): a systematic review and meta-analysis. PLoS One. 2020;15(11):e0241928.
84. Vyas N, Wimberly CE, Beaman MM, Kaplan SJ, Rasmussen LJH, Wertz J, et al. Systematic review and meta-analysis of the effect of adverse childhood experiences (ACEs) on brain-derived neurotrophic factor (BDNF) levels. Psychoneuroendocrinology. 2023;151:106071.
85. Nöthling J, Malan-Müller S, Abrahams N, Hemmings SMJ, Seedat S. Epigenetic alterations associated with childhood trauma and adult mental health outcomes: a systematic review. World J Biol Psychiatry Off J World Fed Soc Biol Psychiatry. 2020;21(7):493–512.
86. Soares S, Rocha V, Kelly-Irving M, Stringhini S, Fraga S. Adverse childhood events and health biomarkers: a systematic review. Front Public Health. 2021;9:649825.
87. Li Z, He Y, Wang D, Tang J, Chen X. Association between childhood trauma and accelerated telomere erosion in adulthood: a meta-analytic study. J Psychiatr Res. 2017;93:64–71.
88. Fries GR, Zamzow MJ, Andrews T, Pink O, Scaini G, Quevedo J. Accelerated aging in bipolar disorder: a comprehensive review of molecular findings and their clinical implications. Neurosci Biobehav Rev. 2020;112:107–16.
89. Sayana P, Colpo GD, Simões LR, Giridharan VV, Teixeira AL, Quevedo J, et al. A systematic review of evidence for the role of inflammatory biomarkers in bipolar patients. J Psychiatr Res. 2017;92:160–82.
90. Sigitova E, Fišar Z, Hroudová J, Cikánková T, Raboch J. Biological hypotheses and biomarkers of bipolar disorder. Psychiatry Clin Neurosci. 2017;71(2):77–103.
91. Fernandes BS, Molendijk ML, Köhler CA, Soares JC, Leite CMGS, Machado-Vieira R, et al. Peripheral brain-derived neurotrophic factor (BDNF) as a biomarker in bipolar disorder: a meta-analysis of 52 studies. BMC Med. 2015;13:289.
92. Rowland T, Perry BI, Upthegrove R, Barnes N, Chatterjee J, Gallacher D, et al. Neurotrophins, cytokines, oxidative stress mediators and mood state in bipolar disorder: systematic review and meta-analyses. Br J Psychiatry J Ment Sci. 2018;213(3):514–25.
93. Rakofsky JJ, Ressler KJ, Dunlop BW. BDNF function as a potential mediator of bipolar disorder and post-traumatic stress disorder comorbidity. Mol Psychiatry. 2012;17(1):22–35.
94. Kauer-Sant' Anna M, Tramontina J, Andreazza AC, Cereser K, da Costa S, Santin A, et al. Traumatic life events in bipolar disorder: impact on BDNF levels and psychopathology. Bipolar Disord. 2007;9(Suppl 1):128–35.

95. Quidé Y, Bortolasci CC, Spolding B, Kidnapillai S, Watkeys OJ, Cohen-Woods S, et al. Association between childhood trauma exposure and pro-inflammatory cytokines in schizophrenia and bipolar-I disorder. Psychol Med. 2019;49(16):2736–44.
96. Moraes JB, Maes M, Barbosa DS, Ferrari TZ, Uehara MKS, Carvalho AF, et al. Elevated C-reactive protein levels in women with bipolar disorder may be explained by a history of childhood trauma, especially sexual abuse, body mass index and age. CNS Neurol Disord Drug Targets. 2017;16(4):514–21.
97. Abi-Dargham A, Moeller SJ, Ali F, DeLorenzo C, Domschke K, Horga G, et al. Candidate biomarkers in psychiatric disorders: state of the field. World Psychiatry Off J World Psychiatr Assoc WPA. 2023;22(2):236–62.
98. Bonanno GA. Loss, trauma, and human resilience: have we underestimated the human capacity to thrive after extremely aversive events? Am Psychol. 2004;59(1):20–8.
99. Imran A, Tariq S, Kapczinski F, de Azevedo CT. Psychological resilience and mood disorders: a systematic review and meta-analysis. Trends Psychiatry Psychother. 2024;46:e20220524.
100. Park JY, Lee CW, Jang Y, Lee W, Yu H, Yoon J, et al. Relationship between childhood trauma and resilience in patients with mood disorders. J Affect Disord. 2023;323:162–70.
101. Choi JW, Cha B, Jang J, Park CS, Kim BJ, Lee CS, et al. Resilience and impulsivity in euthymic patients with bipolar disorder. J Affect Disord. 2015;170:172–7.
102. Chan MK, Chew QH, Sim K. Resilience in bipolar disorder and interrelationships with psychopathology, clinical features, psychosocial functioning, and mediational roles: a systematic review. J Clin Psychiatry. 2023;84(2):22r14431.

Chapter 16
Pharmacotherapy and Latent Bipolar Disorder

Fabiano A. Gomes

16.1 Introduction

Management of individuals at risk of developing bipolar disorder (BD) remains highly controversial despite its relevance and prevalence in clinical settings. As discussed in previous chapters, latent BD refers to diverse situations including individuals with a family history of BD presenting with various unspecific symptoms such as sleep disturbances, internalizing and/or externalizing behaviors, as well as those presenting with depressive symptoms that later evolve into full-blown BD, characterized by the occurrence of manic or hypomanic episodes [11]. This process often unfolds over several years, complicating both the diagnostic process and subsequent treatment strategies. These patients are usually diagnosed with unipolar depression and may be treated solely with antidepressants, which can exacerbate their condition by precipitating manic episodes, which may lead to a more severe and chronic illness course [12]. The management of these complex scenarios seems impossible since one cannot diagnose BD without the presence of a (hypo)manic episode, and there are no reliable clinical or biological markers to predict the diagnostic conversion.

Adding another layer of complexity, individuals with untreated or improperly treated BD frequently present with recurrent depressive and/or manic episodes and their associated psychosocial impairment and reduced quality of life. Moreover, the lack of effective intervention in the early stages is usually associated with a higher incidence of comorbid conditions such as anxiety disorders, substance use disorders, and, tragically, an increased risk of suicide [15].

F. A. Gomes (✉)
Department of Psychiatry and Behavioural Neurosciences, McMaster University, Hamilton, ON, Canada
e-mail: gomesfa@mcmaster.ca

T. de Azevedo Cardoso et al. (eds.), *Latent Bipolar Disorder*,
https://doi.org/10.1007/978-3-032-01297-5_16

This chapter will present a brief review of the scarce literature regarding the pharmacological management of latent BD. It will provide a framework to identify individuals at risk of developing BD and discuss the current pharmacological strategies employed in their treatment. An underlying assumption that should be taken into consideration is that lifestyle and psychosocial interventions should be implemented first in this group of patients, and pharmacological treatment should not be used alone [18].

16.2 Clinical Dilemmas in the Treatment of Latent BD

The treatment of patients who present with depression, anxiety, and other behavioral problems (including externalizing and attention-deficit/hyperactivity disorder (ADHD)-like symptoms) and exhibit potential predictors of latent BD presents significant clinical dilemmas. One of the most contentious issues is whether to initiate treatment with antidepressants and/or stimulants or to start with mood stabilizers or second-generation antipsychotics. While antidepressants are the standard treatment for unipolar depression and stimulants are first-line interventions for ADHD, they carry the risk of triggering (hypo)manic episodes in vulnerable individuals, who may have undiagnosed BD or will eventually develop (hypo)manic episodes but have a first presentation of depression or ADHD. This risk underscores the importance of a comprehensive assessment and monitoring during treatment [19].

The decision-making process regarding treatment initiation must include patients and their families and should consider various factors, including the presence of clinical predictors, the patient's history, and their response to previous treatments. Most clinicians usually choose to prescribe antidepressants, especially if the patient's depressive symptoms are severe or disabling. In these cases, the potential benefits of alleviating depressive symptoms may outweigh the risks, provided that close monitoring for signs of mania or hypomania is implemented. For some clinicians, the cautious approach may involve starting with mood stabilizers or antipsychotics with proven efficacy for bipolar depression, particularly in patients who demonstrate strong predictors of BD, such as a family history of (hypo)mania, early onset of depression, presence of mixed and activation symptoms, and brief recurrent depressive episodes [8].

16.3 Current Management Strategies

16.3.1 Antidepressants

If depressive symptoms are prominent and psychosocial interventions are not effective, the cautious use of antidepressants in individuals with fewer risk factors for latent BD is a common practice [16]. Although current BD guidelines do not recommend monotherapy with standard antidepressants for bipolar depression, there is no clear contra-indication regarding the use of antidepressants in individuals at risk, including those with family history of BD [14, 23]. However, due to the high risk of (hypo)manic and mixed switch, if antidepressants are started in individuals with latent BD, extensive psychoeducation for patients and families about early signs of mania and close clinical monitoring by the treatment team are imperative.

Selective serotonin reuptake inhibitor (SSRI) particularly lower doses of escitalopram and fluoxetine, are usually the preferred initial treatments due to lower rates of affective switch, since tricyclic antidepressants and serotonin-norepinephrin reuptake inhibitor (SNRI) are associated with higher risk [22]. Of note, olanzapine–fluoxetine combination is an Food and Drug Administration (FDA)-approved treatment of bipolar depression in children and adolescents but has not been tested in individuals at high risk [6].

Several studies have shown an increased risk of antidepressant-induced (hypo) mania in the offspring of BD patients treated for a major depressive episode [2, 17, 20], with a nearly 50% rate of activation after antidepressant exposure. Children and youth at higher risk may present with agitation, aggression, and impulsivity when exposed to antidepressants and should be closely monitored.

16.3.2 Mood Stabilizers

Mood stabilizers, including lithium and anticonvulsants, are considered the cornerstone of BD treatment. These medications not only stabilize mood but also have the potential to prevent recurrent depressive and (hypo)manic episodes. A few studies have investigated the use of lithium and valproate in individuals with a family history of BD presenting with behavioral and mood symptoms but no formal diagnosis of BD, with mixed results.

Notwithstanding some positive findings of lithium in reducing depressive symptoms and suicidal ideation in high-risk youth manifesting recurrent depressive episode shown in a recent review [5], a pivotal RCT showed no differences in depressive symptoms when compared to placebo [7]. In the same vein, despite positive findings in improving clinical global impression scores in one study, two other RCTs showed no benefit of valproate in depressive symptoms in youth with familial BD [3]. Despite the lack of studies investigating the effect of lamotrigine in this patient population, it may be a viable option due to its predominant effect on preventing depressive episodes and benefit in bipolar depression [9].

The effect of mood stabilizers in at-risk individuals presenting with hypomanic symptoms has not been investigated in many studies, but preliminary data suggest that they may not be as effective as antipsychotics in preventing the onset of mania [3], as well as in treating manic symptoms in youth with established BD [1]. In the face of these findings, a recommendation for the use of mood stabilizers as a general strategy for the treatment of mood symptoms (particularly depression) and prevention of mania, in at-risk children and youth, cannot be definitively made at this time.

16.3.3 *Atypical Antipsychotics*

The role of second-generation antipsychotics in the treatment of mood disorders has gained popularity in recent years. Recent guidelines have recommended the use of atypical antipsychotics as second-line treatment for major depression (quetiapine monotherapy), adjunctive treatment for treatment-resistant depression (aripiprazole, brexpiprazole, risperidone, olanzapine, quetiapine, and cariprazine) [13], and as monotherapy and/or adjunctive treatment for bipolar depression (cariprazine, lurasidone, olanzapine, and quetiapine) [23]. Second-generation antipsychotics are also first-line treatments for mania and have been recommended as second-line treatments for mixed presentations (asenapine, cariprazine, and lurasidone) [23, 24]. Due to their superior efficacy in the treatment of mania in children and adolescents, atypical antipsychotics are usually recommended as first-line therapy in this patient population and may be suitable options for the treatment of agitation, impulsivity, activation, and sub-threshold hypomanic symptoms in latent BD [1].

Based on a few studies with at-risk populations, the use of atypical antipsychotics may be warranted in individuals with multiple risk factors for latent BD presenting with depressive symptoms. Quetiapine has been the most studied medication showing improvement in both depressive and manic symptoms compared to placebo [4]. Lurasidone is FDA-approved for the treatment of bipolar depression in children and adolescents [10] and showed efficacy in the treatment of mixed unipolar depression compared to placebo [21]. Although not studied in at-risk populations, it may also be an interesting option since mixed presentations are common in this group of patients.

16.4 Conclusion

Managing latent BD requires a careful, individualized approach due to the potential risks of destabilizing and precipitating (hypo)manic episodes. While early identification of at-risk individuals is ideal, the current reliance on inconsistent clinical predictors and the lack of biological markers makes it challenging. Clinicians must remain vigilant for signs of bipolarity, especially in patients with a history of early-onset depression or a family history of BD.

Treatment strategies must balance the potential benefits and risks of antidepressants and mood stabilizers, with careful monitoring for emerging signs of mania. Given the absence of clear guidelines in this area, ongoing research and clinical trials are essential to develop evidence-based strategies for identifying and managing patients who may have latent BD.

References

1. Amerio A, Arduino G, Fesce F, Costanza A, Aguglia A, Amore M, Serafini G. Advances in the management of bipolar disorder in children and adolescents: an update on the literature. Expert Rev Neurother. 2024;24(10):1011–24. https://doi.org/10.1080/14737175.2024.2386429. Epub 2024 Aug 5
2. Bechdolf A, Nelson B, Cotton SM, Chanen A, Thompson A, Kettle J, Conus P, Amminger GP, Yung AR, Berk M, McGorry PD. A preliminary evaluation of the validity of at-risk criteria for bipolar disorders in help-seeking adolescents and young adults. J Affect Disord. 2010;127(1–3):316–20. https://doi.org/10.1016/j.jad.2010.06.016. Epub 2010 Jul 8
3. Del Favero E, Montemagni C, Bozzatello P, Brasso C, Riccardi C, Rocca P. The management of prodromal symptoms of bipolar disorder: available options and future perspectives. Medicina (Kaunas). 2021;57(6):545. https://doi.org/10.3390/medicina57060545. PMID: 34071356; PMCID: PMC8229021
4. DelBello MP, Adler CM, Whitsel RM, Stanford KE, Strakowski SM. A 12-week single-blind trial of quetiapine for the treatment of mood symptoms in adolescents at high risk for developing bipolar I disorder. J Clin Psychiatry. 2007;68(5):789–95. https://doi.org/10.4088/jcp.v68n0520.
5. Duffy A, Grof P. Lithium treatment in children and adolescents. Pharmacopsychiatry. 2018;51(5):189–93. https://doi.org/10.1055/a-0575-4179. Epub 2018 Feb 28
6. Garcia-Rodriguez L, Burton DJ, Leonards CA, Davey CG. Effectiveness of atypical antipsychotics for unipolar and bipolar depression in adolescents and young adults: a systematic review and meta-analysis. J Affect Disord. 2023;339:633–9. https://doi.org/10.1016/j.jad.2023.07.082. Epub 2023 Jul 17
7. Geller B, Cooper TB, Zimerman B, Frazier J, Williams M, Heath J, Warner K. Lithium for prepubertal depressed children with family history predictors of future bipolarity: a double-blind, placebo-controlled study. J Affect Disord. 1998;51(2):165–75. https://doi.org/10.1016/s0165-0327(98)00178-5.
8. Gitlin MJ. Diagnosing latent bipolar disorder: A clinical dilemma. Bipolar Disord. 2018;20(4):300–2. https://doi.org/10.1111/bdi.12648. Epub 2018 Apr 10
9. Haenen N, Kamperman AM, Prodan A, Nolen WA, Boks MP, Wesseloo R. The efficacy of lamotrigine in bipolar disorder: a systematic review and meta-analysis. Bipolar Disord. 2024;26(5):431–41. https://doi.org/10.1111/bdi.13452. Epub 2024 May 15
10. Hobbs E, Reed R, Lorberg B, Robb AS, Dorfman J. Psychopharmacological treatment algorithms of manic/mixed and depressed episodes in pediatric bipolar disorder. J Child Adolesc Psychopharmacol. 2022;32(10):507–21. https://doi.org/10.1089/cap.2022.0035. Epub 2022 Dec 2
11. Kapczinski F, Montezano BB, de Azevedo CT. Latent bipolar disorder. Lancet. 2023;401(10394):2109. https://doi.org/10.1016/S0140-6736(23)00402-6.
12. Keramatian K, Chithra NK, Yatham LN. The CANMAT and ISBD guidelines for the treatment of bipolar disorder: summary and a 2023 update of evidence. Focus (Am Psychiatr Publ). 2023;21(4):344–53. https://doi.org/10.1176/appi.focus.20230009. Epub 2023 Oct 15. PMID: 38695002; PMCID: PMC11058959
13. Lam RW, Kennedy SH, Adams C, Bahji A, Beaulieu S, Bhat V, Blier P, Blumberger DM, Brietzke E, Chakrabarty T, Do A, Frey BN, Giacobbe P, Gratzer D, Grigoriadis S, Habert J, Ishrat Husain M, Ismail Z, McGirr A, McIntyre RS, Michalak EE, Müller DJ, Parikh SV, Quilty LS, Ravindran AV, Ravindran N, Renaud J, Rosenblat JD, Samaan Z, Saraf G, Schade K, Schaffer A, Sinyor M, Soares CN, Swainson J, Taylor VH, Tourjman SV, Uher R, van Ameringen M, Vazquez G, Vigod S, Voineskos D, Yatham LN, Milev RV. Canadian Network

for Mood and Anxiety Treatments (CANMAT) 2023 update on clinical guidelines for management of major depressive disorder in adults: Réseau canadien pour les traitements de l'humeur et de l'anxiété (CANMAT) 2023: Mise à jour des lignes directrices cliniques pour la prise en charge du trouble dépressif majeur chez les adultes. Can J Psychiatry. 2024;69(9):641–87. https://doi.org/10.1177/07067437241245384. Epub 2024 May 6. PMID: 38711351; PMCID: PMC11351064
14. Malhi GS, Bell E, Bassett D, Boyce P, Bryant R, Hazell P, Hopwood M, Lyndon B, Mulder R, Porter R, Singh AB, Murray G. The 2020 Royal Australian and New Zealand College of Psychiatrists clinical practice guidelines for mood disorders. Aust N Z J Psychiatry. 2021;55(1):7–117. https://doi.org/10.1177/0004867420979353.
15. McIntyre RS, Berk M, Brietzke E, Goldstein BI, López-Jaramillo C, Kessing LV, Malhi GS, Nierenberg AA, Rosenblat JD, Majeed A, Vieta E, Vinberg M, Young AH, Mansur RB. Bipolar disorders. Lancet. 2020;396(10265):1841–56. https://doi.org/10.1016/S0140-6736(20)31544-0.
16. Møller C, Miskowiak KW, Kessing LV, et al. Pharmacological treatment of individuals at familial risk for bipolar or major depressive disorders: a scoping review. Curr Treat Options Psych. 2022;9:55–72. https://doi.org/10.1007/s40501-022-00258-2.
17. Nery FG, Wilson AR, Schneider MR, Strawn JR, Patino LR, McNamara RK, Adler CM, Strakowski SM, DelBello MP. Medication exposure and predictors of first mood episode in offspring of parents with bipolar disorder: a prospective study. Braz J Psychiatry. 2020;42(5):481–8. https://doi.org/10.1590/1516-4446-2019-0802. PMID: 32401870; PMCID: PMC7524417
18. Pfennig A, Correll CU, Marx C, Rottmann-Wolf M, Meyer TD, Bauer M, Leopold K. Psychotherapeutic interventions in individuals at risk of developing bipolar disorder: a systematic review. Early Interv Psychiatry. 2014;8(1):3–11. https://doi.org/10.1111/eip.12082. Epub 2013 Aug 22
19. Post RM, Goldstein BI, Birmaher B, Findling RL, Frey BN, DelBello MP, Miklowitz DJ. Toward prevention of bipolar disorder in at-risk children: potential strategies ahead of the data. J Affect Disord. 2020;272:508–20. https://doi.org/10.1016/j.jad.2020.03.025. Epub 2020 Mar 6. PMID: 32553395; PMCID: PMC8986089
20. Strawn JR, Adler CM, McNamara RK, Welge JA, Bitter SM, Mills NP, Barzman DH, Cerullo MA, Chang KD, Strakowski SM, DelBello MP. Antidepressant tolerability in anxious and depressed youth at high risk for bipolar disorder: a prospective naturalistic treatment study. Bipolar Disord. 2014;16(5):523–30. https://doi.org/10.1111/bdi.12113. Epub 2013 Aug 13. PMID: 23937313; PMCID: PMC9435372
21. Suppes T, Silva R, Cucchiaro J, Mao Y, Targum S, Streicher C, Pikalov A, Loebel A. Lurasidone for the treatment of major depressive disorder with mixed features: a randomized, double-blind. Placebo-Controlled Study Am J Psychiatry. 2016;173(4):400–7. https://doi.org/10.1176/appi.ajp.2015.15060770. Epub 2015 Nov 10
22. Yamaguchi Y, Kimoto S, Nagahama T, Kishimoto T. Dosage-related nature of escitalopram treatment-emergent mania/hypomania: a case series. Neuropsychiatr Dis Treat. 2018;14:2099–104. https://doi.org/10.2147/NDT.S168078. PMID: 30147322; PMCID: PMC6103304
23. Yatham LN, Kennedy SH, Parikh SV, Schaffer A, Bond DJ, Frey BN, Sharma V, Goldstein BI, Rej S, Beaulieu S, Alda M, MacQueen G, Milev RV, Ravindran A, O'Donovan C, McIntosh D, Lam RW, Vazquez G, Kapczinski F, McIntyre RS, Kozicky J, Kanba S, Lafer B, Suppes T, Calabrese JR, Vieta E, Malhi G, Post RM, Berk M. Canadian Network for Mood and Anxiety Treatments (CANMAT) and International Society for Bipolar Disorders (ISBD) 2018 guidelines for the management of patients with bipolar disorder. Bipolar Disord. 2018;20(2):97–170. https://doi.org/10.1111/bdi.12609. Epub 2018 Mar 14. PMID: 29536616; PMCID: PMC5947163

24. Yatham LN, Chakrabarty T, Bond DJ, Schaffer A, Beaulieu S, Parikh SV, McIntyre RS, Milev RV, Alda M, Vazquez G, Ravindran AV, Frey BN, Sharma V, Goldstein BI, Rej S, O'Donovan C, Tourjman V, Kozicky JM, Kauer-Sant'Anna M, Malhi G, Suppes T, Vieta E, Kapczinski F, Kanba S, Lam RW, Kennedy SH, Calabrese J, Berk M, Post R. Canadian Network for Mood and Anxiety Treatments (CANMAT) and International Society for Bipolar Disorders (ISBD) recommendations for the management of patients with bipolar disorder with mixed presentations. Bipolar Disord. 2021;23(8):767–88. https://doi.org/10.1111/bdi.13135. Epub 2021 Nov 1

Chapter 17
Psychosocial Interventions and Latent Bipolar Disorder

Kamyar Keramatian, Emma Morton, and Marc Gelineau

17.1 Introduction

Bipolar disorder is a complex and often severe psychiatric condition that typically emerges during adolescence and early adulthood. The disorder can have profound impacts on an individual's day-to-day functioning [1], cognitive capacity [2], and quality of life [3], even in the early stages of the illness, making it the fourth leading cause of disability worldwide among the 10–24-year age group [4]. Unfortunately, despite significant advancements in the pharmacological and psychological treatments of bipolar disorder, these developments have not necessarily translated into improved outcomes for many affected individuals [5].

One of the key contributors to the lack of progress in improving outcomes is the well-recognized observation that bipolar disorder tends to go undiagnosed for several years [6, 7]. Such prolonged delay in diagnosis has been shown to predict poor clinical outcomes, including elevated risk of suicide [8–10]. Additionally, data from prospective studies following a first manic episode suggest that many patients with bipolar disorder continue to show significant cognitive impairment [2], high relapse rates [11], gross structural abnormalities in prefrontal and subcortical limbic brain areas [12], as well as persistent subsyndromal symptoms and functional disability despite receiving timely and comprehensive evidence-based interventions. These findings are consistent with an accumulating body of research suggesting that at least for a subgroup of patients with bipolar disorder, once the diagnosis of bipolar disorder is fully established, it follows a neuroprogressive trajectory, marked by

K. Keramatian (✉) · M. Gelineau
Department of Psychiatry, University of British Columbia, Vancouver, BC, Canada
e-mail: Kamyar.Keramatian@ubc.ca; Marc.Gelineau@ubc.ca

E. Morton
School of Psychological Sciences, Monash University, Clayton, Australia
e-mail: Emma.Morton@monash.edu

T. de Azevedo Cardoso et al. (eds.), *Latent Bipolar Disorder*,
https://doi.org/10.1007/978-3-032-01297-5_17

increasing symptom severity associated with progressive brain changes over time [13–15]. Altogether, these findings underscore the critical need to focus on identifying individuals who are at high risk of developing bipolar disorder and intervening prior to the full manifestation of the illness in order to minimize the burden of the disorder and achieve the best possible outcome.

In recent years, psychosocial interventions, which encompass a wide range of therapeutic approaches, have earned growing attention as a safe and generally well-accepted treatment modality for individuals at risk of bipolar disorder. These include both psychological therapies and support programs and practical assistance with functional and personal recovery. This chapter delves into emerging psychosocial interventions for this population, structured around specific therapeutic targets for intervention, including early recognition, preventing the onset of illness and risk modification, and reducing the severity of symptoms and improving overall functioning and quality of life (Table 17.1).

Table 17.1 Summary of studies on psychosocial interventions for high-risk bipolar disorder

Authors	Target of intervention	Summary of main findings
Goldstein et al. (2014) [36]	Risk factor modification	In a pilot trial of IPSRT for those at high risk of bipolar disorder, it was found that IPSRT was effective in a pre- and post-test design at reducing instances of poor sleep hygiene. No significant differences were found for measures of psychosocial functioning nor for measures of bipolar symptoms.
Goldstein et al. (2018) [37]	Risk factor modification	A randomized clinical trial of IPSRT versus data-informed referral showed that the two groups did not differ in measures of subjective sleep, depression, and self- and parent-rated mood dysfunction. Differences were found for subthreshold manic symptoms, with the IPSRT group exhibiting less symptoms. Actigraphy data revealed that WASO decreased over time in the IPSRT group, which may be indicative of improved sleep hygiene.
Nadkarni and Fristad (2010) [42]	Prevention	A waitlist-controlled trial of MF-PEP illustrated that the control group had a four-times greater rate of conversion to bipolar disorder as compared to the intervention group.
Fristad et al. (2015) [47]	Symptom improvement	In a 2×2 design, a randomized controlled trial found that multi-treatment therapy (Omega 3 + IF-PEP) showed greater improvement in depression scores as compared to the control group (placebo + active monitoring). IF-PEP had greater effects on measures of depression compared to active monitoring. No significant differences were found over time for scores on measures of mania.
Miklowitz et al. (2011) [48]	Symptom improvement	A pilot trial of FFT-HR illustrated that the intervention related to large improvements in psychiatric status ratings for depression scores over time, and moderate improvements to hypomania ratings, even after accounting for medication usage.

(continued)

Table 17.1 (continued)

Authors	Target of intervention	Summary of main findings
Miklowitz et al. (2013) [49]	Symptom improvement	In a randomized clinical trial of FFT-HR versus educational control, patients who were in remission at study end had longer average time-to-recovery in the control group (21.25 weeks) as compared to the FFT-HR group (13 weeks). Those in the FFT-HR group spent a longer time in remission for subthreshold bipolar symptoms and showed greater improvements in manic symptoms as compared to the control group.
Miklowitz et al. (2020) [51]	Symptom improvement	A randomized controlled trial of FFT-HR versus enhanced usual care found no significant differences between groups for time-to-recovery from baseline symptoms. Those in the intervention group showed longer gaps between depressive episodes compared to the control and showed a more favorable course of symptoms at 48-month follow-up.
Garrett et al. (2015) [50]	Symptom improvement	Pre- to post-treatment differences for scores on measures of mania and depression were found to be significant, indicating a reduction of mania and depressive symptomatology.
Weintraub et al. (2022) [52]	Symptom improvement	Secondary analysis of randomized controlled trial data revealed that FFT-HR participants showed greater improvements in family functioning as compared to the control group. Mediation models illustrated that the relationship between FFT-HR intervention and depressive symptoms was mediated by family functioning.
Cotton et al. (2016) [53]	Symptom improvement	A pilot trial of MBCT-C found that anxiety symptoms decreased significantly over the course of the intervention, and clinician-rated anxiety showed that 90% of participants were in remission following the intervention.
Cotton et al. (2020) [54]	Symptom improvement	In a waitlist-controlled trial of MBCT-C, those assigned to the intervention showed greater improvements in clinician-rated anxiety severity over time. Within-group analyses revealed improvements in self-rated anxiety and severity of anxiety symptoms.
Leopold et al. (2020) [55]	Symptom improvement	A randomized controlled trial of CBT versus unstructured group meetings found no significant differences between groups for depression and psychosocial functioning scores. A significant difference for mania symptoms was found only for the baseline to 14-week follow-up.
Keramatian et al. (2025) [26]	Early recognition	In a feasibility trial of a telehealth-based group psychoeducation program for individuals at high risk of bipolar disorder, the intervention was feasible and acceptable, with preliminary improvements in help-seeking intentions and quality of life.

CBT cognitive behavioral therapy, *FFT-HR* Family-Focused Therapy for those at high risk of bipolar disorder, *IF-PEP* Individual-Family Psychoeducational Psychotherapy, *IPSRT* Interpersonal and Social Rhythms Therapy, *MBCT-C* Mindfulness-Based Cognitive Therapy for Children, *MF-PEP* Multifamily Psychoeducational Psychotherapy

17.2 The Role of Psychosocial Interventions in Early Recognition

An accumulating body of evidence over the past two decades indicates that the diagnosis of bipolar disorder is frequently missed, leading to delayed diagnosis and treatment initiation. For instance, in a multicenter naturalistic study, the median delay between the first mood episode and the accurate diagnosis of bipolar disorder in Canada was reported to be 5 years for the adult-onset group and 15 years for the pediatric-onset group [16]. These findings are consistent with a systematic review and meta-analysis that estimated the median delay in diagnosis of bipolar disorder across 20 different studies to be 6.7 years [17]. Such prolonged delay in diagnosis and subsequent treatment initiation has been shown to cause disruption of crucial age-specific developmental tasks [18], greater severity and frequency of mood episodes [19], higher number of hospitalizations [20], higher number of comorbidities including substance use disorders [8, 21], and elevated risk of suicide [8–10, 22] as well as significantly higher healthcare costs [23] and higher indirect costs due to work loss [23, 24].

Reducing delays in the diagnosis and treatment of bipolar disorder in youth and young adults is a complex public health challenge, as it involves different components that can be potentially influenced by a multitude of interconnected illness, patient, social, cultural, provider, and service factors. These potential factors—as outlined in our recently published conceptual framework [25]—include internalized self-stigmatization of mental illness, limited mental health literacy among the general population, symptom overlap with other conditions such as schizophrenia and major depression, underutilization of appropriate screening tools, limited access to specialized mental health services, and long wait times to see a specialist. Although the exact contribution of each factor to the delayed diagnosis and treatment of bipolar disorder remains uncertain, it is nonetheless prudent to proactively develop innovative individual and systems-focused interventions aimed at targeting modifiable factors to enhance the timely recognition and treatment.

One example of such a proactive approach focused on an individual-level contributor to delays in diagnosis is our recent development of a manualized telehealth-based group Psychoeducational and Resilience Enhancement Program for individuals at high risk for bipolar disorder (PREP-BD). By raising awareness of bipolar disorder and reducing stigma, this program aims to improve help-seeking intentions among adolescents and young adults who are at high risk for bipolar disorder. PREP-BD consists of weekly virtual educational sessions focused on providing participants with the tools and knowledge to recognize early symptoms of bipolar disorder and encouraging them to seek help early if those symptoms emerge in the future. A pilot trial of this program has been successfully completed, demonstrating the feasibility and acceptability of this approach as well as preliminary efficacy of this intervention in improving help-seeking intentions among at-risk individuals [26]. Building on these findings, our group is currently planning an efficacy trial to further investigate the effect of PREP-BD in improving help-seeking in high-risk individuals and facilitating early recognition of bipolar disorder.

17.3 The Role of Psychosocial Interventions in Prevention and Risk Factor Modification

While pharmacological treatments can be highly effective in stabilizing acute symptoms and reducing the risk of relapse, many patients continue to experience residual symptoms [27] as well as persistent cognitive decline [2] even during periods of euthymia and despite medication adherence. Moreover, side effects associated with mood stabilizers and antipsychotics can contribute to the higher rates of mortality and add to the overall burden of the disease. Side effects such as sedation, cognitive slowing, weight gain, metabolic syndrome, and teratogenicity, among many others, can lead to additional health conditions, reduce quality of life, impact treatment adherence, and increase stigma. Therefore, there is a need to focus on developing evidence-based preventive interventions aimed at reducing the incidence and burden of bipolar disorder in those who are at risk of developing the illness or are experiencing prodromal symptoms. Psychosocial interventions may be particularly well-positioned to contribute to this goal, as a number of known risk factors of bipolar disorder can be modified through psychological and behavioral intervention. In addition, psychosocial interventions may be more acceptable to people at risk of developing bipolar disorder and their families, as they avoid the risk of side effects and stigma associated with pharmacological interventions. Psychosocial interventions also target transdiagnostic risk factors and may therefore be of benefit for the prevention of mental health disorders in general.

Studies evaluating current preventative psychosocial interventions for bipolar disorder are outlined below, focusing on two main modifiable risk factors: sleep cycle disturbances and social rhythm irregularities and emotion regulation. Preventative studies can take two forms in terms of their outcome assessment. A more direct approach would be to focus on evaluating the rate or timing of conversion to bipolar disorder, investigating whether an intervention can delay or prevent the onset of the disorder in high-risk individuals. Alternatively, studies may assess impacts on known modifiable risk factors, in the hopes that mitigating the impacts of these vulnerabilities would translate to downstream impacts for the development of bipolar disorder.

17.3.1 Sleep Cycle Disturbances and Social Rhythm Irregularities

One factor that has been identified as influencing the course of bipolar disorder is sleep cycle disturbances and social rhythm irregularities. Circadian rhythm disturbances have been implicated in the onset of bipolar episodes [28], and those at high risk for bipolar disorder have been shown to have poorer sleep quality as compared to those not at risk [29]. Indeed, Levenson and colleagues [30] found that circadian rhythm abnormalities such as frequent nighttime awakenings and poor sleep quality predicted the development of bipolar disorder in a sample of high-risk individuals. Similarly, irregular social rhythms have been shown to predict the onset of mood episodes in patients with bipolar disorder [31]. These findings have led to the development of Interpersonal and Social Rhythm Therapy (IPSRT), a psychosocial intervention that is designed to target dysregulation of social and circadian rhythms and is considered a third-line psychosocial intervention in maintenance treatment of bipolar disorder [32, 33].

It has been hypothesized that addressing the maladaptive sleep patterns present in youth at risk for bipolar disorder may be an effective strategy for preventing the emergence of clinically diagnosable bipolar disorder [34, 35]. As such, Goldstein and colleagues at the University of Pittsburgh have undertaken the task of adapting IPSRT for at-risk youth [36]. The adapted version of IPSRT for at-risk youth, which involves both the youth and their parents, is composed of 12 sessions administered over the course of 6 months. The initial phase of the intervention is designated to a psychoeducational component outlining the risks of bipolar disorder, as well as creating an inventory of interpersonal relationships in the adolescent's life and establishing current sleep and social rhythms. In the subsequent sessions, at-risk youth establish target times for sleep and social rhythms and explore the adolescent's feelings regarding having a family member with bipolar disorder, the knowledge that they have an increased risk of bipolar disorder, and how the youth copes with this. The clinician helps the adolescent to form connections between stressful life events, interpersonal relationships, and mood as well as circadian and social rhythms. The final sessions involve identifying strategies for the future management of interpersonal struggles and the potential emergence of bipolar disorder symptoms.

In a sample of adolescents (12–18 years old) with a first-degree relative with a history of bipolar disorder, Goldstein and colleagues [36] conducted a pilot study testing the effects of the adapted IPSRT on social and circadian rhythms. Participants were assessed on sleep hygiene, mood symptomatology, and psychosocial functioning at three timepoints: pre-treatment, 3 months post-treatment, and 6 months post-treatment. At pre-treatment, ratings of mood symptoms were indicative of mild symptoms of bipolar disorder, and there were no significant changes found on any of the scales used to assess bipolar symptoms between pre-treatment and follow-ups. The authors [36] suggest that the reason for the null findings in terms of symptom reduction may have been due to the small sample size (n = 13) and minimal subthreshold symptom severity exhibited by the sample at study intake. For psychosocial functioning, the authors did not find a significant difference between pre-treatment and follow-ups. However, they found that the intervention was effective in mitigating oversleeping and "sleeping-in" on weekends, suggesting that IPSRT had an impact on the sleep irregularities that have been documented in those at high risk for bipolar disorder [29, 30].

However, the sleep-related findings in the initial trial were not replicated in a randomized controlled trial. Goldstein and colleagues [37] conducted a randomized clinical trial investigating the effects of IPSRT versus data-informed referral (i.e., participants were informed of their clinical assessment and offered referrals for treatment). Participants were adolescents aged 12–18 years with a biological parent diagnosed with bipolar disorder. Participant measures were taken at study enrollment, and at 3- and 6-month post-enrollment. Over the course of follow-up, the two groups did not differ in clinician-rated subthreshold depressive symptoms, but did differ in subthreshold hypo/manic symptoms, with the IPSRT group being less likely to display such symptoms. The authors did not find statistically significant effects between groups over time for self- and parent-rated mood dysfunction, nor for measures of subjective sleep. However, data obtained via actigraphy found that wake after sleep onset (WASO) decreased significantly over time in the IPSRT group. The authors suggest that this might be indicative of improved sleep hygiene, thus offering some evidence toward the efficacy of IPSRT in reducing sleep abnormalities in those at-risk for bipolar disorder.

17.3.2 Emotion Regulation

Another psychological factor that has been hypothesized to play a role in the emergence of bipolar disorder in high-risk individuals involves emotional regulation capacity. Emotion regulation inefficiency has been identified as a vulnerability marker in those at high risk for bipolar disorder, wherein individuals who present with subthreshold hypomanic symptoms exhibit heightened emotional reactivity and have more difficulties in down-regulating emotional activity as compared to healthy controls [38]. In addition, given that stressful life events and traumatic experiences have also been implicated in the onset of mood symptoms in youth with a genetic risk of bipolar disorder [39], interventions could potentially mitigate the risk of full conversion to bipolar disorder by regulating the family environment to prevent stressful/traumatic situations that may arise as a product of familial dysfunction. Multifamily psychoeducational psychotherapy (MF-PEP) is a group intervention that combines elements of psychoeducation, family system intervention, and cognitive behavioral therapy (CBT) to target mood symptoms in children and adolescents with depression and bipolar spectrum disorder [40, 41]. The youth in MF-PEP intervention are taught emotion regulation and coping strategies, how to identify the symptoms of mood dysregulation, and ways to modify the negative cognitions that accompany mood symptoms while parents receive information regarding ways that family members can help to manage mood symptoms, options for treatment, and mental health services that can help the family.

In a waitlist-controlled trial, Nadkarni and Fristad [42] investigated the effects of MF-PEP on the conversion rates from unipolar depressive disorders to bipolar disorder in youth aged 8–11 years with both depressive spectrum disorders and transient manic symptoms. The sample was randomized to either the intervention group or a waitlist and followed up over the course of 18 months. Findings indicated that there was a significant difference in conversion rates across groups, with the waitlist control exhibiting a four-times greater conversion rate as compared to the intervention group. Nadkarni and Fristad [42] suggest that the observed differences across groups may be attributed to the family functioning that is bolstered by MF-PEP and the development of crucial emotion regulation skills in youth who participated in the intervention.

The identification and reduction of modifiable risk factors in the progression of bipolar symptoms is crucial to mitigate the risk of conversion to bipolar disorder in at-risk populations. As such, therapies that target risk factors such as circadian rhythm irregularities, emotional regulation inefficiency, and familial dysfunction may provide a valid avenue for the prevention of bipolar conversion in high-risk youth. However, given the dearth of literature on this subject, more research is needed to identify potential therapeutic modalities that can reduce risk factors and prevent conversion to bipolar disorder.

17.4 The Role of Psychosocial Interventions in Symptom Improvement

Many individuals who eventually develop bipolar disorder exhibit subsyndromal mood symptoms prior to the full conversion to bipolar disorder [42, 43], with such symptoms often presenting many years before the clinical threshold for diagnosis [44, 45]. Examples of such subthreshold presentations include depressive symptoms, subthreshold manic symptoms, and mood instability. Research has shown that the risk of developing clinically diagnosable bipolar disorder increases significantly when individuals present with subthreshold bipolar symptoms; youth with a parent with bipolar disorder who are exhibiting such symptoms have a 49% chance of developing diagnosable bipolar disorder, as compared to 6.8% of youth who have a biological parent with bipolar disorder but are not exhibiting subthreshold symptoms [46]. Given that subthreshold symptoms have been demonstrated to be a major predictor of conversion to bipolar disorder, such symptoms have become the target for a number of psychosocial interventions. The purpose of these interventions is to reduce the subsyndromal symptoms of bipolar disorder in order to prevent progression into full bipolar symptomatology.

To date, only a handful of studies have attempted to investigate the effects of psychosocial interventions on symptom reduction in those at high risk of bipolar disorder. As such, we are aware of only four psychosocial interventions that have been tested in the reduction of symptoms in at risk individuals: Psychoeducational Psychotherapy (PEP; [47]), Family-Focused Therapy for those at high risk of bipolar disorder (FFT-HR; [48–52]), Mindfulness-Based Cognitive Therapy for Children (MBCT-C; [53, 54]), and CBT [55]. The design, procedures, and results of these interventions are presented below.

17.4.1 Family-Focused Therapy

Of the psychosocial interventions aimed at symptom improvement in individuals at high risk of bipolar disorder, FFT-HR has the most extensive body of literature. While Family Focused Therapy (FFT) has been demonstrated to be effective in the treatment of diagnosed bipolar disorder based on nearly 40 years of use, the effects of FFT on those at high risk for bipolar disorder are less definitive. A group of researchers headed by David Miklowitz have modified FFT for use with individuals at high-risk of bipolar disorder, and the efficacy of the modified FFT-HR has been preliminarily established. As such, the following description of the FFT-HR intervention is still experimental in nature. The modified intervention takes place over the course of 12 sessions, wherein the goal is to assist high-risk youth and their families in recognizing symptoms, distinguishing between developmentally normative emotions and mood dysregulation, identifying triggers for mood dysregulation, enhancing communication, and developing prevention strategies for symptoms. The first few sessions [1–4] involve a psychoeducation element, wherein clients are informed of the goals of FFT-HR and the signs of mood disorders. These early sessions also involve the parent sharing with the youth about the nature of bipolar disorder and how the parent has coped with the symptoms of the disorder. Also in these initial sessions, the youth identify any current stressors associated with mood dysregulation and develops a mood management plan, where the youth, the parents, and the clinician list medical and behavioral strategies to use if symptoms begin to manifest. Sessions 5–8 involve communication enhancement training, where families are introduced to adaptive communication skills. These skills are reinforced through practice and role-play in order to enhance the quality of communication between family members. The final sessions [9–12] involve problem-solving skill training, where the families identify problems and break them down into smaller issues that can be addressed individually. Lists of solutions for such smaller problems are generated, and the family settles on the most appropriate course of action for a particular issue.

An initial trial of FFT-HR [48] was conducted in a sample of high-risk youth who met criteria for bipolar disorder not otherwise specified (BD-NOS), major depressive disorder (MDD), or cyclothymic disorder and had a biological parent with bipolar disorder. The authors followed the participants for a year, taking measurements of symptom severity every 4 months. Over the course of the follow-ups, it was found that youth showed large improvements in psychiatric status ratings for depression scores over time and moderate improvements to hypomania scores. Even after accounting for medication use as a covariate, the authors still found significant improvements to both depression and hypomania. Similar findings on the effects of FFT-HR have been demonstrated by Garrett and colleagues [50]. Using the same protocol described above as designed by Miklowitz and colleagues [48], Garrett and colleagues [50] found that pre- to post-treatment differences were significant for measures of manic and depressive symptoms, indicating a reduction of subthreshold bipolar symptomatology.

Following the promising results found during the initial test of FFT-HR on the improvement of symptoms in youth, Miklowitz and colleagues [49] conducted a randomized clinical trial with 40 symptomatic youth (ages 9–17 years) who met the criteria for BD-NOS or cyclothymic disorder and had a first-degree relative with diagnosed bipolar disorder. Youth were randomly assigned to either the FFT-HR condition or an educational control and followed over the course of a year. Of the patients who were in remission at the end of the study, the average time for recovery in the FFT-HR group was 13.0 weeks, whereas the average time for recovery in the educational control group was 21.25 weeks. Additionally, youth in the FFT-HR group spent a longer time in remission and showed greater improvements in manic symptoms as compared to the educational control group.

Miklowitz and colleagues [51] followed the previous two studies with a second randomized clinical trial investigating the effects of FFT-HR versus enhanced usual care (i.e., psychoeducation followed by implementation of a mood management system) in a sample of symptomatic youth (ages 9–17 years) with BD-NOS or MDD and a first-degree relative with diagnosed BD. The FFT-HR condition was as described above, whereas the enhanced usual care condition received family-based psychoeducation sessions, followed by monthly youth-only sessions focused on establishing a plan to manage mood dysfunction. Participants were followed for 4 years, with measures of depression and mania taken every 4 months in the first year, and every 6 months in the following 3 years. Contrary to the Miklowitz et al. [49] study, no significant differences between groups were found for time to recovery from baseline symptoms. However, the authors did find that youth assigned to the FFT-HR group who recovered from baseline symptoms experienced longer gaps between subsequent depressive episodes as compared to the enhanced care condition, indicating longer periods of well-being in the FFT-HR group. In the 48-month follow-up period, youth in the FFT-HR group showed a more favorable course of symptoms as compared to the control group.

Adding to the work of Miklowitz and colleagues [48, 49, 51] outlined above, Weintraub et al. [52] sought to determine if the mood improvements described by Miklowitz and colleagues [48, 49, 51] were mediated by psychosocial functioning. Using the same sample and procedure as Miklowitz et al. (50; described above), the authors found that youth in the FFT-HR condition reported greater improvements to family functioning as compared to youth in the control condition, which remained significant even when controlling for depression and mania scores. Social-emotional functioning improved in both groups over time, which was associated with decreasing depressive symptoms. The authors also found a mediation effect of family functioning on the relationship between FFT-HR and depressive symptoms at post-treatment, and that the mediation effect increased in magnitude over follow-ups. Additionally, post hoc analyses indicated that youth with a comorbid anxiety disorder or an externalizing disorder (ADHD/conduct disorder/oppositional defiant disorder) who were a part of the FFT-HR condition demonstrated greater improvements to family functioning over time as compared to the control group.

17.4.2 Psychoeducational Psychotherapy

Another psychosocial intervention that has shown efficacy in the reduction of subthreshold bipolar symptoms is PEP. While PEP (described above) has been demonstrated to be effective in the prevention of conversion from unipolar depression to bipolar disorder [42], it has also been shown to reduce symptoms in high-risk individuals. In a randomized controlled trial conducted by Fristad and colleagues [47], youth aged 7–14 years with BD-NOS or cyclothymic disorder were randomized to receive Individual-Family Psychoeducational Psychotherapy (IF-PEP) and Omega 3, IF-PEP and active monitoring, active monitoring and Omega 3, or placebo and active monitoring. The sample was assessed at study enrollment and multiple times over the course of 12 weeks. The findings of the trial conducted by Fristad and colleagues [46] demonstrated that combined therapy (Omega 3 + IF-PEP) showed greater improvements in scores on depression over time as compared to placebo + active monitoring and Omega 3 + active monitoring groups. The effect of IF-PEP on depression compared to active monitoring ranged from medium to large effect sizes. All groups decreased over time in terms of mania scores, but no significant differences between groups were found.

17.4.3 Mindfulness-Based Cognitive Therapy for Children

In addition to PEP and FFT-HR, the effects of MBCT-C [56] for reducing symptoms in youth at high-risk of bipolar disorder have been investigated. While MBCT-C has been largely established as a psychotherapy that is efficacious in the treatment of anxiety symptoms, its use in the context of youth at-risk for bipolar disorder has garnered far less attention. As such, the use of MBCT-C for high-risk youth remains experimental for the time being, until more research can verify its efficacy. MBCT-C is a 12-session program made up of three phases. In the initial phase, clients are given an overview and introduction to mindfulness and mindful practice, with facilitators encouraging the youth to cultivate mindfulness through mindful breathing exercises and bodily awareness. The second phase involves sensory-based practices, wherein clients are informed how somatic sensations can contribute to the heightening or mitigation of anxiety symptoms. The final phase of the intervention is focused on integrating mindfulness into everyday life and maintaining the skills taught in sessions across contexts.

In a pilot trial of MBCT-C for youth (aged 9–17 years) with a diagnosed anxiety disorder and a biological family member with bipolar disorder, Cotton and colleagues [53] took measures of emotion regulation, mindfulness, state and trait anxiety, and clinician-rated anxiety weekly throughout the course of the intervention. In the initial pilot phase, Cotton and colleagues [53] found promising results, with anxiety scores decreasing significantly over the course of the intervention.

Examining pre- and post-test measures revealed that emotion regulation scores increased significantly after the MBCT-C intervention. In addition, scores on clinician-rated anxiety revealed that 90% of the participants were in remission following being administered the intervention. The optimistic findings of the initial trial led Cotton and colleagues [54] to conduct a waitlist-controlled trial of MBCT-C. A sample of youth aged 9–18 years who met diagnostic criteria for a DSM-IV-TR anxiety disorder and had a biological family member with a bipolar disorder diagnosis were randomized to either receive the intervention or to be waitlisted while receiving psychoeducation in the interim, and both groups were assessed using a pre- and post- test design. The authors found a significant difference between the waitlist and MBCT-C groups, wherein MBCT-C showed greater improvements in clinician-rated illness severity over time. They also found significant improvements in within-group analyses for self-reported anxiety and clinical severity of anxiety symptoms for the MBCT-C group.

17.4.4 Cognitive Behavioral Therapy

The fourth and final therapeutic modality that has been tested in the context of symptom reduction in a sample of youth at high-risk for bipolar disorder is CBT. CBT in the context of at-risk youth has but one efficacy trial published to date, wherein the authors [55] modified traditional CBT to include elements of psychoeducation and mindfulness. As such, the modified intervention has yet to be empirically validated as being efficacious. The intervention is based on classic CBT interventions, where participants were trained in problem-solving strategies, cognitive bias modification, identification of critical behaviors, and sensitization for a balanced life rhythm. Participants also received information about handling early warning signs and were encouraged to make a plan for use when in crisis.

Leopold and colleagues [55] conducted a randomized controlled trial to investigate the effects of this modified group CBT versus a control of unstructured group meetings in a sample of young adults (ages 15–30 years) presenting with subthreshold bipolar disorder symptoms (mania, depression, and cyclothymia). Participants were followed across 5 time points up to 78 weeks. Overall, the authors found that both conditions exhibited decreases in depressive symptoms and the severity of manic symptoms over the follow-ups. No significant differences were found between groups for scores on depression measures nor in measures of psychosocial functioning. A significant difference was found for manic symptoms only for the baseline to 14-week follow-up, but not beyond that.

17.4.5 Efficacy of Psychosocial Therapies for Symptom Reduction

While many of the above intervention studies aimed at the reduction of symptoms in individuals at high risk of bipolar disorder seem promising, more research is needed to establish a model of best practice. Of the aforementioned interventions, FFT-HR has the most substantial amount of literature lending evidence to the efficacy of reducing subsyndromal symptoms in those at high risk of bipolar disorder. However, this does not discount the other therapeutic modalities, as the above evidence illustrates a promising future in the use of psychosocial interventions for the purpose of reducing subsyndromal symptoms in those at high risk of bipolar disorder. Importantly, however, the efficacy of a particular intervention relies heavily upon the at-risk individuals' perceptions of the intervention. By qualitatively investigating the participants' experiences while taking part in interventions, researchers can help to identify qualities of such interventions that encourage participation and, in turn, enhance efficacy. For instance, Jones and colleagues [57] documented the experiences of participants who partook in a CBT-based intervention for those at high risk of bipolar disorder. The authors found that the flexibility of the research team, the relevance of the materials, and the personalization of procedures encouraged the participants to fully embrace the intervention. As such, researchers who use specific interventions should incorporate qualitative elements in their research findings to further refine the interventions and increase the effectiveness of these psychosocial programs. By doing so, researchers may be able to bolster the effects of their interventions in reducing subthreshold bipolar symptomatology.

In sum, research on psychosocial interventions targeting symptom reduction in those at high risk of bipolar disorder has demonstrated the preliminary efficacy of various therapeutic modalities in reducing the subthreshold manic and depressive symptoms that characterize bipolar disorder [47–51], as well as reducing symptoms of comorbid conditions such as anxiety disorders [53, 54]. While such results offer encouraging evidence toward the use of psychosocial interventions for the reduction of symptoms in those at high risk of bipolar disorder, these interventions have yet to be adopted for use by clinicians in clinical settings. Therefore, there is a need for implementation research that examines how to close the gap between evidence-based best practices and routine clinical care for this population.

17.5 Conclusion and Future Directions

Psychosocial interventions are well-positioned to improve outcomes for young people at risk of or with subthreshold presentations of bipolar disorder. Here, we have argued for the existence of multiple points of intervention where psychosocial treatments may be of benefit, including enhancing help-seeking and consequent timely diagnosis and early intervention, reducing known psychological vulnerabilities for conversion to full bipolar disorder, and reducing symptoms in at-risk or subthreshold groups. Several psychosocial interventions have preliminary evidence to support their application; however, more evidence is still required to support their translation into usual care. Further large-scale randomized controlled trials, long-term follow-up studies, and implementation studies in real-world settings are needed to build confidence in the clinical application of these therapies.

Other areas for future development in this field include applying psychosocial interventions to understudied risk factors for bipolar disorder. For example, one potentially modifiable risk factor for bipolar disorder is the use of tobacco, alcohol, or other substances [58]. This can be treated using psychosocial approaches and indeed is a component of psychoeducation interventions for diagnosed bipolar disorder. Other interventions have been developed to specifically target this comorbidity [59]; however, the benefits of this have not yet been examined for prevention of bipolar disorder in at-risk groups or for symptom reduction in prodromal phases.

Our chapter has focused on the potential benefits of psychosocial interventions for clinical outcomes in at-risk and subthreshold presentations of bipolar disorder. However, we note that these types of interventions also have relevance for broader aspects of functioning and quality of life impacted by the symptoms of this condition. Given that the onset of bipolar disorder is typically in adolescence or early adulthood, these symptoms can have a profound impact on the developmental trajectories of young people, including social relationships, educational outcomes, employment, and transition to independent living [60]. The development of a sense of self and identity is also a key aspect of the psychological maturation that occurs in this phase of life, and the stark changes in mood and behavior associated with mood episodes can disrupt this critical developmental task [61]. Such outcomes are understudied in this group, despite youth with bipolar disorder expressing interest in interventions that specifically target social recovery and stigma [62, 63]. Recovery-focused interventions, which focus on both relapse reduction and personal recovery, have shown some benefits in recent onset bipolar disorder (within the past 5 years) and may be an ideal form of psychosocial intervention to adapt for the needs and concerns of individuals at risk or experiencing subthreshold symptoms [64]. Future efforts should therefore focus not only on improving the evidence base for psychosocial interventions, as well as intervention development, in partnership with community members, to optimize the ability of psychosocial interventions to address patient-valued outcomes.

Finally, we note that, in order to refer individuals who would benefit from such psychosocial interventions to appropriate forms of early intervention, individuals, their families or supports, and clinicians must be equipped to detect the presence of risk factors or potentially problematic prodromal symptoms, and be aware of and willing to engage with appropriate avenues for help-seeking. Our pilot evaluation of a psychoeducation intervention to promote help-seeking was the first of its kind to be applied in bipolar disorder; however, our conceptual framework of contributors to delays in diagnosis and treatment in bipolar disorder suggests several other key modifiable barriers [25]. Advances to psychosocial interventions for this group will therefore be most effective when paired with public health interventions to build awareness and reduce stigma [65], as has been attempted to increase uptake of early psychosis services [66, 67]. As with interventions for bipolar disorder more broadly, a systems perspective is required to improve pathways to care.

17.6 Clinical Considerations

- The diagnosis of bipolar disorder is frequently missed, leading to inadequate or inappropriate treatment and negative functional and clinical outcomes.
- Help-seeking adolescents and young adults presenting with mood symptoms and behavioral changes, as well as those with a family history of bipolar disorder, are especially at risk of developing bipolar disorder.
- Clinicians in outpatient settings and emergency departments should consider the diagnosis of bipolar disorder by obtaining a thorough history that would include inquiring about manic symptoms, family psychiatric history, and response to previous treatments, and offer follow-up visits and treatment with mood-stabilizing agents if clinically indicated.
- Providing education to at-risk individuals who do not meet the criteria for bipolar disorder and their families may improve help-seeking in those who will develop bipolar disorder.
- Many patients with bipolar disorder experience mood symptoms characteristic of depression, emotional dysregulation, and subthreshold manic symptoms prior to the onset of full manic or hypomanic episodes.
- An individualized treatment plan for individuals who present with subthreshold mood symptoms, especially those who are identified to be at risk for bipolar disorder, should include considering the use of evidence-based psychosocial interventions, along with ongoing monitoring for conversion to bipolar disorder.

References

1. Kauer-Sant'Anna M, Bond DJ, Lam RW, Yatham LN. Functional outcomes in first-episode patients with bipolar disorder: a prospective study from the systematic treatment optimization program for early mania project. Compr Psychiatry [Internet] 2009 [cited 2023 Jan 8];50(1):1–8. Available from: https://pubmed.ncbi.nlm.nih.gov/19059506/.
2. Keramatian K, Torres IJ, Yatham LN. Neurocognitive functioning in bipolar disorder: What we know and what we don't. Dialogues Clin Neurosci [Internet]. 2022 [cited 2023 Jan 8];23(1):29–38. Available from: https://pubmed.ncbi.nlm.nih.gov/35860174/.
3. Michalak EE, Yatham LN, Lam RW. Quality of life in bipolar disorder: a review of the literature. Health Qual Life Outcomes [Internet] 2005 [cited 2024 Sep 14];3. Available from: https://pubmed.ncbi.nlm.nih.gov/16288650/.
4. Gore FM, Bloem PJN, Patton GC, Ferguson J, Joseph V, Coffey C, et al. Global burden of disease in young people aged 10–24 years: a systematic analysis. Lancet [Internet]. 2011 [cited 2023 Jan 8];377(9783):2093–2102. Available from: https://pubmed.ncbi.nlm.nih.gov/21652063/.

5. Geddes JR, Miklowitz DJ. Treatment of bipolar disorder. Lancet [Internet] 2013 [cited 2024 Sep 14];381(9878):1672–1682. Available from: https://pubmed.ncbi.nlm.nih.gov/23663953/.
6. Fritz K, Russell AMT, Allwang C, Kuiper S, Lampe L, Malhi GS. Is a delay in the diagnosis of bipolar disorder inevitable? Bipolar Disord [Internet]. 2017 Aug 1 [cited 2023 Jan 8];19(5):396–400. Available from: https://pubmed.ncbi.nlm.nih.gov/28544121/.
7. Keramatian K, Pinto J V., Schaffer A, Sharma V, Beaulieu S, Parikh S V., et al. Clinical and demographic factors associated with delayed diagnosis of bipolar disorder: Data from Health Outcomes and Patient Evaluations in Bipolar Disorder (HOPE-BD) study. J Affect Disord [Internet]. 2022 [cited 2023 Jan 8];296:506–13. Available from: https://pubmed.ncbi.nlm.nih.gov/34606817/.
8. Altamura AC, Dell'Osso B, Berlin HA, Buoli M, Bassetti R, Mundo E. Duration of untreated illness and suicide in bipolar disorder: a naturalistic study. Eur Arch Psychiatry Clin Neurosci [Internet]. 2010 [cited 2023 Feb 18];260(5):385–91. Available from: https://pubmed.ncbi.nlm.nih.gov/19911248/.
9. Drancourt N, Etain B, Lajnef M, Henry C, Raust A, Cochet B, et al. Duration of untreated bipolar disorder: missed opportunities on the long road to optimal treatment. Acta Psychiatr Scand [Internet]. 2013 [cited 2023 Feb 18];127(2):136–44. Available from: https://pubmed.ncbi.nlm.nih.gov/22901015/.
10. Nery-Fernandes F, Quarantini LC, Guimarães JL, De Oliveira IR, Koenen KC, Kapczinski F, et al. Is there an association between suicide attempt and delay of initiation of mood stabilizers in bipolar I disorder? J Affect Disord [Internet]. 2012 [cited 2023 Aug 26];136(3):1082–7. Available from: https://pubmed.ncbi.nlm.nih.gov/22138284/.
11. Gignac A, McGirr A, Lam RW, Yatham LN. Course and outcome following a first episode of mania: four-year prospective data from the Systematic Treatment Optimization Program (STOP-EM). J Affect Disord [Internet]. 2015 [cited 2024 Jan 14];175:411–7. Available from: https://pubmed.ncbi.nlm.nih.gov/25678174/.
12. Keramatian K, Dhanoa T, McGirr A, Lang DJ, Honer WG, Lam RW, et al. Structural brain changes in first episode mania with and without psychosis: data from the systematic treatment optimization program for early mania (STOP-EM). World J Biol Psychiatry. 2018;19(sup2):S30–S40. Available from: https://pubmed.ncbi.nlm.nih.gov/27762161/.
13. Berk M. Neuroprogression: pathways to progressive brain changes in bipolar disorder. Int J Neuropsychopharmacol [Internet]. 2009 [cited 2024 Apr 17];12(4):441–5. Available from: https://pubmed.ncbi.nlm.nih.gov/18922203/.
14. Kozicky JM, McGirr A, Bond DJ, Gonzalez M, Silveira LE, Keramatian K, et al. Neuroprogression and episode recurrence in bipolar I disorder: a study of gray matter volume changes in first-episode mania and association with clinical outcome. Bipolar Disord. 2016;18(6):511.
15. Fries GR, Pfaffenseller B, Stertz L, Paz AVC, Dargél AA, Kunz M, et al. Staging and neuroprogression in bipolar disorder. Curr Psychiatry Rep [Internet] 2012 [cited 2024 Sep 14];14(6):667–675. Available from: https://pubmed.ncbi.nlm.nih.gov/23090632/.
16. Keramatian K, Pinto J V., Schaffer A, Sharma V, Beaulieu S, Parikh S V., et al. Clinical and demographic factors associated with delayed diagnosis of bipolar disorder: Data from Health Outcomes and Patient Evaluations in Bipolar Disorder (HOPE-BD) study. J Affect Disord [Internet]. 2022 [cited 2024 Apr 17];296:506–13. Available from: https://pubmed.ncbi.nlm.nih.gov/34606817/.
17. Scott J, Graham A, Yung A, Morgan C, Bellivier F, Etain B. A systematic review and meta-analysis of delayed help-seeking, delayed diagnosis and duration of untreated illness in bipolar disorders. Acta Psychiatr Scand [Internet]. 2022 [cited 2024 Apr 17];146(5):389–405. Available from: https://pubmed.ncbi.nlm.nih.gov/36018259/.
18. Berk M, Hallam K, Malhi GS, Henry L, Hasty M, MacNeil C, et al. Evidence and implications for early intervention in bipolar disorder. J Ment Health [Internet]. 2010 [cited 2024 Apr 17];19(2):113–26. Available from: https://pubmed.ncbi.nlm.nih.gov/20433320/.
19. Post RM, Leverich GS, Kupka RW, Keck PE, McElroy SL, Altshuler LL, et al. Early-onset bipolar disorder and treatment delay are risk factors for poor outcome in adulthood. J Clin

Psychiatry [Internet]. 2010 [cited 2023 Jan 8];71(7):864–872. Available from: https://pubmed.ncbi.nlm.nih.gov/20667291/.
20. Altamura AC, Buoli M, Caldiroli A, Caron L, Cumerlato Melter C, Dobrea C, et al. Misdiagnosis, duration of untreated illness (DUI) and outcome in bipolar patients with psychotic symptoms: A naturalistic study. J Affect Disord [Internet]. 2015 [cited 2023 Jan 8];182:70–5. Available from: https://pubmed.ncbi.nlm.nih.gov/25978716/.
21. Lagerberg TV, Larsson S, Sundet K, Hansen CB, Hellvin T, Andreassen OA, et al. Treatment delay and excessive substance use in bipolar disorder. J Nerv Ment Dis [Internet] 2010 [cited 2023 Feb 18];198(9):628–633. Available from: https://pubmed.ncbi.nlm.nih.gov/20823723/.
22. Keramatian K, Pinto JV, Tsang VWL, Chakrabarty T, Yatham LN. Duration of untreated or undiagnosed bipolar disorder and clinical characteristics and outcomes: systematic review and meta-analysis. Br J Psychiatry. 2025;1–11. Available from: https://pubmed.ncbi.nlm.nih.gov/40337852/.
23. Shi L, Thiebaud P, McCombs JS. The impact of unrecognized bipolar disorders for patients treated for depression with antidepressants in the fee-for-services California Medicaid (Medi-Cal) program. J Affect Disord [Internet]. 2004 [cited 2023 Jan 8];82(3):373–83. Available from: https://pubmed.ncbi.nlm.nih.gov/15555688/.
24. Birnbaum HG, Shi L, Dial E, Oster EF, Greenberg PE, Mallett DA. Economic consequences of not recognizing bipolar disorder patients: a cross-sectional descriptive analysis. J Clin Psychiatry [Internet] 2003 [cited 2023 Jan 8];64(10):1201–1209. Available from: https://pubmed.ncbi.nlm.nih.gov/14658969/.
25. Keramatian K, Morton E. Barriers to timely identification of bipolar disorder in youth: a multidimensional perspective. Frontiers in Child and Adolescent Psychiatry [Internet]. 2023:2. Available from: https://www.frontiersin.org/articles/10.3389/frcha.2023.1186722/abstract
26. Keramatian K, Levit A, Chavoshi-Nejad H, Westwell-Roper C, Nunez JJ, Forbes A, Morton E, Michalak EE, Vieta E, Yatham LN. Early psychoeducational intervention for youth and young adults at risk for bipolar disorder: a feasibility study: intervention psychoéducative précoce pour les adolescents et les jeunes adultes à risque de trouble bipolaire: Une étude de faisabilité. Can J Psychiatry [Internet] 2025 [cited 2025 May 20]. Available from: https://pubmed.ncbi.nlm.nih.gov/40390541/.
27. Samalin L, de Chazeron I, Vieta E, Bellivier F, Llorca PM. Residual symptoms and specific functional impairments in euthymic patients with bipolar disorder. Bipolar Disord [Internet]. 2016 [cited 2024 Sep 14];18(2):164–73. Available from: https://onlinelibrary.wiley.com/doi/full/10.1111/bdi.12376.
28. Wals M, Hillegers MH, Reichart CG, Verhulst FC, Nolen WA, Ormel J. Stressful life events and onset of mood disorders in children of bipolar parents during 14-month follow-up. J Affect Disord [Internet]. 2005; [cited 2024 Sep 15];1;87(2-3):253–63. Available from: https://pubmed.ncbi.nlm.nih.gov/15979149/
29. Zanini MA, Castro J, Cunha GR, Asevedo E, Pan PM, Bittencourt L, Coelho FM, Tufik S, Gadelha A, Bressan RA, Brietzke E. Abnormalities in sleep patterns in individuals at risk for psychosis and bipolar disorder. Schizophrenia Res [Internet] 2015 [cited 2024 Sep 15];169(1–3):262–267. Available from: https://pubmed.ncbi.nlm.nih.gov/26391284/.
30. Levenson JC, Axelson DA, Merranko J, Angulo M, Goldstein TR, Mullin BC, Goldstein BI, Brent DA, Diler R, Hickey MB, Monk K. Differences in sleep disturbances among offspring of parents with and without bipolar disorder: association with conversion to bipolar disorder. Bipolar Disord [Internet]. 2015 [cited 2024 Sep 15];17(8):836–848. Available from: https://www.ncbi.nlm.nih.gov/pmc/articles/PMC4734929/.
31. Shen GH, Alloy LB, Abramson LY, Sylvia LG. Social rhythm regularity and the onset of affective episodes in bipolar spectrum individuals. Bipolar Disord [Internet]. 2008 [cited 2024 Sep 18];10(4):520–9. Available from: https://www.ncbi.nlm.nih.gov/pmc/articles/PMC4090015/.
32. Yatham LN, Kennedy SH, Parikh SV, Schaffer A, Bond DJ, Frey BN, Sharma V, Goldstein BI, Rej S, Beaulieu S, Alda M, MacQueen G, Milev RV, Ravindran A, O'Donovan C, McIntosh D, Lam RW, Vazquez G, Kapczinski F, McIntyre RS, Kozicky J, Kanba S, Lafer B, Suppes

T, Calabrese JR, Vieta E, Malhi G, Post RM, Berk M. Canadian Network for Mood and Anxiety Treatments (CANMAT) and International Society for Bipolar Disorders (ISBD) 2018 guidelines for the management of patients with bipolar disorder. Bipolar Disord [Internet]. 2018 [cited 2024 Sep 18];20(2):97–170. Available from: https://www.ncbi.nlm.nih.gov/pmc/articles/PMC5947163/.

33. Keramatian K, Chithra NK, Yatham LN. The CANMAT and ISBD Guidelines for the treatment of bipolar disorder: summary and a 2023 Update of Evidence. Focus (Am Psychiatr Publ) [Internet]. 2023 [cited 2024 Sep 18];21(4):344–53. Available from: https://pubmed.ncbi.nlm.nih.gov/38695002/.
34. McNamara RK, Nandagopal JJ, Strakowski SM, DelBello MP. Preventative strategies for early-onset bipolar disorder: towards a clinical staging model. CNS drugs [Internet]. 2010 [cited 2024 Sep 18];24:983–96. Available from: https://pubmed.ncbi.nlm.nih.gov/21090835/.
35. Conus P, Ward J, Hallam KT, Lucas N, Macneil C, McGorry PD, Berk M. The proximal prodrome to first episode mania–a new target for early intervention. Bipolar Disord [Internet]. 2008 [cited 2024 Sep 18];10(5):555–565. Available from: https://pubmed.ncbi.nlm.nih.gov/18657240/.
36. Goldstein TR, Fersch-Podrat R, Axelson DA, Gilbert A, Hlastala SA, Birmaher B, Frank E. Early intervention for adolescents at high risk for the development of bipolar disorder: pilot study of Interpersonal and Social Rhythm Therapy (IPSRT). Psychotherapy [Internet]. 2014; [cited 2024 Sep 4];51(1):180. Available from: https://psycnet.apa.org/record/2013-45431-001
37. Goldstein TR, Merranko J, Krantz M, Garcia M, Franzen P, Levenson J, Axelson D, Birmaher B, Frank E. Early intervention for adolescents at-risk for bipolar disorder: A pilot randomized trial of Interpersonal and Social Rhythm Therapy (IPSRT). J Affect Disord [Internet]. 2018 [cited 2024 Sep 4];235:348–56. Available from: https://www.ncbi.nlm.nih.gov/pmc/articles/PMC5951768/.
38. Heissler J, Kanske P, Schönfelder S, Wessa M. Inefficiency of emotion regulation as vulnerability marker for bipolar disorder: evidence from healthy individuals with hypomanic personality. J Affect Disord [Internet]. 2014 [cited 2024 Sep 15];152:83–90. Available from: https://pubmed.ncbi.nlm.nih.gov/23948633/.
39. Wals M, Hillegers MH, Reichart CG, Verhulst FC, Nolen WA, Ormel J. Stressful life events and onset of mood disorders in children of bipolar parents during 14-month follow-up. J Affect Disord [Internet] 2005 [cited 2024 Sep 15];87(2–3):253–63. Available from: https://pubmed.ncbi.nlm.nih.gov/15979149/.
40. Fristad MA, Ackerman JP, Nick EA. Adaptation of Multi-Family Psychoeducational Psychotherapy (MF-PEP) for adolescents with mood disorders: preliminary findings. Evid Based Pract Child Adolesc Ment Health [Internet]. 2018 [cited 2024 Sep 18];3(4):252–62. Available from: https://pubmed.ncbi.nlm.nih.gov/30854463/.
41. Fristad MA, Verducci JS, Walters K, Young ME. Impact of multifamily psychoeducational psychotherapy in treating children aged 8 to 12 years with mood disorders. Arch Gen Psychiatry [Internet] 2009 [cited 2024 Sep 6];66(9):1013–1021. Available from: https://jamanetwork.com/journals/jamapsychiatry/fullarticle/210303.
42. Nadkarni RB, Fristad MA. Clinical course of children with a depressive spectrum disorder and transient manic symptoms. Bipolar Disord [Internet] 2010 [cited 2024 Sep 4];12(5):494–503. Available from: https://onlinelibrary.wiley.com/doi/abs/10.1111/j.1399-5618.2010.00847.x.
43. Axelson DA, Birmaher B, Strober MA, Goldstein BI, Ha W, Gill MK, Goldstein TR, Yen S, Hower H, Hunt JI, Liao F. Course of subthreshold bipolar disorder in youth: diagnostic progression from bipolar disorder not otherwise specified. J Am Acad Child Adolesc Psychiatry [Internet]. 2011 [cited 2024 Sep 14];50(10):1001–1016. Available from: https://pubmed.ncbi.nlm.nih.gov/21961775/.
44. Egeland JA, Hostetter AM, Pauls DL, Sussex JN. Prodromal symptoms before onset of manic-depressive disorder suggested by first hospital admission histories. J Am Acad Child Adolesc Psychiatry [Internet]. 2000 [cited 2024 Sep 14];39(10):1245–1252. Available from: https://www.sciencedirect.com/science/article/pii/S0890856710601013.

45. Shaw JA, Egeland JA, Endicott J, Allen CR, Hostetter AM. A 10-year prospective study of prodromal patterns for bipolar disorder among Amish youth. J Am Acad Child Adolesc Psychiatry [Internet]. 2005 [cited 2024 Sep 14];44(11):1104–11. Available from: https://psycnet.apa.org/record/2005-13523-004.
46. Hafeman DM, Merranko J, Axelson D, Goldstein BI, Goldstein T, Monk K, Hickey MB, Sakolsky D, Diler R, Iyengar S, Brent D. Toward the definition of a bipolar prodrome: dimensional predictors of bipolar spectrum disorders in at-risk youths. Am J Psychiatry [Internet] 2016 [cited 2024 Sep 12];173(7):695–704. Available from: https://psychiatryonline.org/doi/full/10.1176/appi.ajp.2015.15040414.
47. Fristad MA, Young AS, Vesco AT, Nader ES, Healy KZ, Gardner W, Wolfson HL, Arnold LE. A randomized controlled trial of individual family psychoeducational psychotherapy and omega-3 fatty acids in youth with subsyndromal bipolar disorder. J Child Adolesc Psychopharmacol [Internet] 2015 [cited 2024 Sep 2];25(10):764–774. Available from: https://www.liebertpub.com/doi/abs/10.1089/cap.2015.0132.
48. Miklowitz DJ, Chang KD, Taylor DO, George EL, Singh MK, Schneck CD, Dickinson LM, Howe ME, Garber J. Early psychosocial intervention for youth at risk for bipolar I or II disorder: a one-year treatment development trial. Bipolar Disord [Internet]. 2011 [cited 2024 Sep 4];13(1):67–75. Available from: https://onlinelibrary.wiley.com/doi/full/10.1111/j.1399-5618.2011.00890.x.
49. Miklowitz DJ, Schneck CD, Singh MK, Taylor DO, George EL, Cosgrove VE, Howe ME, Dickinson LM, Garber J, Chang KD. Early intervention for symptomatic youth at risk for bipolar disorder: a randomized trial of family-focused therapy. J Am Acad Child Adolesc Psychiatry [Internet]. 2013 [cited 2024 Sep 4];52(2):121–131. Available from: https://www.sciencedirect.com/science/article/pii/S0890856712007757.
50. Garrett AS, Miklowitz DJ, Howe ME, Singh MK, Acquaye TK, Hawkey CG, Glover GH, Reiss AL, Chang KD. Changes in brain activation following psychotherapy for youth with mood dysregulation at familial risk for bipolar disorder. Progress in Neuro-Psychopharmacology and Biological Psychiatry [Internet]. 2015 [cited 2024 Sep 4];56:215–20. Available from: https://www.sciencedirect.com/science/article/pii/S0278584614001833.
51. Miklowitz DJ, Schneck CD, Walshaw PD, Singh MK, Sullivan AE, Suddath RL, Borlik MF, Sugar CA, Chang KD. Effects of family-focused therapy vs enhanced usual care for symptomatic youths at high risk for bipolar disorder: a randomized clinical trial. JAMA Psychiatry [Internet] 2020 [cited 2024 Sep 4];77(5):455–463. Available from: https://jamanetwork.com/journals/jamapsychiatry/article-abstract/2758325.
52. Weintraub MJ, Schneck CD, Posta F, Merranko JA, Singh MK, Chang KD, Miklowitz DJ. Effects of family intervention on psychosocial functioning and mood symptoms of youth at high risk for bipolar disorder. J Consult Clin Psychol [Internet]. 2022; [cited 2024 Sep 6];90(2):161. Available from: https://psycnet.apa.org/fulltext/2022-23731-001.html
53. Cotton S, Luberto CM, Sears RW, Strawn JR, Stahl L, Wasson RS, Blom TJ, Delbello MP. Mindfulness-based cognitive therapy for youth with anxiety disorders at risk for bipolar disorder: a pilot trial. Early Intervent Psychiatry [Internet] 2016 [cited 2024 Sep 4];10(5):426–434. Available from: https://onlinelibrary.wiley.com/doi/full/10.1111/eip.12216.
54. Cotton S, Kraemer KM, Sears RW, Strawn JR, Wasson RS, McCune N, Welge J, Blom TJ, Durling M, Delbello MP. Mindfulness-based cognitive therapy for children and adolescents with anxiety disorders at-risk for bipolar disorder: A psychoeducation waitlist controlled pilot trial. Early Intervent Psychiatry [Internet]. 2020 [cited 2024 Sep 4];14(2):211–9. Available from: https://onlinelibrary.wiley.com/doi/full/10.1111/eip.12848.
55. Leopold K, Bauer M, Bechdolf A, Correll CU, Holtmann M, Juckel G, Lambert M, Meyer TD, Pfeiffer S, Kittel-Schneider S, Reif A. Efficacy of cognitive-behavioral group therapy in patients at risk for serious mental illness presenting with subthreshold bipolar symptoms: Results from a prespecified interim analysis of a multicenter, randomized, controlled study. Bipolar Disord [Internet] 2020 [cited 2024 Sep 4];22(5):517–529. Available from: https://onlinelibrary.wiley.com/doi/full/10.1111/bdi.12894.

56. Lee J, Semple RJ, Rosa D, Miller L. Mindfulness-based cognitive therapy for children: Results of a pilot study. Journal of Cognitive Psychotherapy [Internet]. 2008 [cited 2024 Sep 9];22(1). Available from: https://psycnet.apa.org/record/2009-10559-003.
57. Jones WT, Peters S, Byrne RE, Shiers D, Law H, Parker S. "It felt very special, it felt customised to me"—a qualitative investigation of the experiences of participating in a clinical trial of CBT for young people at risk of bipolar disorder. Psychol Psychother Theory Res Pract [Internet] 2021 [cited 2024 Sep 9];94(3):686–703. Available from: https://bpspsychub.onlinelibrary.wiley.com/doi/full/10.1111/papt.12313.
58. Lalli M, Brouillette K, Kapczinski F, de Azevedo Cardoso T. Substance use as a risk factor for bipolar disorder: A systematic review. J Psychiatr Res [Internet]. 2021 [cited 2024 Sep 19];144:285–95. Available from: https://pubmed.ncbi.nlm.nih.gov/34710665/.
59. Richardson TH. Substance misuse in depression and bipolar disorder: a review of psychological interventions and considerations for clinical practice. Mental Health and Substance Use [Internet]. 2013 [cited 2024 Sep 19];6(1):76–93. Available from: https://www.tandfonline.com/doi/abs/10.1080/17523281.2012.680485.
60. Macneil CA, Hasty MK, Berk M, Henry L, Evans M, Redlich C, Daglas R, McGorry PD, Conus P. Psychological needs of adolescents in the early phase of bipolar disorder: implications for early intervention. Early Intervent Psychiatry [Internet] 2011 [cited 2024 Sep 19];5(2):100–107. Available from: https://pubmed.ncbi.nlm.nih.gov/21535422/.
61. Inder ML, Crowe MT, Moor S, Luty SE, Carter JD, Joyce PR. "I actually don't know who I am": the impact of bipolar disorder on the development of self. Psychiatry [Internet] 2008 [cited 2024 Sep 19];71(2):123–133. Available from: https://pubmed.ncbi.nlm.nih.gov/18573034/.
62. Noack K, Elliott NB, Canas E, Lane K, Paquette A, Lavigne JM, Michalak EE. Credible, centralized, safe, and stigma--free: What youth with bipolar disorder want when seeking health information online. UBC Med J [Internet] 2016 [cited 2024 Sep 19];8(1). Available from: https://web.p.ebscohost.com/ehost/detail/detail?vid=0&sid=bd7679ea-ca82-4005-b25b-ffc8df4de5dc%40redis&bdata=JnNpdGU9ZWhvc3QtbGl2ZQ%3d%3d#AN=117888940&db=a9h.
63. Nicholas J, Boydell K, Christensen H. Self-management in young adults with bipolar disorder: Strategies and challenges. Journal of affective disorders [Internet]. 2017 [cited 2024 Sep 19];209:201–8. Available from: https://pubmed.ncbi.nlm.nih.gov/27930913/.
64. Jones SH, Smith G, Mulligan LD, Lobban F, Law H, Dunn G, Welford M, Kelly J, Mulligan J, Morrison AP. Recovery-focused cognitive–behavioural therapy for recent-onset bipolar disorder: randomised controlled pilot trial. Br J Psychiatry [Internet] 2015 [cited 2024 Sep 19];206(1):58–66. Available from: https://pubmed.ncbi.nlm.nih.gov/25213157/.
65. Jain V, Rebeiz A, Ritchie K, Cotton S, Hasty M, Shelton C, Ratheesh A, Macneil C. Advancing early intervention for bipolar disorder. Daymark Foundation [Internet] 2023 [cited 2024 Sep 19]. Available from: https://www.orygen.org.au/Training/Resources/Bipolar-Disorder/.
66. Lloyd-Evans B, Sweeney A, Hinton M, Morant N, Pilling S, Leibowitz J, Killaspy H, Tanskanen S, Totman J, Armstrong J, Johnson S. Evaluation of a community awareness programme to reduce delays in referrals to early intervention services and enhance early detection of psychosis. BMC Psychiatry [Internet]. 2015 [cited 2024 Sep 19];15:1–3. Available from: https://pubmed.ncbi.nlm.nih.gov/25934413/.
67. Yeo M, Berzins S, Addington D. Development of an early psychosis public education program using the PRECEDE–PROCEED model. Health Educ Res [Internet] 2007 [cited 2024 Sep 19];22(5):639–47. Available from: https://academic.oup.com/her/article/22/5/639/563832.

Correction to: Bipolar Disorder Offspring Cohorts: Clinical Implications

Maj Vinberg

Correction to:
Chapter 3 in: T. de Azevedo Cardoso et al. (eds.), *Latent Bipolar Disorder*, https://doi.org/10.1007/978-3-032-01297-5

Owing to an unfortunate oversight in the author name of chapter 3, a preliminary version of the book was inadvertently published.

Correct Name of the author is : Maj Vinberg.

The updated version of this chapter can be found at
https://doi.org/10.1007/978-3-032-01297-5_3

T. de Azevedo Cardoso et al. (eds.), *Latent Bipolar Disorder*,
https://doi.org/10.1007/978-3-032-01297-5_18

Index

T. de Azevedo Cardoso et al. (eds.), *Latent Bipolar Disorder*,
https://doi.org/10.1007/978-3-032-01297-5

MIX
Papier aus verantwortungsvollen Quellen
Paper from responsible sources
FSC® C105338

If you have any concerns about our products,
you can contact us on
ProductSafety@springernature.com

In case Publisher is established outside the EU,
the EU authorized representative is:
Springer Nature Customer Service Center GmbH
Europaplatz 3, 69115 Heidelberg, Germany

Printed by Libri Plureos GmbH
in Hamburg, Germany